Viruses, Immunity, and Immunodeficiency

University of South Florida International Biomedical Symposia Series

VIRUSES, IMMUNITY, AND IMMUNODEFICIENCY
Edited by Andor Szentivanyi and Herman Friedman

A Continuation Order Plan is available for this series. A continuation order will bring delivery of each new volume immediately upon publication. Volumes are billed only upon actual shipment. For further information please contact the publisher.

Viruses, Immunity, and Immunodeficiency

Edited by
Andor Szentivanyi
and
Herman Friedman
University of South Florida College of Medicine
Tampa, Florida

PLENUM PRESS • NEW YORK AND LONDON

Library of Congress Cataloging in Publication Data

University of South Florida International Symposium in the Biomedical Sciences
(1st: 1984: Tampa, Fla.)
    Viruses, immunity, and immunodeficiency.

    (University of South Florida international biomedical symposia series)
    "Proceedings of the University of South Florida International Symposium in the
Biomedical Sciences, held April 23–25, 1984, in Tampa, Florida" — T.p. verso.
    Includes bibliographies and index.
    1. Immunological deficiency syndromes — Congresses. 2. Immunosuppression —
Congresses. 3. Virus diseases — Immunological aspects — Congresses. I. Szentivanyi,
Andor. II. Friedman, Herman, 1931–   III. Title. IV. Series. [DNLM: 1. Im-
munity — congresses. 2. Immunologic Diseases — immunology — congresses. 3.
Viruses — immunology — congresses. W3 UN97 1st 1984v/QW 160 U58 1984v]
    QR188.35.U55   1984   616.97′9   86-3263
    ISBN-13:978-1-4612-9286-9   e-ISBN-13:978-1-4613-2185-9
    DOI: 10.1007/978-1-4613-2185-9

Proceedings of the University of South Florida International Symposium
in the Biomedical Sciences, held April 23–25, 1984, in Tampa, Florida

© 1986 Plenum Press, New York
Softcover reprint of the hardcover 1st edition 1986

A Division of Plenum Publishing Corporation
233 Spring Street, New York, N.Y. 10013

PREFACE

   This publication, "Viruses, Immunity and Immunodeficiency," is based
on the first symposium in a series of International Biomedical Symposia
sponsored by the College of Medicine of the University of South Florida in
Tampa, Florida. There is an explosive interest concerning the effects of
viruses on the immune response, especially the immunosuppressive effects of
viral infection. This has come about because of the recognition that the
Acquired Immunodeficiency Syndrome, which has taken biomedical scientists
and the public in general by surprise, is just one of the many examples
that viruses can influence the immune response system and, under appropriate
circumstances, alter immunity in such a way that an infected individual
becomes highly susceptible to a variety of other organisms to which normal
individuals would be resistant.

   This symposium series, sponsored by the University of South Florida
College of Medicine, brings to the biomedical community topics of current
interest. We thank the members of the faculty of various departments of
the College of Medicine and the administration of the College for their
support and encouragement in having these symposia at this medical school.
This volume, based on this symposium on viruses and immunity is a good example of the interdisciplinary nature of modern immunobiology and modern
biomedical science in general. Many investigators with many different back-
grounds and training experiences, including microbiologists, immunologists,
biochemists, oncologists, and physicians, are interested in how and why
viruses influence the immune response system. We believe that bringing
this topic to a wide audience of biomedical scientists through this symposium is of value to the medical community. It is anticipated by the editors
of this volume and the editors of future volumes based on other symposia
that the proceedings will provide for the international biomedical community
the newest information concerning many topics of interest to a wide variety
of biomedical specialists.

                                   Andor Szentivanyi, M.D.
                                   Dean of the College of Medicine
                                   Deputy Vice President for
                                     Medical Affairs

                                   Herman Friedman, Ph.D.
                                   Professor and Chairman
                                   Department of Medical Microbiology
                                     and Immunology
                                   University of South Florida
                                   Tampa, Florida

                                   October 30, 1985

CONTENTS

III. TUMOR VIRUS INFECTIONS AND IMMUNE RESPONSES

IV. MECHANISMS OF VIRUS ASSOCIATED IMMUNODEREGULATION

V. IMMUNE RESTORATION IN VIRUS INFECTIONS

INTRODUCTION AND HISTORICAL PERSPECTIVES

Andor Szentivanyi and Herman Friedman

Departments of Pharmacology and Medical Microbiology
and Immunology, University of South Florida
College of Medicine
Tampa, Florida

It is almost axiomatic that practically every field of biomedicine today has some relationship with the expanding knowledge and interest in immunology. Numerous symposia, meetings and conferences deal with modern aspects of immunology and how this subject interacts with almost all areas of biology. Indeed, immunology is considered to be both the "grandfather" and the "grandchild" of modern biomedical science. However, there is almost no question that the recent widespread interest in acquired immunodeficiencies induced by infectious agents such as viruses has brought even greater attention to the subject of immunology. Nevertheless, it should be noted that it was first recognized that viruses may influence the immune response about 80 years ago when Von Pirquet first described the phenomenon of "anergy" in cutaneous hypersensitivity of children to tuberculin when they developed measles. It was observed that even those children who had pre-existing hypersensitivity to tuberculin extracts lost such reactivity when they developed measles, even though it was not known at the time that measles was a viral illness.

Much work has been performed over the last few years which has shown that the measles virus is markedly immunosuppressive and when the virus infects lymphocytes involved in delayed (i.e. cell mediated) hypersensitivity reactions there is a finite but non-specific suppression of pre-existing cell mediated immunity to a wide variety of agents, including microbial antigens such as those present in the tubercle bacillus. However, it was not until the 1960's that it was first recognized that leukemia viruses, besides causing transformation of lymphocytes to leukemic cells, also produce marked immunosuppression. It was first thought that such immunosuppression induced by leukemia virus in experiments with animals may be the result of a "crowding out" of normal lymphoid cells by nonfunctional leukemic cells in the lymphoid organs of the infected individual. Indeed, such immunosuppression was noted clinically 20 or 30 years earlier when clinicians observed that patients who had large numbers of white blood cells in their peripheral blood as they went through the various stages of leukemia and lymphoma showed marked anergy to a variety of antigens and an inability to respond with a normal immune response. Actually, based on such clinical observations, it was predicted in the 1920's that lymphocytes play no role in immune responses since an increase in lymphocytes during leukemia resulted in a corresponding decrease in antibody formation. Hence, lymphocytes could "obviously not be involved in antibody formation." Although such conclusions were erroneous at the time, the basic observations were correct, i.e., those individuals with leukemia, even before the advent of chemotherapy showed marked immuno-suppression.

Experimental work with animals indicated that leukemia viruses, especially the retroviruses, profoundly suppress immune responses long before there is a significant infiltration of lymphoid organs and appearance of blood with cells recognized as leukemic cells. As is apparent from this volume, there has been much work concerning leukemia, viruses, and retroviruses in general, in terms of immunosuppression. Indeed, in the early 1950's Dr. Robert Good and his associates published findings showing the Gross passage A virus could result in a "biologic thymectomy" of newborn mice and induce in the mice a marked immunodeficiency; such mice could be used as recipients of tissue grafts which they would normally reject. Such "thymectomy" with the Gross leukemia virus at birth was used as a model system similar to surgical thymectomy. It was not until the mid- and late 1960's that a number of investigators started to use leukemia viruses as models to begin to dissect the complexities of immune mechanisms and to examine the alteration of immunity induced by these viruses. However, not until the discovery of the human T cell leukemia viruses, and the rapid explosion of interest due to the emergence of the acquired immunodeficiency syndrome that worldwide attention has become focused on how such viruses suppress immunity. In retrospect, it should be apparent to immunologists and microbiologists that infections with many agents, especially viruses, may predispose an individual to a variety of opportunistic infections. Indeed, it is now recognized that during the great influenza pandemic of 1918, a major cause of death was bacterial pneumonia that frequently followed this viral illness.

The great strides that have been made in the ability to combat opportunisitic diseases have resulted in less interest in the growing risk of individuals to these agents. However, it is now known that many viruses have the ability to mediate suppression of the immune system. It seems, furthermore, that different viruses are able to cause different types of immune suppression due to a wide variety of mechanisms. Indeed, there does not appear to be a single mechanisms by which viral agents or any other infectious agent cause immune suppression. Some viral infections may induce a disordered regulation of immune responses, including increase in one arm of the response and decrease in the other arm, or actually a hyperreactivity of both arms of the immune network.

In the first section of this volume, the role of natural resistance mechanisms, both cellular and humoral, to viruses is described. Attention is focused on the role of natural killer cells and macrophages in resisting viral infections. Various specific viral infections, and how they influence immunity, are then discussed in the second section of this volume. Epstein-Barr virus, cytomegalovirus, herpes simplex, hepatitis B virus, and coxsackievirus infection in both man and experimental animals is discussed in detail by various experts in the field.

The third section of the volume discusses tumor virus infections and immune responses. There are chapters dealing with mammary tumor viruses, retroviruses of man, as well as of mice and cats, and using this particular framework, several reviews concerning action of both tumor and nontumor viruses on the host immune response. The fourth section of this volume concentrates on mechanisms of virus induced immunoderegulation. Chapters are presented concerning genetics and immunosuppression by viruses, molecular mimicry, pharmacological regulatory effects, aging, and a number of other mechanisms whereby viruses affect immune responses.

The fifth section of this volume deals with contemporary methods to restore immune responses in individuals with viral infections. Biological response modifiers used for restoring immunodeficiencies, including those induced by viruses, are discussed as well as chapters dealing with substances such as interferon, interleukins, leukocyte dialysis factors, histamine$_2$ receptor blockers, etc. Also, specific vaccines in modifying immune suppression in virally infected individuals are described. Following the fifth section, a final chapter provides an overview on viruses, immunity, immunodeficiency, and cancer.

As can be seen from the wide variety of topics presented, it is evident that there is much interest concerning viral induced immunodeficiency, especially those which cause malignancy. There are now sufficient suggestions and studies pertaining to the mechanisms involved so that rational approaches to therapy of both the viral infection as well as the immunoderegulation induced by such viruses, are being made by a number of laboratories and clinical investigators. It appears that the AIDS problem has not only electrified the biomedical community to study the mechanisms whereby viruses affect immunity and how such immunodeficiencies can be restored, but has also reminded the biomedical community that there are many viruses which can affect immunity. Many model systems have been studied in experimental situations for the last half century or more. It is anticipated by the editors of this volume that publication of this material will provide a level of new information which can be utilized, both experimentally and clinically, for future investigations of how viruses affect immunity and cause immunodeficiency.

I. CELLULAR AND HUMORAL IMMUNE MECHANISMS

IN VIRAL RESISTANCE

NATURAL RESISTANCE MECHANISMS IN HERPESVIRUS INFECTIONS

Carlos Lopez

Sloan-Kettering Institute for Cancer Research
Cornell Graduate School of Medical Sciences
1275 York Avenue
New York, New York

INTRODUCTION

Natural resistance mechanisms require no presensitization and are ready
to immediately respond against an invading microorganism (1). Although other
barriers may participate in such responses against herpesvirus infections,
macrophages, natural killer (NK) cells, and the rapid production of interferon appear to play central roles in host defense. Since the role of macrophages will be covered elsewhere in this book by Soren Mogensen, this chapter
will concentrate on the role of NK cells and interferon.

Host defense systems may interact with a herpesvirus infection on any
of several different levels. After contracting a primary infection, defense
mechanisms may be required to limit the replication and spread of virus at
the site of infection. These systems may also limit the dissemination of
virus from the site of infection to other parts of the body, in particular
the viscera and central nervous system. As distinct from most other viruses,
herpesvirus almost always develop into latent infections which can later be
reactivated to cause disease. Thus, host defense system may also restrict
this aspect of the pathogenesis of infection. Once a primary infection has
become established, an immune response is required for clearing that infection. Similarly, host defense systems are probably required for sequestering
and clearing reactivated herpesvirus infections.

Although natural resistance mechanisms would be thought to be most
important to the host during primary infections, it is also possible that
these systems are required for reducing the incidence of latent virus infections and/or for controlling reactivated infections. For example, by reducing primary infections natural resistance systems may limit the amount of
virus capable of establishing a latent infection and therefore the amount
of virus which might be reactivated. Natural resistance systems may also
have a direct effect to limit spread of virus to the neuron which is the
site of latent infections for herpes simplex viruses. Natural resistance
systems may also have either a direct or indirect effect on reactivated
latent herpesvirus infections and thus be required for resistance to recrudescent disease, as well.

Several different approaches have been taken in studies attempting to
define the host defense systems required for resistance to and recovery

from herpesvirus infections. For example, certain patients with primary or secondary immunodeficiencies have been found to be unusually susceptible to severe disease caused by herpesviruses (2-6). Since these individuals were usually found to be more deficient of cell mediated rather than humoral immune capacity, the former was thought to play the dominant role in host defense against these infections. However, the cell mediated immune response is complex and no one deficiency has been selectively associated with susceptibility to herpesvirus infections. Recent progress in this arena derives from the study of models of genetic resistance to herpesvirus infections in the mouse.

GENETIC RESISTANCE TO HSV-1 IN THE MOUSE

A model of genetic resistance to herpes simplex virus-type 1 (HSV-1) has been developed in order to determine the host defense mechanisms responsible for resistance (7). This model has at least two advantages when compared to studies of HSV-1 infections in outbred mice. First, it allows the use of genetic tools for determining the mechanisms involved in resistance. Thus, resistance mechanisms can be evaluated to determine whether they are found in resistant versus susceptible mice and whether they segregate with genetic resistance in backcrossed mice. Second, since the mice are genetically homogeneous and characterized with respect to the major histocompatibility complex, cell transfer and bone marrow transplantation experiments can be carried out which will help define the mechanisms involved.

There is, however, the possibility that this animal model is a laboratory artifact with nothing to do with resistance to herpesvirus infections in man. Herpesviruses are highly species specific and appear to have evolved with their host. Since HSV-1 is indigenous to man and not the mouse, resistance mechanisms of the mouse may not be the same as those required in man. Fortunately, the data generated to date indicate that the natural resistance mechanisms required in the mouse are also necessary for resistance to HSV-1 in man.

For the initial studies, adult, male mice were challenged intraperitoneally (IP) with ten-fold dilution of a virulent strain of HSV-1 (2931) and the amount of virus required to kill half of the mice (LD_{50}) was determined (7). Resistant strains of mice survived 10^6 plaque forming units (PFU) of virus, moderately resistant mice had LD_{50}'s of 10^3-10^4 PFU, and susceptible mice had LD_{50}'s of 10^1-10^2 PFU. For subsequent studies, C57Bl/6 mice were the prototype resistant strain, BALB/c were the moderately resistant strain, and A/J mice were the susceptible strain. We have carried out most of our studies with HSV-1 (2931) but have found similar results with eleven other strains of HSV-1 (8). Similarly, Kirchner and his colleagues (9) have found comparable results using other strains of HSV-1 and Armerding et al. (10) have found that genetic resistance to HSV-2 was similar to genetic resistance to HSV-1 in distribution of resistance among inbred strains of mice. Genetic resistance to HSV-1 was determined to be a dominant genetic trait governed by two non-H2, independently segregating loci (11).

Genetic resistance to HSV-1 appears to be dependent on host defense mechanisms which inhibit spread of virus to the target organ, the central nervous system for this virus (12). Mice genetically resistant to 10^6 PFU of HSV-1 when challenged IP, were found to be as susceptible to challenge by the intracerebral route as genetically susceptible mice. Also treatments of mice to reduce host defense systems were found to reduce genetic resistance of C57Bl/6 mice. In contrast, bone marrow transplantation from resistant into susceptible strains of mice yielded chimeras resistant to HSV-1 challenge, indicating that resistance was mediated by effector cells descendent from bone marrow stem cells.

4

Studies of strontium-89 (^{89}Sr)-treated mice indicate that a marrow-dependent mechanism is required for resistance against HSV-1 in the mouse (13). Thus, treatment of genetically resistant mice with ^{89}Sr resulted in mice as susceptible to HSV-1 as the genetically most susceptible strains. Since Bennett (14) showed that ^{89}Sr-treatment of mice abrogated allogenic resistance without significantly affecting their capacity to reject skin grafts, genetic resistance to HSV-1 was probably mediated by mechanisms similar to those mediating allogenic resistance to marrow allografts.

Studies were also carried out which indicated that normal T-cell function was not required for resistance to an IP challenge with HSV-1 (12,15). Thus, athymic nude mice were found to be as resistant to challenge with HSV-1 as were the euthymic litter mates. Similarly, thymectomized and anti-thymocyte treated mice were found to be as resistant to IP challenge with HSV-1 as were untreated mice if the studies were carried out after the inhibitory effects on macrophage function had dissipated (16).

Similar studies of genetic resistance to lethal HSV-1 infections have been carried out using other routes of inoculation. Inbred strains of mice have been challenged by the intravenous (8), intraocular (17), and intra-vaginal (18) routes with results similar to those generated by IP challenge In each case, C57Bl/6 mice were more resistant than other strains and resistance to the virus infection could be reduced by cyclophosphamide, irradiation, or ^{89}Sr-treatment.

NATURAL KILLER CELLS

Natural killer (NK) cells were described in 1975 as effector cells capable of lysing certain tumor cells in culture (19). NK cells were recognized to be different from T-cells, B-cells, or macrophages and were detected in non-sensitized hosts. Because of these properties, it was postulated that these effectors might have a major role in surveillance against arising neoplasia. It has become evident in the intervening years that other cells can also be targets for NK cytolysis. Thus, primitive hematopoietic cells and virus infected targets have been found to be lysed by NK effectors. More recent evidence suggests that NK cells play an important role in host resistance against certain virus infections.

In studies of man and mouse, NK cells have been shown to be both derived from bone marrow stem cells (20) and to be dependent on a normal bone marrow microenvironment (21). Thus, mice of the low NK responder phenotype were transplanted with bone marrow from high NK responder mice and the resulting chimeras were found to be high responders. In comparable human studies, transplantation of low NK responder individuals, with bone marrow of donors with normal NK phenotype resulted in transplant recipients with normal NK capacity. Bone marrow dependence has been demonstrated in mice treated with ^{89}Sr or estradiol which destroy bone marrow and cause severe aplasia. In addition, mice with osteopetrosis, an inherited condition in which bone matrix obliterates the marrow cavity, were also found to have markedly diminished NK capacity associated with destruction of the marrow cavity.

All three major classes of interferons have been found to augment NK function (22). Pre-treatment of effectors with alpha, beta, or gamma interferon usually results in significantly increased lysis of poor as well as good NK targets. This pre-treatment appears to both recruit pre-NK cells into functional effectors and to make functioning NK cells even more efficient.

Infection of mice with many different RNA or DNA viruses, including HSV-1, is followed rapidly by increased NK activity of cells in vitro (23).

When evaluated serially, the mice were found to generate peak serum interferon levels just prior to maximum induction of NK activity.

Virus infection of target cells is usually associated with those cells being better targets for NK cytolysis than the uninfected cells (24-26). Lysis of virus infected cells does not require presensitization of the host to viral antigens. In addition, the effector cells which lyse virus infected targets are not mature T-cells, B-cells or macrophages.

Studies of NK effector cells have clearly demonstrated heterogeneity among the effector cells (27,28). Subpopulations of cells differed with respect to susceptibility to in vivo ^{89}Sr-treatment, cell surface markers, and target structures recognized. These studies also showed that the subpopulations of effector cells evaluated depended on the target cell used in the assay.

In more recent studies, heterogeneity has been described for human effector cells. Thus, adsorption to tumor cell monolayers and cell surface determinants have been used to describe different subpopulations of effector cells which lyse tumor targets. More recent studies in our laboratory have indicated that the effector cells which lyse the commonly used K562 erythroleukemia target cells are different than the cells which lyse HSV-1 infected fibroblasts [NK(HSV-Fs)] (29). Although the effectors for both targets are large granular lymphocytes which express Leu-11a on their cell surface, they can be differentiated on the basis of other cell surface determinants and cold target inhibition. The latter studies indicate that different subpopulations of NK cells recognize different structures on target cells.

In addition to being different subpopulations of effectors, recent evidence suggests that the two subpopulations of NK cells are also regulated independently (29). Thus patients have been found whose peripheral blood mononuclear cells consistently lyse one of the targets normally while lysis of the other was very low (greater than two standard deviations below the normal mean). Examples of preferential lysis of each of these targets have been detected indicating that this finding cannot be attributed to one target being more easily lysed than the other.

Trinchieri and Santoli (30) first noted that interferon was generated during lysis of many cells which were good targets for NK effectors. Since interferon has been shown to dramatically augment the lysis of cells which are good targets for NK as well as cells which are poor targets, these workers postulated that selective lysis of virus infected over uninfected targets depended on the generation of interferon during the assay and the non-specific augmentation of lysis of available targets. Our studies clearly showed that interferon was not responsible for selective lysis of HSV-1 infected fibroblasts versus uninfected cells (31). Thus, the amount of interferon generated during each assay did not correlate with the level of lysis attained in the same wells. Addition of enough antibody to neutralize all the antiviral activity in each well failed to significantly diminish the lytic activity. Lastly, we have found a number of patients whose peripheral blood mononuclear cells were capable of lysing these target cells even though only very small or undetectable amounts of interferon were generated concurrently. These results clearly indicated that the cytotoxic activity of NK cells is independent of interferon generation and that these two functions are governed independently.

The studies of ^{89}Sr-treated mice were the first indication that NK effector cells might play an important role in resistance to HSV-1 (13). Clearly ^{89}Sr-treated mice had very low NK lytic activity and greatly diminished resistance to HSV-1. In other experiments, estradiol-treatment of mice and the beige mutation were associated with diminished NK capacity and reduced resistance to infection.

Because of the results which indicated a role for NK cells in resistance to HSV-1 in mice, studies were undertaken to determine whether NK function was also required for resistance to infection in man (32). For these studies, HSV-1 infected fibroblasts were used as targets. Two patient groups were studied because they are known to be susceptible to unusually severe disease caused by herpesvirus infections; newborns and patients with Wiskott-Aldrich syndrome (WAS). Cord bloods were evaluated as an indication of the newborns' NK capacity. Only 30% of the cord bloods tested demonstrated normal NK(HSV-Fs) responses. We have also evaluated the capacity of peripheral blood cells from nine premature infants and found that they also had responses greater than two standard deviations below the normal mean (32). These results suggest that most newborns have NK(HSV-Fs) capacity which is significantly below normal which correlates with their increased susceptibility to severe disease caused by HSV-1 and HSV-2. We have also evaluated six patients with WAS and found that low NK(HSV-Fs) in these individuals correlated with increased susceptibility to infection.

The difficulty with studies of newborns and patients with WAS is that they have been described to have other deficiencies which might also contribute to their susceptibility to infection (33-35). In order to study patients without this difficulty, we have evaluated a number of patients known to be highly susceptible to infection because of the unusually severe nature of their herpesvirus infections, but individuals with no known primary or secondary immunodeficiency which might account for their susceptibility (32). A total of nine such individuals have been studied and were found to have low NK(HSV-Fs) responses. Two of these were also evaluated in between periods of clinically evident infection and both were found to have equally low responses during this period, as well. Four of the patients were evaluated for NK(K562) and two of the four demonstrated normal responses. These studies suggest that the heterogeneity of NK effectors may be important since different subpopulations may have different biological roles. That is, NK(HSV-Fs) may be important in resistance to herpesvirus infections while NK(K562) may have other biologic functions.

More recent studies indicate that NK(HSV-Fs) lytic effectors are capable of lysing target cells early enough in the replication cycle to reduce the amount of virus generated by those infected targets (Fitzgerald et al., submitted). This activity was attributed to the lytic effectors rather than the interferon generating cells since carrying out this experiment in the presence of anti-interferon did not diminish the reduction of virus replication. Also, Leu-11a positive cells, which are lytic but do not generate interferon, were capable of reducing virus yield. These results indicate that NK cytolytic effectors can reduce virus load early in an infection and thus retard the dissemination of infection.

INTERFERON

Approximately thirty years ago, Isaacs and Lindenmann (36) described a factor made by virus infected cells which caused uninfected cells to be resistant to virus infection. Since these early observations, interferon has been found to have a number of different biological roles; all of which appear to be the result of the interaction of interferon with the cell membrane (37). Three major forms of interferon have been described; interferon-alpha is made by leukocytes, interferon-beta is made by fibroblasts and interferon-gamma is made by pre-sensitized T-cells. Most (if not all) of the genes for the human interferons have been cloned and the gene product generated in bacterial cultures (37). Further, the species of interest has been made in large quantities, purified to homogeneity and compared with the others, and evaluated for its various biological functions. Mass-produced interferon has also been used in several clinical trials.

From the outset, interferons have been thought to be important to host defense against virus infections because of their ability to inhibit viral replication. In addition, more recent observations indicate that interferon might act against virus infections by augmenting natural resistance systems (37). Thus, interferons have been shown to augment NK cells and make them lyse virus infected targets even more efficiently (22). Also, interferon has been shown to augment the lytic activity of macrophage against herpesvirus infected targets (38) and to enhance the capacity of macrophages to limit replication and spread of virus. Finally, interferon has been shown to be an enhancer of interferon generation, that is, it regulates its own production (37).

The studies of Gresser et al. (39) indicate that interferon plays an important role in defense of the host against many virus infections, including HSV-1. Thus, producing an interferon deficiency state by treating mice with anti-interferon resulted in mice being much more susceptible to infection than were mock-treated mice. Much lower doeses of virus were lethal to treated mice and they died more rapidly. Kirchner's (40) group has provided evidence that the early production of interferon by HSV-1 infected mice was associated with genetic resistance to HSV-1. The interferon generated was alpha/beta and appeared to precede the augmentation of the NK response.

As noted above, interferon-alpha is generated during the NK(HSV-Fs) assay (31). Although there are several similarities between the NK(HSV-Fs) cytolytic effector cells and the cells which generate interferon-alpha, recently developed data indicate that these are different subpopulations (41, 42, Fitzgerald et al., in preparation). Like NK(HSV-Fs) cells, the interferon-alpha generating cells were found to be enriched in Percoll gradient fractions containing large granular lymphocytes. However, the interferon-alpha generating cell expresses Ia which is only found on a subpopulation of cytolytic effector cells. We have found a number of patients with normal cytolytic capacity but greatly diminished capacity to generate interferon-alpha in the same assay. Others, with interferon generating capacity but greatly diminished NK(HSV-Fs) have also been detected. Thus, the interferon-alpha generating cells and NK(HSV-Fs) cells are independently regulated and probably represent another aspect of the heterogeneity of large granular lymphocytes.

As with the mouse, studies in man suggest that a deficiency of interferon-alpha generating capacity is associated with diminished resistance to herpesvirus infections. Thus, Virelizier et al. (43) showed that patients with inherited deficiencies of interferon generation were susceptible to life-threatening infections caused by herpesvirus.

We have been studying patients with acquired immune deficiency syndrome (AIDS) in order to determine the cause for their susceptibility to infection (44). Patients with AIDS have been found to be susceptible to obligate and facultative intracellular pathogens including ulcerative HSV-1 and HSV-2 infections. The variety and severity of the infections found in patients with AIDS is similar to those found in patients with severe immunodeficiency induced for bone marrow transplantation. Although other deficiencies have been recorded in these patients, the best correlate of their susceptibility to opportunistic infections was a deficiency of interferon-alpha generation (45). Patients with opportunistic infections when first studied as well as patients who shortly thereafter developed such infections were found to generate a geometric mean of less than 30 international units (IU) of

8

interferon-alpha while heterosexual and homosexual controls made 1700 IU. Fifteen patients have been found with this deficiency two to sixteen months prior to their developing an opportunistic infection and it may indicate those patients at greatest risk of developing an infection.

CONCLUSIONS

NK cells and interferon are aspects of natural resistance which have been recently found to play important roles in resistance to herpesvirus infections. In theory, natural resistance mechanisms are especially important during the earliest phases of infection and are probably responsible for sequestering the infection and preventing it from disseminating. It is also possible that these mechanisms are required to control reactivated herpesvirus infection and the recrudescent disease associated with them.

Natural resistance systems are an important barrier to herpes and other viral pathogens. A deficiency of one of these systems would allow the primary infection to spread to viscera and the central nervous system long before the adaptive immune response was capable of responding. Understanding natural resistance systems and how they are regulated will be an important first step to developing ways of manipulating them to the advantage of the patient.

ACKNOWLEDGMENTS

This work was supported in part by CA 08748, CA 34989, CA 23766 and ACS FRA 193.

REFERENCES

1. A. C. Allison, J. S. Harington and M. Birbeck, An examination of the cytotoxic effects of silica on macrophages, J. Exp. Med. 124:141 (1966).
2. A. J. Nahmias and B. Roizman, Infection with herpes-simplex viruses 1 and 2, part 1, part 2, part 3, New Eng. J. Med. 289:667,719,781 (1973).
3. S. E. Bloomfield and C. Lopez, Herpes infections in the immunosuppressed host, Am. Acad. of Ophthal. 87:1226 (1980).
4. J. D. Meyers, N. Fluornoy, and E. D. Thomas, Infection with herpes simplex virus and cell-mediated immunity after marrow transplant, J. Infect. Dis., 142:338 (1980).
5. R. E. Stiehm, The human neonate as an immunocompromised host, in: "Pathogenesis, Prevention and Therapy," J. Verhoef, P. K. Petterson, and P. G. Quie, eds., Elsevier/North Holland, p. 77 (1980).
6. P. S. Morahan, E. R. Kern, and L.A. Glasgow, Immunomodular-induced resistance against herpes simplex virus, Proc. Soc. Exp. Biol. Med. 154:615 (1977).
7. C. Lopez, Genetics of natural resistance to herpesvirus infections in mice, Nature 258:152 (1975).
8. C. Lopez, Resistance to herpes simplex virus-type 1 (HSV-1) in: "Current Topics in Microbiology and Immunology," Vol. 92, O. Haller, ed., p.15 (1981).
9. H. M. Hochen Kirchner, J. M. Hirt, and K. Munk, Immunological studies of HSV infections of resistant and susceptible inbred strains of mice, Z. Immunitätsforsch. 154:147 (1978).
10. D. Armerding, P. Mayer, M. Scriba, A. Hren, and H. Rossiter, In vivo modulation of macrophage functions by herpes simplex virus type 2 in resistant and sensitive inbred mouse strains, Immunobiol. 160:217 (1981).

11. C. Lopez, Resistance to HSV-1 in the mouse is gover ed by two major, independently segregating non-H-2 loci, _Immunogenetics_ 11:87 (1980).

12. C. Lopez, Immunological nature of genetic resistance of mice to herpes simplex virus type 1 infection, _in_: "Oncogenesis and Herpesviruses," G. de-Thé, R. Henle, and F. Rapp, eds., W.H.O., Lyon, France p. 775 (1978).

13. C. Lopez, R. Ryshke and M. Bennett, Marrow dependent cells depleted by ^{89}Sr mediate genetic resistance to herpes simplex virus 1 infection, _Infec. Immun._ 28:1028 (1980).

14. M. Bennett, Prevention of marrow allograft rejection with radioactive strontium: evidence for marrow-dependent effector cells, _J. Immunol._ 110:510 (1973).

15. R. Zawatzky, J. Hilfenhaus, and H. Kirchner, Resistance of nude mice to herpes simplex virus and correlation with in vitro production of interferon, _Cell. Immunol._ 47:424 (1979).

16. A. J. Schlabach, D. Martinez, A. K. Field, and A. A. Tytell, Resistance of C57 mice to primary systemic herpes simplex virus infection, macrophage dependence and T-cell independence, _Infect. Immun._ 26:615 (1979).

17. R. W. Price, and J. Schmitz, Reactivation of latent herpes simplex virus infection of the autonomic nervous system by postganglion neurectomy, _Infect. Immun._ 19:523 (1978).

18. K. E. Schneweis and V. Saftig, The vaginal herpes simplex virus infection of resistant (C57 BL) mice, _Int. Herpes Virus Workshop_, p. 144 (1981).

19. R. B. Herberman, ed., "Natural Cell-Mediated Immunity Against Tumors," Academic Press (1980).

20. R. Kiessling and O. Haller, Natural killer cells in the mouse, an alternative immune surveillance mechanism, _Contemp. Top. Immunobiol._ 8:171 (1978).

21. O. Haller and H. Wigzell, Suppression of natural killer cell activity, with radioactive strontium: effector cells are marrow dependent, _J. Immunol._ 119:1503 (1977).

22. M. Gidlund, A. Orl, H. Wigzell, A. Senik, and I. Gresser, Enhanced NK cell activity in mice injected with interferon and interferon inducers, _Nature_ 273:759 (1978).

23. R. M. Welch, Mouse natural killer cells: induction, specificity and function, _J. Immunol._ 121:1631 (1978).

24. R. D. Diamond, R. Keller, G. Lee, and D. Finkel, Lysis of cytomegalovirus-infected human fibroblasts and transformed human cells by peripheral blood lymphoid cells from normal human donors (39650), _Proc. Soc. Exp. Biol. Med._ 154:259 (1977).

25. M. J. Anderson, Innate cytotoxicity of CBA mouse spleen cells to Sendai-virus infected L-cells, _Infect. Immun._ 20:608 (1978).

26. D. Santoli, G. Trinchieri, and F. S. Lief, Cell-mediated cytotoxicity against virus-infected target cells in humans. I. Characterization of the effector lymphocyte. _J. Immunol._ 121:526 (1978a).

27. V. Kumar, J. Ben-Ezra, M. Bennett, and G. Sonnenfeld, Natural killer cells in mice treated with ^{89}Sr: normal target binding cell numbers but inability to kill even after interferon administration, _J. Immunol._, 123:1832 (1979).

28. J. A. Lust, V. Kumar, R. C. Burton, S. P. Bartlett, and M. Bennett, Heterogeneity of natural killer cells in mouse, _J. Exp. Med._ 154:306 (1981).

29. P. A. Fitzgerald, R. Evans, D. Kirkpatrick and C. Lopez, Heterogeneity of human NK cells: comparison of effectors that lyse HSV-1-infected fibroblasts and K562 erythroleukemia targets. _J. Immunol._ 130:1663 (1983).

30. G. Trinchieri and D. Santoli, Antiviral activity induced by culturing lymphocytes with tumor-derived or virus-transformed cells. Enhancement of human natural killer cell activity by interferon and

antagonistic inhibition of susceptibility of target cells to lysis, J. Exp. Med. 147:1299 (1978).

31. P. A. Fitzgerald, V. von Wussow and C. Lopez, Role of interferon in natural kill of HSV-1 infected fibroblasts. J. Immunol. 129:819 (1982).

32. C. Lopez, D. Kirkpatrick, S. Read, P. A. Fitzgerald, J. Pitt, S. Pahwa, C. Y. Ching, and E. M. Smithwick, Correlation between low natural kill of HSV-1 infected fibroblasts, NK(HSV-1) and susceptibility to herpesvirus infections, J. Infect. Dis. 147:1030 (1983).

33. M. Miller, Phagocyte function in the neonate: selected aspects, Pediatrics 64:709 (1979).

34. M. Blaese, W. Strober, and T. A. Waldman, Immunodeficiency in the Wiscott-Aldrich Syndrome in: "Immunodeficiency in Man and Animals," D. Bergsma, R. A. Good, and J. Finstad, eds., Sinauer Assoc., Inc., Sunderland, Maryland, p. 250 (1975).

35. M. D. Cooper, H. P. Chase, J. T. Lawman, W. Krivit, and R. A. Good, Wiscott-Aldrich syndrome: an immunologic deficiency disease involving the afferent limb of immunity, Amer. J. Med. 44:499 (1968).

36. A. Isaacs and J. Lindemann, Virus interference. I. The interferons, Proc. Roy. Soc. Ser. B 147:258 (1956).

37. E. R. Stiehm, L. H. Kronenberg, H. M. Rosenblatt, Y. Bryson, and T. C. Merigan, Interferon: immunobiology and clinical significance, Ann. Int. Med. 96:80 (1982).

38. T. L. Stanwick, D. E. Campbell, and A. J. Nahmias, Spontaneous cytotoxicity mediated by human monocyte-macrophages against human fibroblasts infected with herpes simplex virus--augmentation by interferon, Cell. Immunol. 53:413 (1980).

39. I. Gresser, M. G. Tovey, C. Maury and M.-T. Bandu, Role of interferon in the pathogenesis of virus diseases in mice as demonstrated by the use of anti-interferon serum. II. Studies with herpes simplex, Maloney sarcoma, vesicular stomatitis, Newcastle disease, and influenza viruses, J. Exp. Med. 144:1316 (1976).

40. H. Engler, R. Zawatzky, A. Goldbach, C. H. Shroder, C. Weyand, G. J. Hammerling, and H. Kirchner, Experimental infection of inbred mice with herpes simplex virus. II. Interferon production and activation of natural killer cells in the peritoneal exudate, J. Gen. Virol. 55:25 (1981).

41. H. H. Peter, H. Dallugge, R. Zawatzky, S. Euler, W. Leibold, and H. Kirchner, Human peripheral null lymphocytes. II. Producers of type 1 interferon upon stimulation with tumor cells, herpes simplex virus and Corynebacterium parvum, Eur. J. Immunol. 10:547 (1980).

42. J. D. Djeu, N. Stocks, and K. Zoom, Positive self regulation of cytotoxicity upon exposure to influenza and herpes viruses, J. Exp. Med. 156:1222 (1982).

43. J.-L. Virelizier, Viral infections in patients with selective disorders of the interferon system, Fifth Int. Congress of Virology, p. 152, (1981).

44. F. P. Siegal, C. Lopez, G. S. Hammer, A. E. Brown, S. J. Kornfeld, J. Gold, J. Hassett, S. Z. Hirchman, C. Cunningham-Rundles, B. R. Adelsberg, D. M. Parham, M. Siegal, S. Cunningham-Rundles, and D. Armstrong, Severe acquired immunodeficiency in male homosexuals, manifested by chronic perianal ulcerative herpes simplex lesions, New Eng. J. Med. 305:1439 (1981).

45. C. Lopez, P. A. Fitzgerald, and F. P. Siegal, Severe acquired immunodeficiency syndrome in male homosexuals: diminished capacity to make interferon alpha in vitro is associated with susceptibility to severe opportunistic infections, J. Infect. Dis. 148:962 (1983).

MACROPHAGES AND GENETICALLY DETERMINED
NATURAL RESISTANCE TO VIRUS INFECTIONS

Søren C. Mogensen

Institute of Medical Microbiology
University of Aarhus, Denmark

INTRODUCTION

A wide variety of host defense mechanisms are involved in resistance
against virus infections. Although it has become increasingly clear that
the potential means of defense work in concert during a virus infection and
that the outcome will reflect a delicate and dynamic interaction between
the invading virus and the defense mechanisms mounted by the host, their
relative roles may vary in different virus infections and also in different
phases of a particular infection.

In primary virus infections, nonspecific host resistance factors represent the main line of defense during the first few days. They are either
present in the uninfected host or they are induced early in the course of
the infection. The nonspecific resistance mechanisms may have important
implications for the course of an infection by interfering with the invasion
and early dissemination of the virus in the body. However, the final recovery from a fully established virus infection is mediated through the
immunological response elicited by the infection and directed specifically
against the infecting virus.

Animal models of virus infections have been widely used to study the
pathogenesis of virus infections and to dissect the relative roles of the
host defense armamentarium against these infections. An important aspect
of many viral infections in experimental animals has been the finding of a
great variation in natural or innate resistance of animals from the same
species, indicating that the genetic constitution of the animal plays an
important role in the phenomenon (1). Because of the availability of
numerous inbred and congenic mouse strains most studies made on factors
controlling genetically determined resistance to viral infections have been
conducted in mice. Such studies of genetically determined resistance have
been offered unique opportunities to define more precisely the mechanisms
behind resistance, because the genetic analysis may indicate whether a
putative resistance factor cosegregates with resistance in crosses and
backcrosses between resistant and susceptible individuals.

Most studies have found genetically determined defense mechanisms
against virus infections to be operative early in the infection before the
advent of specific immunity (2). Among potential factors associated with
hereditary resistance interest has been focused on the role of macrophages

(1,3), interferon (2,4) and natural killer (NK) cells (2,5). Although they represent different resistance mechanisms, host defense in the early stage of infection probably depends to a major degree on a close collaboration between these (and possibly other) antiviral principles.

The present review will focus on the role played by cells of the mononuclear phagocyte system (monocytes/macrophages) in genetically determined natural resistance to virus infections.

THE MONONUCLEAR PHAGOCYTE SYSTEM

The term "macrophage" was introduced by Metchnikoff (6) who classified phagocytic cells as "macrophages" and "microphages" (polymorphonuclear leucocytes) on morphological and functional grounds. Mononuclear phagocytic cells resident in various organs and tissues were, according to Metchnikoff, closely related and belonged to a "macrophage system." This system was further elaborated by Aschoff (7), who grouped reticular cells of the spleen and lymph nodes, endothelial cells of the lymph and blood sinuses as well as histiocytes, splenocytes and blood monocytes in a unifying cell system called the "reticuloendothelial system," a term which has since been widely accepted and used. However, the current knowledge of phagocytic mononuclear cells has prompted reevaluation of the classification of these cells. On the basis of morphology, function, and kinetics of development, all highly phagocytic mononuclear cells and their precursors fit into one cell lineage called the "mononuclear phagocyte system" (8). Mononuclear phagocytes originate from precursor cells of the bone marrow. Following maturation of these cells into promonocytes and monocytes, the monocytes are transported via the blood to organs and tissues, where they finally develop into macrophages.

From an anatomical point of view, macrophages are well suited to function as a barrier against invasion of infectious agents, including viruses (9). They are long-lived and strategically placed at the portal of entry of many infections (e.g., alveolar macrophages of the lung) and are widely distributed in most organs of the body in close contact with the circulating blood (e.g., Kupffer cells of the liver), thus encountering the virus early in the infection. From a functional point of view, the ability of macrophages to restrict virus replication internally and externally may prevent the access of virus to susceptible cells and reduce the amount of virus produced in these cells, if they are infected. Furthermore, the ability of the mononuclear phagocyte system to provide an influx of new cells from the bone marrow and blood monocyte compartments into foci of infection and the potential of these newly arrived and activated cells to exert various antiviral functions may also be decisive in determining the outcome of a virus infection.

INDICATIONS FOR A ROLE OF MACROPHAGES IN

NATURAL RESISTANCE TO VIRUS INFECTIONS

In a number of virus infections evidence has accumulated that the early virus-macrophage interaction may be of vital importance for the final outcome of a virus infection (3,10). The following will give examples of the kind of observations that have led to this concept.

1) Macrophages can Exert Intrinsic Restriction of Virus Replication

Macrophages may either be intrinsically resistant (nonpermissive) or susceptible (permissive) to virus replication (3). In the nonpermissive situation, macrophages may take up and destroy the virus or the infection may be aborted in the cells. In both instances the macrophage represents a blind alley for propagation of the infection. On the other hand, if the virus is able to replicate efficiently in macrophages, infection may spread to susceptible cells resulting in extensive destruction of organs and tissues. Furthermore, by their migration through the body, infected monocytes and macrophages may serve as a vehicle for dissemination of the infection (9).

In analyzing macrophage intrinsic restriction of virus replication, it is important to realize that a number of variables in the experimental approach may influence the outcome of the virus-macrophage interaction. First, macrophages from different anatomical compartments may differ in permissiveness for a virus (11). Second, the widespread use of nonspecific irritants to increase macrophage yields may also influence permissiveness. Thus, Lopez and Dudas (12) found peritoneal macrophages elicited with thioglycollate much more susceptible to replication of herpes simplex virus type 1 (HSV-1) than normal resident or proteose-peptone stimulated macrophages. Third, culture conditions may influence the result. This was also illustrated by Lopez and Dudas (12), who found that precultivation of macrophages for three to seven days considerably increased their permissiveness for HSV-1. Also blood monocytes from adult humans become more susceptible to HSV replication upon culture for several days (13). Among other culture conditions that influence virus-macrophage interactions, mention may be made of the type and concentration of serum used (14). The presence of antiviral antibody has in some instances been found to enhance the replication of a virus in macrophage cultures (15), presumably because of an Fc receptor-mediated promotion of virus uptake into the cells (16).

Macrophages are generally more restrictive for virus replication than other cell types (3). Therefore, it is often necessary to use indirect measures such as infectious center assays to detect virus replication. This kind of assays indicate the number of macrophages in a culture that support virus replication, but give no information on the amount of virus produced in each cell. In some virus-macrophage systems virus replication has been measured directly by titration of extracellular or intracellular virus. However, in many of these instances the virus has been adapted to grow in macrophages or special elicitation or culture procedures favoring productive replication are employed, thereby making their relevance for the natural situation more questionable.

2) Macrophages can Exert Extrinsic Antiviral Activity

Macrophage extrinsic antiviral activity is defined as the ability of macrophages to affect the virus or virus replication in the surroundings (10). Generally, this is measured in vitro by adding macrophages to infected monolayers of permissive cells and observing reduced cytopathic effect, plaque-reduction or reduced amounts of intracellular or extracellular virus. Morahan and Morse (10) have outlined the various ways in which macrophages might theoretically interfere with virus replication in permissive cells. The vulnerable stage of the infection will depend on the specific virus-host cell interaction. Special interest has focused on the question, whether interferon production or direct macrophage cytotoxicity toward infected cells are involved. In the HSV system, which has been studied in detail, this does not seem to be the case. Rather, some disturbance of host cell macromolecular synthesis, which requires macrophage-cell contact, is at work (17,18). Alternatively, Wildy et al. (19) have suggested that arginase produced by activated macrophages might be responsible for the extrinsic inhibition of HSV and vaccinia virus multiplication by depleting the medium of arginine, which is essential for virus replication. This effect does not require cell-contact.

Extrinsic antiviral activity is generally not a prominent feature of normal, unstimulated macrophages (10,17), although it has been reported in some instances (20,21). Therefore, extrinsic restriction of virus replication can probably not be considered a ready-to-function barrier to the establishment of virus infections in the sense that has been described for intrinsic restriction. However, since macrophage activation is an early event in many virus infections (10), extrinsic activity of activated macrophages accumulating in established foci of infection might be important to diminish further spread of the infection.

3) Transfer of Macrophages Increases Resistance to Virus Infections

Most studies on the effect of macrophage transfer have been conducted in inbred mice, where cells have been transferred from resistant adult mice to more susceptible young or suckling mice of the same inbred strain (3). Protection of the recipient mice against subsequent infection can be ascribed to the transferred cells. In most instances an effect, as measured by higher survival rates, has only been achieved after transfer of stimulated or activated macrophages. However, we in our laboratory have observed reduced virus titers in the liver of HSV-2-infected young mice after intravenous transfer of resident macrophages from resistant adult mice (22). One reason for this good rate of protection with normal macrophages is probably that death of the animal is a less sensitive marker of macrophage protection than is the degree of early virus replication in a selected target organ. Furthermore, the intravenous route of transferring cells may be especially suited to protect the liver from subsequent infection, since it has been shown that approximately 60% of peritoneal macrophages injected intravenously in mice are localized in the liver within a few hours post-inoculation (23).

4) Macrophage Blockade Decreases Resistance to Virus Infections

Another way of determining the role of macrophages in host resistance to viruses is to impair macrophage functions by antimacrophage serum or chemical agents that are more or less selectively toxic to macrophages. Among the macrophage toxic agents, silica has been most widely used. It was originally described by Allison and coworkers (26) to be selectively toxic to monocytes/macrophages, but in recent years it has been realized that the function of other cell populations may also be adversely affected (27). When using silica, it is important to look for an effect during the early phases of the infection, since the agent may cause a late rebound effect with recruitment of monocytes from the bone marrow (28). It has also been reported that silica treatment may be followed by an augmented antibody response to viruses, probably due to an increased antigenic stimulus or, alternatively, because macrophages are involved in antibody-depressing mechanisms (29).

5) Macrophage Activation Increases Resistance to Virus Infections

It has been documented with a number of viruses that induced or naturally occurring nonspecific activation of macrophages is accompanied by increased resistance to virus infections, indicating a role for the mononuclear phagocyte system in the natural defense against the infection.

Mice treated with immunomodulators like pyran and bacterial adjuvants such as C. parvum or BCG exhibit enhanced resistance to virus infections together with augmented extrinsic and intrinsic antiviral activity of their macrophages (10). However, the sole role of macrophages in this augmented resistance may be questioned. First, immunomodulators are known to activate other potential defense systems, for instance interferon production, which might exert an antiviral activity in its own right or through activation of

16

NK cells (10,4). Second, it has been found that pyran and C. parvum still induce resistance in ^{89}Sr-marrow-ectomized mice, which are severely monocyto-penic (30). Third, resistance induced by these two immunomodulators is not reversed by treatment with silica (30).

Further evidence of the potential importance of nonspecifically acti-vated macrophages in resistance to viral infections has emerged from studies in nude mice. These mice are severely immunodeficient and yet have been shown to exhibit increased early natural resistance to some infections (3). Thus, nude mice beyond the age of four to five weeks are considerably more resistant than their normal littermates to the induction of hepatitis by HSV-2 (31). Studies of the course of infection showed that nude mice were able to restrain virus multiplication in the liver far better during the first five days of the infection than were normal mice. Macrophages from nude mice were found to exhibit enhanced intrinsic restriction of the virus, and silica treatment was able to abolish the augmented resistance. Probably, an increased intestinal bacterial flora of nudes is responsible for a sus-tained nonspecific macrophage activation, since macrophages from nude mice raised under germfree conditions or treated with antibiotics do not possess activated macrophages (3).

6) Virus Virulence Correlates with Macrophage Restriction

In some instances a difference in virulence of closely related virus types or virus strains is reflected in the interaction of macrophages with the viruses, indicating that this interaction may be an important host resistance determinant (3). For instance, the marked difference in mouse hepatotropism between the two types of HSV (HSV-2 readily induces focal necrotic hepatitis in mice, which is not the case with HSV-1) is correlated with a far better restriction of HSV-1 than of HSV-2 in macrophages from the mice (32). Further evidence in support of the participation of macro-phages in the pathogenic distinction between liver infections with the two virus types was obtained by blocking the macrophage function of the animals by silica, which was able to almost completely eliminate the difference, allowing HSV-1 also to induce liver necrosis (33).

7) Age-related Resistance to Virus Infections Correlates with Macrophage Restriction

The ability of many viruses to replicate productively in macrophages from animals and humans has been found to dramatically decrease with age (3). Likewise, extrinsic antiviral activity has also been found to be age-related (20,17). This maturation of macrophage antiviral potencies has been found to occur concomitant with the well-known age-dependent increase in resistance, which is seen in most virus infections. Of course, the macrophage system is not the only potential antiviral defense system which is undergoing a maturation during this period. However, additional support for a role of macrophages in age-related resistance development comes from studies on macrophage depletion or macrophage transfer as outlined above (3).

8) Genetically Determined Resistance to Virus Infections Correlates with Macrophage Restriction

In a number of virus infections, in which a genetic basis for resistance or susceptibility has been demonstrated, the outcome of the infection has been shown to correlate with the outcome of the early virus-macrophage inter-action, suggesting that macrophages may be important determinants in the phenomenon (3). This aspect of the role of macrophages in natural resistance to virus infection will be discussed in more detail in the following section.

MACROPHAGES AND GENETICALLY DETERMINED

NATURAL RESISTANCE TO VIRUS INFECTIONS

The earliest reports on a genetic basis for resistance to animal virus infections were published half a century ago (34,35,36). Since then, the inheritability of resistance to virus infections has been demonstrated in several animal model systems and the genetics behind the variation has been explored (1). In some instances a single dominant gene has been found to make a major impact on resistance or susceptibility. The classical examples of this are the resistance of mice to flaviviruses and the susceptibility of mice to mouse hepatitis virus type 2 (MHV-2), both of which are inherited as monogenic autosomal dominant characteristics (Fig. 1). In other instances the trait has been found to be under polygenic control, which generally makes an evaluation of the mechanism of resistance more difficult. The following will give some examples of virus infections in which macrophages have been found to express at the cellular level the genetic resistance seen in vivo.

1) Flaviviruses

During the thirties, Webster (36) developed by selective breeding, strains of mice which differed greatly in resistance to two flaviviruses, St. Louis and louping ill viruses. Genetic analysis indicated that resistance was dominant and unifactorial (Fig. 1a). In the fifties, Sabin (37) extended this work on nonselected PRI and C_3H strains of mice and found PRI mice resistant and C_3H mice susceptible to yellow fever and a number of other flaviviruses. The work of Sabin also indicated that resistance operated on the level of individual cells.

In extensive studies in the sixties with West Nile virus, Goodmann and Koprowski (38) concluded that the cells representing the phenotypic expression of the gene for flavivirus resistance belong to the reticuloendothelial system. Thus, cultures of peritoneal and splenic macrophages from resistant and susceptible mice were found to differ greatly in permissiveness for the virus, and this trait segregated as expected in macrophage cultures from backcross mice. Also macrophages from cogenic resistant C_3HRV mice, only differing from susceptible C_3H mice at the gene for flavivirus resistance expressed the resistance phenotype in vitro. The depressed flavivirus replication in cells from resistant mice was found in the original reports to involve macrophages selectively. Later studies have found other cell types, for instance brain cells and fibroblasts, also to express flavivirus

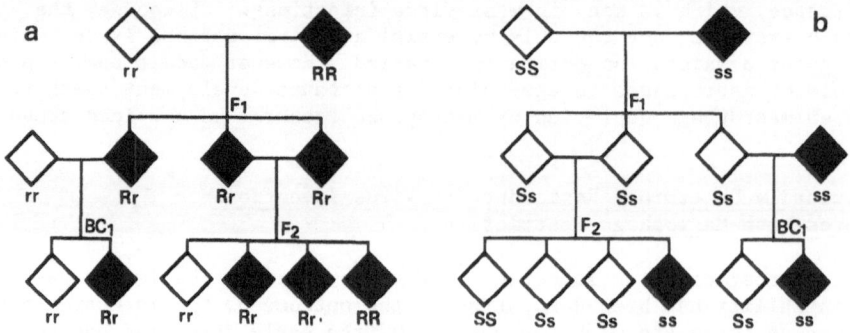

Figure 1. Autosomal dominant inheritance of resistance (a) or susceptibility (b) to virus infections. The symbols indicate both female and male individuals and resistant (◆) or susceptible (◇) phenotype.

resistance (39,40). However, this does not rule out a role for the macrophage barrier in resistance, but only implies that the resistance gene also operates, if the barrier has been broken.

The mechanism of action of the flavivirus resistance gene is not fully understood. Neither differential interferon production nor interferon sensitivity seem to play any particular role (40). Studies by Darnell and Koprowski (39) have indicated that production of defective interfering particles by resistant cells is of importance, although this may not constitute the only or major mechanism by which virus replication is blocked in resistant cells.

2) Mouse Hepatitis Viruses

Infection of mice with mouse hepatitis viruses provides the best example of susceptibility inherited as a dominant,monogenic trait (Fig. 1b). Studies over two decades by Bang and coworkers (1) on mouse resistance to MHV-2 have yielded evidence that macrophages represent a cellular barrier to virus access to the liver. Genetic analyses of several strains of mice have shown a complete agreement between mouse and macrophage susceptibility to the virus. It is interesting to notice that the same two strains of mice (PRI and C_2H) have been used in studies of the genetics of macrophage resistance to MHV-2 and flaviviruses and that the strain susceptible to MHV-2 is resistant to flaviviruses and vice versa. This indicates that virus-macrophage interactions require individual assessment with each virus-host system.

Susceptibility of mouse macrophages to MHV-3 has also been found to parallel the susceptibility of mice of different strains to infection (41). With this virus most strains of mice (including C57BL, which is generally resistant to most other viruses) and macrophages from these mice are highly susceptible, whereas A/J mice and their macrophages are resistant. The virus-macrophage interaction also reflects the in vivo situation in "semiresistant" C_3H mice, in that macrophages from these mice show an intermediate level of virus replication.

Several attempts have been made to elucidate the mechanism of macrophage restriction of MHVs (1,4). Resistance is clearly expressed at the level of individual cells and interferon production by macrophages does not seem to be important. Although various manipulations of macrophage cultures (transfer of extracts from susceptible to resistant cultures, cortisone-treatment and addition of supernatants from allogeneic mixed lymphocyte cultures or Con A-stimulated lymphocytes) have been found to modify the virus-macrophage interaction, these studies have not clarified the situation. On the basis of studies with anti-interferon treatment Virelizier (41) has suggested that endogenous interferon production in response to the MHV-3 infection in question and also to past exposure to bacterial infections may be essential for the acquisition of the ability of macrophages to restrict virus replication, and that the efficiency of interferon to do this varies in different mouse strains.

3) Herpesvirus

Herpes simplex virus (HSV) exists in two closely related antigenic types HSV-1 and HSV-2. Studies of inbred mouse strains have revealed a marked difference in resistance among various strains to both HSV-1 and HSV-2. Thus, Lopez (42) found resistance to HSV-1-induced encephalitis to be dominant and governed by at least two independent non-H-2-linked genes, whereas we found resistance to hepatitis induction by HSV-2 to be influenced by one major X-linked dominant gene (43). The X-linkage of resistance was revealed in the F_1 generation of crosses between resistant GR male and susceptible BALB/c female mice (Fig. 2), where the characters for susceptibility and resistance segregated between male and female mice (males susceptible, females resistant).

With both types of HSV, macrophages from resistant strains of mice exert higher intrinsic restriction of virus replication than macrophages from susceptible strains, a difference which is not seen in fibroblast cultures. In the case of HSV-2 we found macrophage restriction of virus replication to correlate with resistance in the F_1 generation. This has been confirmed by Armerding et al. (44). Furthermore, we found segregation of high and low restriction close to a 1:1 ratio in macrophage cultures prepared from individual mice in the BC_1 generation, indicating that a single gene is at work. With HSV-1, Lopez and Dudas (12) were unable to relate the genetics of macrophage restriction of virus replication to resistance. Although F_1 mice were found to be resistant to HSV-1 infection, macrophages from these mice replicated the virus as well as did macrophages from the susceptible parent. One reason for the different results obtained with the two virus types might well be found in the experimental approaches used. The results with HSV-2 were obtained with normal peritoneal macrophages infected in vivo or the day after plating in culture, whereas the results with HSV-1 were derived with thioglycollate-induced or four-day-cultured macrophages, which have lost much of the native restriction capability against the virus.

Suggestions for alternative mechanisms behind the genetically determined resistance to HSV in the mouse have included NK cells and interferon production. Thus, Lopez (45) described an association between resistance and natural killing of HSV-1-infected targets by spleen cells. The nature of the effector cell(s) in the mouse has not been determined, but studies in humans have pointed to precursors of the monocyte-granulocyte series (46). Data from the laboratory of Kirchner (4) have indicated that genetically determined resistance to HSV-1 is related to very early interferon production, which is in part governed by an X-linked gene (47). We have also shown that infection of resistant mice with high doses of HSV-2 elicits an early interferon response, which shows the same pattern of inheritance (X-linked, dominant) as macrophage-related resistance, suggesting an association between interferon induction and macrophage restriction (48). Since interferon is known to activate NK cells and macrophages, early interferon induction may well be a central feature in genetically determined resistance to HSV. Whether the link turns out to be genetically determined interferon production by macrophages, or interferon-induced, genetically determined activation of monocytes/macrophages to virus restriction or nonspecific cytotoxicity is not clear at the moment.

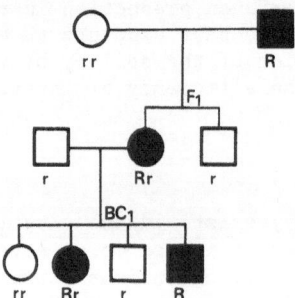

Figure 2. X-linked dominant inheritance of resistance
to virus infection in females (circles) and
males (squares) with resistant (closed symbols)
and susceptible (open symbols) phenotypes.

20

Genetic control of resistance of mice to another herpesvirus, murine cytomegalovirus (MCMV), was described by Selgrade and Osborn (49). They also found that resistance was the dominant feature, but it was independent of resistance to HSV-1 infection. Thus, C57BL mice were resistant to HSV-1 and susceptible to MCMV, whereas CBA mice were susceptible to HSV-1 and resistant to MCMV. Although transfer and blockade experiments suggested some importance of macrophages in resistance, infection in vitro of macrophages from resistant mice was no less productive than was infection of cells from susceptible mice. These findings do not support the concept of a simple barrier function of macrophages in genetic resistance to this infection.

Concerning other herpesviruses macrophages have also been found to be restrictive for replication of Marek's disease virus (MDV) of chickens (50) and infectious bovine rhinotracheitis (IBR) virus of cattle (51). However, there was no correlation between macrophage intrinsic restriction of MDV and genetic resistance of chickens to infection. With IBR virus, no data on genetic resistance of macrophages are available.

4) Myxoviruses

Mice of the A2G strain have been found to express a pronounced and selective resistance to various orthomyxoviruses (2). Resistance has been attributed to a single dominant gene designated Mx. For many years the phenotypic expression of Mx gene was an enigma. In 1978 it was shown that peritoneal macrophages and Kuppfer cells from A2G and F_1 mice, as opposed to macrophages from a number of susceptible mouse strains, resisted replication of influenza virus (52). Furthermore, resistance and susceptibility of individual mice and their macrophages cosegregated in a ratio close to 1:1 in backcrosses between resistant F_1 mice and susceptible mice, indicating that resistance in vivo and macrophage restriction of virus replication were related. However, in elegant studies with radiation chimeras it was later found that lethally irradiated Mx+ mice substituted with macrophage precursors from susceptible Mx- mice and vice versa expressed the resistance phenotype of the recipient, in spite of the fact that their macrophages expressed the phenotype of the donor (53). Thus, macrophage resistance and resistance of the intact animal did not seem to be causally related. Instead, evidence has been presented that the Mx-gene influences the sensitivity of individual cells, including macrophages but also parenchymal cells, to an influenza virus-specific antiviral action of interferon (54).

CONCLUDING REMARKS

Studies reviewed here have revealed the existence of a genetic basis for natural resistance to a number of virus infections and focused on the role of macrophages in this phenomenon. Most of these studies have been conducted in mice, where the availability of inbred and congenic strains has facilitated the genetic analysis. Although not directly transferable to man, the results obtained may give important directions for the search for potential resistance determinants being involved in the individual variation in susceptibility to viral diseases observed in otherwise healthy humans.

REFERENCES

1. F. B. Bang, Genetics of resistance of animals to viruses: I. Introduction and studies in mice, Adv. Virus Res. 23:270 (1978).
2. O. Haller, Natural resistance to tumors and viruses, Curr. Top. Microbiol. Immunol. 92 (1981).

3. S. C. Mogensen, Role of macrophages in natural resistance to virus in-
    fections, Microbiol. Rev. 43:1 (1979).
4. H. Kirchner, "Immunobiology of Infection with Herpes Simplex Virus,"
    Karger, Basel (1982).
5. R. M. Welsh, Natural cell-mediated immunity during viral infections,
    Curr. Top. Microbiol. Immunol. 92:83 (1981).
6. E. Metchnikoff, "Leçons sur la Pathologie Comparée de l'Inflammation,"
    Masson, Paris (1892).
7. L. Aschoff, Das reticulo-endotheliale system, Ergeb. Inn. Med. Kinder-
    heilkd. 26:1 (1924).
8. R. van Furth, A. Cohn, J. G. Hirsch, J. H. Humphrey, W. G. Spector, and
    H. L. Langevoort, The mononuclear phagocyte system: a new classifica-
    tion of macrophages, monocytes, and their precursor cells, Bull.
    W.H.O. 46:845 (1972).
9. C. A. Mims, Aspects of pathogenesis of virus diseases, Bacteriol. Rev.
    28:30 (1964).
10. P. S. Morahan and S. S. Morse, Macrophage-virus interactions, in:
    "Virus-Lymphocyte Interactions: Implications for Disease," M. R.
    Proffitt, ed., Elsevier/North Holland Publishing Co., New York
    (1979).
11. S. Plaeger-Marshall, L. A. Wilson, and J. JW. Smith, Permissiveness of
    rabbit monocytes and macrophages for herpes simplex virus type 1,
    Infect. Immun. 35:151 (1982).
12. C. Lopez and G. Dudas, Replication of herpes simplex virus type 1 in
    macrophages from resistant and susceptible mice, Infect. Immun. 23:
    432 (1979).
13. C. A. Daniels, E. S. Kleinerman, and R. Snyderman, Abortive and produc-
    tive infections of human mononuclear phagocytes by type 1 herpes
    simplex virus, Am. J. Pathol. 91:119 (1978).
14. G. C. Lavelle and F. B. Bang, Influence of type and concentration of
    sera in vitro on susceptibility of genetically resistant cells to
    mouse hepatitis virus, J. Gen. Virol. 12:233 (1971).
15. S. B. Halstead and E. J. O'Rourke, Dengue viruses and mononuclear phago-
    cytes. I. Infection enhancement by non-neutralizing antibody, J. Exp.
    Med. 146:201 (1977).
16. J. J. Schlesinger and M. W. Brandriss, Growth of 17 D yellow fever virus
    in a macrophage-like cell line, U 937: role of Fc and viral receptors
    in antibody-mediated infection, J. Immunol. 127:659 (1981).
17. K. Hayashi, T. Kurata, T. Morishima, and T. Nassery, Analysis of the
    inhibitory effect of peritoneal macrophages on the spread of herpes
    simplex virus, Infect. Immun. 28:350 (1980).
18. S. S. Morse and P. S. Morahan, Activated macrophages mediate, Cell.
    Immunol. 58:72 (1981).
19. P. Wildy, P. G. H. Gell, J. Rhodes, and A. Newton, Inhibition of herpes
    simplex virus multiplication by activated macrophages: a role for
    arginase? Infect. Immun. 37:40 (1982).
20. A. J. Schlabach, D. Martinez, A. K. Field, and A. A. Tytell, Resistance
    of C58 mice to primary systemic herpes simplex virus infection:
    macrophage dependence and T-cell independence, Infect. Immun. 26:
    615 (1979).
21. S. A. Stohlman, J. G. Woodward, and J. A. Frelinger, Macrophage anti-
    viral activity: extrinsic versus intrinsic activity, Infect. Immun.
    36:672 (1982).
22. S. C. Mogensen, Genetics of macrophage-controlled resistance to hepati-
    tis induced by herpes simplex virus type 2 in mice, Infect. Immun.
    19:46 (1978).
23. B. Roser, The distribution of intravenously injected peritoneal macro-
    phages in the mouse, Aust. J. Exp. Biol. Med. Sci. 43:553 (1965).
26. A. C. Allison, J. S. Harington, and M. Birbeck, An examination of the
    cytotoxic effects of silica on macrophages, J. Exp. Med. 124:141
    (1966).

27. J. J. Wirth, W. P. Carney, and E. F. Wheelock, The effect of particle size on the immunodepressive properties of silica, J. Immunol. Meth. 32:357 (1980).

28. H. duBuy, Effect of silica on virus infections in mice and mouse tissue culture, Infect. Immun. 11:996 (1975).

29. A. Knoblich, J. Gortz, V. Harle-Grupp, and D. Falke, Kinetics and genetics of herpes simplex virus-induced antibody formation in mice, Infect. Immun. 39:15 (1983).

30. P. S. Morahan, P. H. Coleman, S. S. Morse, and A. Volkman, Resistance to infections in mice with defects in the activities of mononuclear phagocytes and natural killer cells: effects of immunomodulators in beige mice and ^{89}Sr-treated mice, Infect. Immun. 37:1079 (1982).

31. S. C. Mogensen and H. K. Anderson, Role of activated macrophages in resistance of congenitally athymic nude mice to hepatitis induced by herpes simplex virus type 2, Infect. Immun. 19:792 (1978).

32. S. C. Mogensen, Role of macrophages in hepatitis induced by herpes simplex virus types 1 and 2 in mice, Infect. Immun. 15:686 (1977a).

33. S. C. Mogensen and H. K. Anderson, Effect of silica on the pathogenic distinction between herpes simplex virus type 1 and 2 hepatitis in mice, Infect. Immun. 17:274 (1977).

34. J. W. Gowen and R. H. Schott, Genetic constitution in mice as differentiated by two diseases, pseudorabies and mouse typhoid, Am. J. Hyg. 18:674 (1933).

35. C. J. Lynch and T. P. Hughes, The inheritance of susceptibility to yellow fever encephalitis in mice, Genetics 21:104 (1936).

36. L. T. Webster, Inheritance of resistance of mice to enteric bacterial neurotropic virus infections, J. Exp. Med. 65:261 (1937).

37. A. B. Sabin, Nature of inherited resistance to viruses affecting the nervous system, Proc. Natl. Acad. Sci. 38:540 (1952).

38. G. T. Goodmann and H. Koprowski, Study on the mechanism of innate resistance to virus infection, J. Cell. Comp. Physiol. 59:333 (1962).

39. M. B. Darnell and H. Koprowski, Genetically determined resistance to infection with group B arboviruses. II. Increased production of interfering particles in cell cultures from resistant mice, J. Infect. Dis. 129:248 (1974).

40. M. A. Brinton, Genetically controlled resistance to flavivirus and lactate-dehydrogenase-elevating virus-induced disease, Curr. Top. Microbiol. Immunol. 92:1 (1981).

41. J.-L. Virelizier, Role of macrophages and interferon in natural resistance to mouse hepatitis virus infection, Curr. Top. Microbiol. Immunol. 92:53 (1981).

42. C. Lopez, Genetics of natural resistance to herpesvirus infection in mice, Nature 258:152 (1975).

43. S. C. Mogensen, Genetics of macrophage-controlled resistance to hepatitis induced by herpes simplex virus type 2 in mice, Infect. Immun. 17:268 (1977b).

44. D. Armerding, P. Mayer, M. Scriba, A. Hren, and H. Rossiter, In vivo modulation of macrophage functions by herpes simplex virus type 2 in resistant and sensitive inbred mouse strains, Immunobiol. 160:217 (1981).

45. C. Lopez, Resistance to herpes simplex virus-type 1 (HSV-1), Curr. Top. Microbiol. Immunol. 92:15 (1981).

46. C. Lopez, D. Kirkpatrick, P. A. Fitzgerald, C. Y. Ching, R. Pahwa, R. A. Good, and E. M. Smithwick, Studies of the cell-lineage of the effector cells that spontaneously lyse HSV-1 infected fibroblasts [NK(HSV-1)], J. Immunol. 129:824 (1982).

47. R. Zawatzky, H. Kirchner, J. DeMaeyer-Guignard, and E. DeMaeyer, An X-linked locus influences the amount of circulating interferon induced in the mouse by herpes simplex virus type 1, J. Gen. Virol. 63:325 (1982).

48. E. B. Pederson, S. Haahr, and S. C. Mogensen, X-linked resistance of mice to high doses of herpes simplex virus type 2 correlates with early interferon production, Infect. Immun. 42:740 (1983).

49. M. K. Selgrade and J. E. Osborn, Role of macrophages in resistance to murine cytomegalovirus, Infect. Immun. 10:1383 (1974).

50. K. Haffer, M. Sevoian, and M. Wilder, The role of the macrophage in Marek's disease: in vitro and in vivo studies, Int. J. Cancer, 23: 648, (1979).

51. A. J. Forman, L. A. Babiuk, V. Misra, and F. Baldwin, Susceptibility of bovine macrophages to infectious bovine rhinotracheitis virus infection, Infect. Immun. 35:1048 (1982).

52. J. Lindenmann, E. Deuel, S. Fanconi, and O. Haller, Inborn resistance of mice to myxoviruses: macrophages express phenotype in vitro, J. Exp. Med. 147:531 (1978).

53. O. Haller, H. Arnheiter, J. Lindenmann, Natural, genetically determined resistance toward influenza virus in hemopoietic mouse chimeras. Role of mononuclear phagocytes, J. Exp. Med. 150:117 (1979).

54. O. Haller, H. Arnheiter, J. Lindenmann, and I. Gresser, Host gene influences sensitivity to interferon action selectively for influenza virus, Nature 283:660 (1980).

VIRUS INTERACTIONS WITH THE IMMUNE DEFENSE SYSTEM

Herman Friedman, Andor Szentivanyi, Steven Specter and
Mauro Bendinelli

Department of Medical Microbiology and Immunology, and
Department of Pharmacology and Therapeutics,
University of South Florida College of Medicine
Tampa, Florida and Institute of Hygiene and Microbiology
University of Pisa, Faculty of Medicine, Pisa, Italy

Viruses, which are obligate intracellular parasites, are not only cyto-lytic for target cells, but also may affect many physio-pharmacologic and immunologic parameters of the host. In particular, viruses may influence humoral or cellular immune defenses that develop as protective mechanisms against microbial infection (24,31,33,37,38,40). In this context, viruses have developed various strategies to survive in harmony with a host in which they replicate. One such mechanism is the ability to subvert or impair immune responses, especially those, which may be detrimental to the survival of the virus (2,4,10,17-20). The methods whereby viruses may affect immunity, either in a positive or a negative manner, are still not clear. In general, modification of host immune responses may be manifested by altered humoral or cellular immunity, or both, as well as altered suscep-tibility to infection by the same or other microorganisms.

GENERAL CHARACTERISTICS OF VIRUS INTERACTION WITH THE IMMUNE SYSTEM

The type as well as strain of a virus, the genetic and phenotypic char-acter of the host, are important determinants in establishment of a virus infection, either overt or subclinical (2,12,15,17,37,40). Viruses have a strong affinity for certain cell types. Although specific receptors on various cell populations are important for initiating the process resulting in virus replication (14), various nonspecific factors may also influence resistance vs. susceptibility. For example, factors as divergent as the temperature of the host, pH of the body fluids, general environmental niche of both the host and virus, etc., serve an important role in delineating the host/parasite relationship in virus infections. There are also a series of effectors, both specific and nonspecific, which are specialized in nature and probably evolved to counteract viruses and other invading agents. For example, phagocytosis is considered an important aspect of host defenses to viruses (2,21,24,33,40) together with nonspecific antiviral serum factors, including enzymes such as lysozyme, the complement system, etc. As far as specific immunity is concerned, it is widely accepted that antibody responses to specific viral antigens are important in limiting viral invasion. Thus, lymphocytes sensitized with specific antibody as well as T lymphocyte re-sponses during cell mediated immunity are considered essential components

of resistance to most viruses (2,39,40). Humoral mediators, that is lymphokines, monokines, and cytokines, including interferons and interleukins,
have important roles in antiviral immunity. Many of these agents are produced not only by lymphocytes and macrophages but also by other cell types
which may serve as a target for virus infection.

VIRUS INDUCED IMMUNOMODULATION

Viral infections may suppress or enhance one or more components of the
immune system (3,5,8-11,17-23) while under certain circumstances no detectable effect may occur. The virus infection may induce specific immune paralysis, especially when infectious to a newborn or fetus as well as nonspecific
immune suppression, either finite or permanent (17-20). It is the latter
type of suppression which has attracted much attention in recent years,
especially with recognition that certain retroviruses may suppress immunity
not only in experimental animals but also in man.

Conversely, viruses may stimulate specific as well as nonspecific cellular and humoral immune responses to the virus itself or to its components.
Enhancement of cellular and humor immunity mostly occurs through direct
stimulation of lymphoid elements or through altering the secretion or
formation of immunoactive substances by these cells.

Table 1. Major Effects of Viruses on Humoral vs. Cellular Immune
Responses and Cells of the Immune System.

Virus	Immune System Affected		Cell Type Affected		
	Cell-Mediated	Humoral	Macro-phages	T cells	B cells
Adenovirus	+	+		+	+
Coxsackievirus	+	+			+
Cytomegalovirus	+	+	+		+
Dengue	+	+	+	+(±)	+
Echovirus	+	+	+	+(±)	
Epstein-Barr	+			+	
Hepatitis A	+		+	?	?
Hepatitis B	+		+	+	
Herpex Simplex	+	+	+	+(±)	+(±)
Influenza	+	+	+	+(±)	
Lymphocytic choriomeningitis			+	+	
Measles	+	+	+	+	+
Mumps	+			+	+
Poliovirus	+		+	+(±)	
Retrovirus	+	+	+	+	+
Rabies	+		+	+	
Rubella	+	+	+	+	
Smallpox	+		+	+(±)	
Vaccinia	+		+		
Varicella-Zoster	+		+	+	
Yellow Fever	+				

Table 1 lists the major effects of viruses on humoral and cellular immune reactivities and the cell types that participate in the organization of these responses. Table 2 presents some of the cell classes or parameters of immunologic responsiveness which have been found suppressed during viral infections. The mechanisms whereby such suppression occurs are still ill-defined and probably highly diversified, but from studies concerning many different viral infections some generalizations are now possible. In most, if not all instances where some insights into mechanisms have been obtained immunological impairment appears due mainly to functional alterations of immunocompetent cells. This may occur because of direct interactions of immunocompetent cells with a virus and/or less frequently by substances produced by cells as a consequence of viral infection (2-5,17-20). As indicated in Table 1, a large number of viruses have been found to replicate in lymphoid cells, including T and B lymphocytes and macrophages. Such replication may affect the functional activity of the lymphoid cells and the general immunocompetence of the individuals (Tables 3, 4, and 5). Alteration of cell mediated immunity may be due to effects of a virus on T lymphocytes or macrophages, or both, as well as related to products produced by B cells. Humoral immunity can be affected not only by the influence of virus on B lymphocytes, but also on helper or regulatory T lymphocytes as well as accessory macrophages necessary for antibody responsiveness.

Because of functional complexities, the immune system can be affected by viruses that influence different levels of the response system. Such functional alterations do not necessarily presuppose extensive damage to lymphoid tissue itself. Indeed, hypoplastic changes may occur but, as a rule, substantially few, if any, histologic alterations of lymphoid tissues become evident during many viral infections (2,17-20). Nevertheless, in some virus infections lymphatic tissues show usually limited lesions which may resemble the cytopathic effects characteristic of the infecting virus in vitro. For instance, in measles infection typically polynucleated giant cells develop in various lymphoid organs beginning at the very early stages of infection. Furthermore, in certain viral infections various degrees of cellular depletion may occur which affect distinct areas within the lymphoid tissue.

Table 2. Parameters of Immunological Responsiveness Suppressed During Viral Infections

Virus	Immune Parameter
Congenital Rubella	Ig levels in serum
Junin	Antibody-dependent hypersensitivity
Reovirus, selected retroviruses	Circulating autoantibody
Lactic dehydrogenase virus	Spontaneous autoimmune lesions
Lactic dehydrogenase virus	Lymphocyte and antigen trapping by spleen
Polio, Coxsackie B, Mumps, Measles, Epstein-Barr	Contact sensitivity, cell-mediated hypersensitivity
Retroviruses	T cell-mediated cytotoxicity
Cytomegalovirus, Marek	Skin allograft rejection
Dengue	Graft-versus-host induction
Lymphocytic choriomeningitis	Immunological maturation
Venezuelan equine encephalitis, lymphocytic choriomeningitis	Tolerance induction
Cytomegalovirus, influenza, measles, parainfluenza	Resistance to superinfection

The structural integrity of lymphoid tissue does not prevent immunocompetent cells from exhibiting profound manifestations of functional deficiency. A typical example is reduced in vitro blastogenic responsiveness of lymphocytes to specific antigens, mitogens, and alloantigens which is readily reproducible in experimentally infected animals (17-22,25,27). Tables 4 and 5 list some of the alterations in lymphoid classes which have been noted during virus infections in vivo or, in experimental situations, in vitro when individuals or cells are infected with a particular virus. For instance, B lymphocyte number and function can be markedly altered by viruses, either in a positive or negative manner both in vivo and in vitro. T cells are also readily affected. In addition, viruses affect other lymphoid cells, including null cells, K cells, NK cells, etc. Traffic of infected lymphocytes may also be affected by virus infection (1,2). This may be due to cell surface changes which reduce the ability of cells to interact with endothelial cells or to "home" to appropriate target organs.

Altered peripheral lymphocytes may also occur in many viral diseases. It is widely known that infections induced by measles, rubella, varicella, poliomyelitis, adenovirus or arbor viruses markedly alter lymphocyte number and function. Such changes are often transient. For example, lymphopenia may be present in early stages of certain infections or may become pronounced later, affecting all or only selected cells or subpopulations of lymphocytes.

Major effects of virus infection may be associated either directly or indirectly with mediators of immunological mechanisms (5-7,16). A direct

Table 3. Possible Mechanisms of Virus Induced Immunosuppression

---

Inactivates or modifies (binds) Ig, including antibody and
antibody forming cells.

Inactivates complement or complement producing cells.

Directly infects antibody producing B cells.

Directly affects effector and/or helper/suppressor T cells
or their functions.

Affects precursor T or B cells or stem cells.

Affects macrophages and their function.

Induces suppressor T cells or macrophages.

Indirect effects on B or T cells or macrophages by products
induced by other cells, either lymphoid or non-lymphoid.

Induces immunomodulatory soluble substances such as lymphokines, monokines,
prostaglandins, leukotriens, specific kinins, the amine mediators
(histamine, serotonin, acetylcholine, the catecholamines) etc.

Suppressor Ag (virus)/antibody complexes.

Direct or suppressive effects by virus components.

Direct or indirect suppressive effects by products of virus
infected cells (suppressor molecules).

Table 4.   Alterations in Lymphocyte Function or Activity
          by Viruses

B Lymphocytes:

Peripheral blood number	Increase or decrease
Surface Ig expression	Decrease mainly
Surface Ig capping	Decrease mainly
Proliferation, spontaneous	Increase mainly
Mitogen induced blastogenesis	Decrease mainly
Polyclonal Ig synthesis	Decrease or increase
Specific antibody formation	Decrease mainly

T Lymphocytes:

Peripheral blood number	Increase or decrease
E-rosette formation	Decrease mainly
Thy-antigen expression	Increase or decrease
Proliferation - spontaneous	Decrease or increase
Mitogen induced blastogenesis	Decrease mainly
Antigen-induced blastogenesis	Increase mainly
Lymphokine production	Decrease mainly
Cytotoxicity	Decrease mainly
Antibody dependent cytolysis	Decrease mainly
B-cell helper activity	Decrease mainly
Suppressor cell activity	Increase or decrease

Uncharacterized Lymphocytes:

Peripheral blood number	Increase or decrease
Leukocyte circulation and migration	Increase or decrease
Proliferation - spontaneous	Increase mainly

K and NK Activity:

Natural cytolysis of target cells	Increase or decrease
Antibody dependent cytolysis	Decrease mainly
Interferon production	Decrease mainly
Response to cytokines	Decrease mainly

action of a virus may affect mediator formation or storage, especially during
cytolytic infection of leukocytes, although it is to be noted that certain
viruses do not replicate within leukocytes. Nevertheless, various studies
have permitted recognition of cellular classes and sometimes specific sub-
classes of lymphoid cells capable of replicating viruses. Experiments in
vitro have shown that many lymphoid cells may be targets of virus infections,
in general, and macrophages in particular (3-5,13,17-22). While the latter
are often restricted in susceptibility to infection by viruses, these cells
may undergo changes in their susceptibility once nonspecifically activated
through signals emitted by lymphocytes. As is apparent in Table 5, macrophages and monocytes in general may show functional alterations following
viral infections.

It is interesting to note that despite the repeated observations that
certain cells of the lymphoid system may have innate susceptibility to
virus infection, activation of lymphocytes by nonspecific means, such as

mitogenic or antigenic stimulation, may alter their susceptibility (2-5). It is important to note that in vitro a variety of viruses may cause unsensitized lymphocytes to undergo polyclonal activation and/or blastogenesis. This does not appear to be experimental artifacts because lymphocytes from subjects in the acute phases of measles or rubella infection, when cultured in vitro, often show a high degree of spontaneous proliferation. Furthermore, during mononucleosis caused by EB virus extremely large numbers of activated lymphocytes appear in the patient's circulation. It is not clear whether such effects of viruses on lymphocytes are related to functional alterations. However, it should be noted that as a result of direct contact of viruses with lymphocytes in vitro immunocompetent cells may develop similar defects as those observed following in vivo experimental or clinical infections. Nevertheless, virus induced changes do not necessarily require that the virus replicates in the infected cells since in some instances inactivated viruses or purified viral components also produce in similar alterations (Table 6).

Many observations suggest that in a large proportion of cases where immune depression occurs during viral infection the mechanism may be related to the ability of a virus to interact directly with cells of the immune system and/or replicate selectively in those cell populations actively engaged in immunologic reactions (10,13,17,29,30). As seen in Table 6, indirect effects of viruses on immunocompetent cells have been observed repeatedly. Soluble substances toxic for lymphocytes have been found in patients during acute phases of viral infections. Furthermore, it has been found that serum factors that nonspecifically inhibit cell-mediated immune responses or humoral antibody formation may occur in patients with infections such as hepatitis, mononucleosis, etc. These factors include antigen-antibody complexes and a large variety of substances potentially released during viral infections such as lymphokines, monokines, specific kinins, prostaglandins, leukotrienes, the so-called amine-mediators (catecholamines, acetylcholine, histamine, serotonin) etc.

LEUKEMIA VIRUS INDUCED IMMUNOSUPPRESSION

There is much current interest concerning immunodepression induced by retroviruses. The explosive interest revolving around human T cell leukemia viruses have focused attention on the nature and mechanism whereby leukemia viruses may affect the immune response in general. There are numerous studies concerning feline, murine, and human leukemia viruses, as well as

Table 5. Effects of Viruses on Macrophage/Monocyte Function or Activity

Number in peripheral blood	Increase mainly
Attachment/spreading on surfaces	Increase or decrease
Motility/chemotaxis	Decrease mainly
Phagocytosis	Increase or decrease
Phagosome-lysosome fusion	Decrease mainly
Microbe or particle ingestion	Decrease
Cytolysis/cytostasis	Increase or decrease
Antigen/presentation	Increase
Ia antigen expression	Decrease
Suppressor cell activity	Increase
Soluble mediator formation	Increase or decrease
Interferon production	Decrease

Table 6. Some Mechanisms, Other than Immunosuppression, that Allow
         Viruses to Elude Host Immune Defenses

Examples	Mechanisms
Papovaviruses, retroviruses	Integration in unexpressed form into host cell DNA
Herpes simplex, varicella-zoster	Intracytoplasmic latency with occasional reactivation concomitant with declines in host resistance
Herpes simplex, cytomegalovirus	Direct cell-to-cell spread
Coronaviruses	Budding on intracellular membranes
Influenza, visna	Antigenic drift
Defective retroviruses	Deletion of virion envelope gene
Putative viroids (rheumatoid arthritis)	Propagation as naked genomes
Retroviruses	Incorporation of host antigens in virion envelope
Unconventional viruses (spongiform encephalopathies)	Lack of stimulation of immune responses
Lymphocytic choriomeningitis, rubella	Partial tolerance
Lactic dehydrogenase virus, dengue, reoviruses	Induction of non-neutralizing antibodies that hinder neutralization of facilitate viropexis
Hepatitis B	Production of excess soluble antigens that compete with virions for immune effectors
Cytomegalovirus, lymphocytic choriomeningitis, selected retroviruses	Depression of response to interferon induction
Adenoviruses	Low sensitivity to interferon
Junin virus	Induction of anticomplementary factors
Papilloma, mumps, Creutzfeld-Jacob, KB, measles	Invasion of body districts in which immune effectors are weak (skin, exocrine glands, kidney, CNS)

the avian leukemia and leukosis viruses (2-4,17,20-22,35). The murine
leukemia viruses in particular have been studied in great depth in regard
to biochemistry, epidemiology and pathogenesis and there is an expanding
literature on the nature and mechanism whereby leukemia viruses suppress
immune function. The latter may directly affect the function of immunocompetent cells, and they also induce altered lymphoid cell surfaces resulting
in auto-immune type responses of the host to the altered cells. The systemic
antitumor virus immunity may result in the release of relatively high levels
of immunosuppressive factors. Tumor virus antigen/antibody complexes may
also serve as nonspecific immunosuppressants.

Viral antigens or inactivated virus may affect antigen processing cells
such as macrophages, and the virus itself, or its antigens, may affect antibody precursor cells as antigen reactive cells, etc. Many of these mechanisms have been studied in great detail in recent years. Among these studies

have been those concerning immunosuppression induced by the Friend leukemia virus (FLV) complex. During the early 1960's it was observed that Swiss mice infected by FLV showed depressed immune responses to an antigen such as sheep red cells (2-4,17-20). Stemming from this observation are the extensive investigations concerning the mechanisms involved. A complex series of interactions occur following infections of a susceptible mouse with this virus, resulting in marked splenomegaly, hepatomegaly, and blood cell dyscrasia, culminating in erythroleukemia and death of the animal (28,32,36). Besides direct immunosuppression, heightened susceptibility to infection with other viruses, bacteria, and fungi also occurs (34).

Studies on immunosuppression induced by FLV have dealt with the effects of the virus on both antibody formation and cell mediated immunity, especially to nonmicrobial antigens. As is evident in Table 7, following infection of susceptible BALB/c mice with FLV a marked increase in spleen weight occurs, concomitant with a marked decrease in antibody formation, both primary and secondary, to a T-dependent antigen like sheep red cells or a T-independent gram negative bacterium. The level of immunosuppression is related to the dose of virus used for infection as well as the type and form of antigen used for challenge. Suppression of antibody response also occurs for protein antigens, bacteria and other viruses (2-4,17,20-22). Mice infected with FLV also show decreased delayed hypersensitivity reactions and allograft immunity. Examination of the antibody responsiveness of FLV infected mice has provided information concerning the possible mechanisms involved. Although it was felt initially that the virus may compete with antigen for a

Table 7. Effects of Friend Leukemia Virus (FLV) Infection on Antibody Responses in Vivo to Sheep RBC's and E. coli LPS

Day After Infection[B]	Spleen Weight (mg)	Antibody response (PFC[A]/Spleen)[*]			
		AntiSRBC[C]			Anti E. Coli[D]
		Primary (IgM)	Secondary IGM	IgG	
None (control)	122± 13	42,500	38,750	97,500	65,300
- 1	129± 11	46,300	30,300	66,300	70,100
- 3	136± 22	31,400	15,500	44,400	51,300
- 5	158± 30	12,900	10,300	21,500	32,100
- 8	197± 43	5,310	6,500	12,300	19,400
-15	1640±380	1,500	2,100	3,100	2,400

[*]Individual Spleens for 3-5 mice per group.

[A]Plaque Forming Cells (PFC)

[B]Groups of BALB/c mice injected i.p. with ID_{850} FLV on day indicated relative to day of immunization with 4×10^8 SRBC or 10^8 heat killed E. coli.

[C]Average number of hemolytic PFC to SRBC per spleen for 3-5 mice per group four days after primary or secondary immunization of mice with SRBC; IgG PFC's detected by antiglobulin facilitation procedure using mice primed four weeks earlier with same dose of erythrocytes.

[D]Number of bacteriolytic PFC to E. coli in spleen of 3-5 mice four days after primary immunization with E. coli.

32

finite number of precursor cells, deviating them into the pathway of leukemogenesis, it appears likely that the mechanism of immunosuppression is much more complex. Electron micrographic studies revealed that lymphoid cells from FLV infected mice exhibited both replicating virus and antibody formation at the individual cell level (29,30). Thus it did not appear that virus infection per se inhibited antibody synthesis. B lymphocytes involved in antibody production seemed most suppressed at the single cell level. T lymphocytes also showed some defect but usually later in the infection. Budding viruses could also be seen on the surface of both B and T lymphocytes (29,30). Functional assays showed that although B lymphocytes were markedly markedly suppressed early after viral infection, helper T cell function was also inhibited within a short time after infection.

It is apparent in Table 8 that bone marrow cells derived from FLV infected animals are markedly depressed in their ability to reconstitute the immune response of irradiated animals receiving thymocytes from normal mice. In contrast, thymocytes from early infected (i.e., seven days) animals reconstituted the immune response of irradiated animals given optimal numbers of marrow cells from normal mice. However, the competency of thymocytes after infection was quite finite; within 10 days to two weeks after FLV infection

Table 8. Effect of FLV[*] Infection on the Capability of Bone Marrow or Thymus Cells to Collaborate in Anti-SRBC Response When Used to Reconstitute PFC[**] Responsiveness of Irradiated Recipient

Cells Transferred[a]	PFC per Recipient Spleen[b]	
	Day +5	Day +10
None (control)	100	180± 62
Spleen cells – normal	3580±560	4900±730
Spleen cells – FLV infected	290± 40	386± 90
Thymus cells – normal plus normal marrow cells	3500±800	3950±765
Thymus cells – normal plus FLV marrow cells	176± 38	250± 69
Thymus cells – FLV infected plus normal marrow cells	2950±640	3250±178

* Friend Leukemia Virus

** Plaque Forming Cells

a Indicated suspension of cells (5×10^6) from normal or FLV infected donor BALB/c mice injected i.p. into groups of x-irradiated (750R) recipient mice five or ten days before i.p. immunization with 4 x 10^8 SRBC; infected donor injected with 100 ID_{50} FLV ten days before cell transfer.

b Average number of anti-SRBC PFC ± SE for individual spleen of 3-5 mice five or ten days after challenge immunization with SRBC.

the thymocytes lost their ability to serve as helper cells for antibody formation in irradiated animals.

Thus selected cell populations are involved in immunosuppression induced by FLV. Further analysis showed that suppressor activity was evident when cells from infected animals were co-cultured with normal spleen cells (Table 9). The major suppressor cell population appeared to be FLV transformed cells (13,29,30,35). However, cell free supernatants from these leukemic cells also had marked immunosuppressive activities, both in vivo and in vitro (Table 10). In addition, suppressor macrophages as well as an occasional suppressor T cell were also evident late after FLV infection (26,30, 35). Restoration of immune responsiveness in FLV infected mice could be accomplished with syngeneic macrophages (Table 11). Furthermore, soluble factors released from normal macrophages stimulated in vitro with bacterial lipopolysaccharide had marked immunorestorative activities for FLV suppressed spleen cell cultures in vitro (2,6,16,23,35).

DISCUSSION AND CONCLUSIONS

Many unanswered questions remain as to the role of virus induced immuno-suppression in the development of the primary infection and how it contrib-

Table 9. Effect of Spleen Cells from FLV[*]-infected Mice on the Antibody Responsiveness of Normal Spleen Cells in Vitro

Spleen Cell Source[a]		Antibody Response[b] PFC/10^6 Spleen Cells	Percent of Control
Normal (control)		865±76	--
FLV-infected	0 day	730±32	84%
	+3 days	510±45	59%
	+7 days	320±30	37%
	+12 days	235±65	27%
	+20 days	140±38	16%

[*]Friend Leukemia Virus

[a]Spleen cells (2×10^5) from indicated donor mice added to cultures of 5×10^7 normal spleen cells immunized in vitro with 2×10^6 SRBC; infected mice injected with 100 ID$_{50}$ FLV on day indicated.

[b]Average direct PFC response ± S.E., for 3-6 cultures per group five days after in vitro immunization.

utes to subsequent pathology. Although generalizations are not possible, the contribution of immunopathology to virus induced damages is quite consistent. In some infections, both the experimental and naturally acquired pathologic lesions appear to be due solely to an immune response against antigens of the infecting virus and/or against host structure(s) modified by the virus. The classic example of such disorders is the disease caused by lymphocytic choriomeningitis virus in mice (2,4). Similarly, immunopathology may contribute to the liver damage caused by hepatitis B and yellow fever viruses. Moreover, immune complexes are also found in many viral infections (4,17,18, 37-40). These may contribute to the development of skin lesions in measles, and other viral exanthemata, and represent a pathogenic basis for some of the related complications or sequellae such as polyarthritis nodosa, urticaria, and vasculitis.

Immunopathologic mechanisms triggered by virus infections have been implicated in the genesis of chronic gloumerulonephritis and other autoimmune diseases. This may suggest that at least in some circumstances immunologic impairment caused by a virus, even if it facilitates the spreading of the virus and causes a delay in recovery, nevertheless may be beneficial to the individual by containing the immunologically mediated damage caused by the virus infection. On the other hand, immunosuppression associated

Table 10. Effect of FLV-containing Cell-free Extracts on Antibody Response of Normal Spleen Cell Cultures

Addition to Source[a]	Antibody Response[b] $PFC/10^6$ Spleen Cells	Percent of Control
Normal (control)	955±73	--
Spleen extracts – normal	1030±80	108%
– FLV + 5 days	438±72	46%
+15 days	310±50	33%
+25 days	180±32	19%
Ascites fluid –		
FLV + 5 days	573±68	60%
+10 days	210±42	22%

[a] Indicated extract, in 0.1 ml quantities, added to cultures of 5×10^7 normal mouse spleen cells immunized in vitro with 2×10^6 SRBC; infected donor mice injected with 100 ID_{50} FLV on day indicated prior to testing.

[b] Average direct PFC response, ± S.E., for 3-6 cultures per group five days after in vitro immunization.

Table 11. Effect of Normal Peritoneal Exudate (PE) Cells or LPS Stimulated PE Cell Supernatants on Antibody Responsiveness of Normal or FLV-infected Spleen Cell Cultures.

Addition to Spleen Cell Cultures[a]	Antibody Response (PFC/10^6 Spleen Cells)[c]	
	Normal Cultures	FLV-infected Cultures
None (control)	738± 65	285±36
PE cells 10^3	782± 95	398±76
10^4	810±140	435±69
10^5	720± 78	630±88
10^6	630± 53	686±73
PE cell supernatant[b]		
0.1 ml	790± 48	435±60
0.2 ml	890± 76	595±38

[a]Indicated material added to cultures of 5×10^7 spleen cells from normal or 10-day infected mice.

[b]Supernatant obtained 48 hours after in vitro incubation of 10^6

with retroviruses, such as leukemia viruses in experimental animals, and now apparently acquired immunodeficiency in man may be important in reducing the immune competence of an individual, at least at the initial site of virus infection (2-4,17).

Replication of the virus and transformation of target lymphoid cells may occur despite the concomitant appearance in the cells of virus associated antigens that are either unrecognized or undisturbed by the host immune response. This may enable the initial virus transformation of cells to result in a rapidly replicating mass of tumor cells. Furthermore, the virus may specifically delete certain important cells necessary for normal immunocompetence, such as helper T lymphocytes as in the case of HTLV. B lymphocytes or their precursors are affected very early after infection with murine leukemia virus, whereas helper T cells at a somewhat later time (17-20). Macrophages may also be suppressed during virus infections, including leukemia virus infections (2-4).

There have been many attempts to reverse virus induced immunosuppression by various immunomodulating agents (2-4,35). In this regard it must be taken into account that some of these agents may enhance the number of target lymphoid cells, resulting in greater rather than less virus replication. Many believe that immune responses can be restored in virus suppressed individuals. This could contribute to control of the infection, but is is also possible that this may actually augment the infection. Knowledge concerning the mechanism of the immune response to viruses, including the role of different cell classes and the importance of antibody vs. other humoral factors, such as interferons and interleukins, are necessary to develop useful strategies for treating not only the virus infection itself but the immunoderegulation caused by the infection. It seems difficult at the present time to develop rational approaches to potentiate natural defenses to viral infection and limit the damage done to or by the immune response.

SUMMARY

Many viruses interact with cells of the immune response system. Both enhancement and suppression of immunity may occur during virus infection and such effects may be related to the time of virus infection relative to the time of assay, the dose of virus, etc. Suppression in general may be due to direct effects of a virus on end stage effector lymphocytes or their precursors. Viruses may also affect stem cells or selected cell populations such as antibody producing plasma cells or B lymphocyte precursors, T lymphocytes involved in cellular immunity as effector cells and regulatory T cells such as helper or suppressor cells. Equally important, however, may be the effect of virus infections on macrophages. Both the number and functions of these cells, as well as their secretory and/or regulatory function, may be affected, usually by suppression but sometimes by enhancement. Viruses may also stimulate nonspecific suppressor activity by macrophages or T cells and thus influence the control of immune responsiveness of the host. Recent studies concerning humoral factors involved in immunity have shown that some viruses, especially the retroviruses, may induce various lymphoid and non-lymphoid cells to produce soluble substances, probably immunoregulatory lymphokines, prostaglandins, etc. Furthermore, interferon production by virus affected cells may also have marked immunoregulatory activity. Thus it is apparent that virus infections markedly influence a wide variety of immune parameters. The complexity of the interaction of viruses with the immune system indicates that further studies are necessary to dissect and understand the mechanisms involved.

REFERENCES

1. D. R. Bainbridge and M. Bendinelli, Circulation of lymphoid cells in mice infected with Friend leukemia virus, J. National Cancer Institute 49:773 (1972).
2. M. Bendinelli, Mechanisms and significance of immunodepression in viral diseases, Clin. Immunol. Newsletter 2:75 (1981).
3. M. Bendinelli, W. I. Cox, S. Specter, and H. Friedman, Interferon induced augmentation of natural killer cell activity by splenocytes from leukemia virus-immunosuppressed mice, and DMSO-induced enhancement of Friend leukemia cell susceptibility to natural cytolysis, Current Chemotherapy and Immunology 1121 (1982).
4. M. Bendinelli, D. Matteucci, and H. Friedman, Virus induced immunosuppression, Adv. Cancer Res. in press (1985).
5. M. Bendinelli, D. Matteucci, A. Toniolo, and H. Friedman, Macrophage involvement in leukemia virus-induced tumorigenesis, Adv. Exper. Med. 121B:493 (1979).
6. R. C. Butler and H. Friedman, Leukemia virus induced immunosuppression: reversal by subcellular factors, Ann. N.Y. Acad. Sci. 332:451 (1979).
7. R. C. Butler, J. M. Frier, M. S. Chapekar, M. O. Graham, and H. Friedman, Role of antibody response helper factors in immunosuppressive effects of Friend leukemia virus, Infec. Immun. 39:1200 (1983).
8. W. S. Ceglowski and H. Friedman, Suppression of the primary antibody plaque response of mice following infection with Friend disease virus, Proc. Soc. Exp. Biol. Med. 126:662 (1967).
9. W. S. Ceglowski and H. Friedman, Immunosuppressive effects of Friend and Rauscher leukemia disease viruses on cellular and humoral antibody formation, J. Nat. Cancer Inst. 40:983 (1968).

10. W. S. Ceglowski and H. Friedman, Murine virus leukemogenesis. Relationship between susceptibility and immunodepression, Nature, 224:1318 (1969).

11. W. S. Ceglowski and H. Friedman, Immunosuppression by leukemia viruses. I. Effect of Friend disease virus on cellular and humoral hemolysin responses of mice to a primary immunization with sheep erythrocytes, J. Immunol. 101:594 (1968).

12. A. M. Denman, B. K. Pleton, D. Appleford, and M. Kinsley, Virus infections of lympho-reticular cells and autoimmune diseases, Transpl. Reviews 31:79 (1976).

13. P. Farber, S. Specter, and H. Friedman, Leukemia virus induced immunosuppression: scanning electron microscopy of infected spleen cells, in: "Regulatory Immune Reactivity," V. P. Eijsvogel, D. Ross, and W. P. Zeijlemaker, eds., Academic Press, New York (1976).

14. A. Fontana and H. L. Weiner, Interaction of REOvirus with cell surface receptors. II. Generation of suppressor T cells by the hemagglutinin of REOvirus type 3, J. Immunol. 125:2660 (1980).

15. S. Specter, W. S. Ceglowski, and H. Friedman, Genetic control of the effects of leukemia viruses on immune responses, in: "Infection, Immunity and Genetics," H. Friedman, T. J. Linna, and J. Prier, eds., University Park Press, Baltimore (1978).

16. S. Specter, R. C. Butler, and H. Friedman, Bacterial lipopolysaccharide induced enhancement of antibody formation by leukemia virus suppressed mouse spleen cells, in: "Immunomodulation by Microbial Products and Related Synthetic Compounds," Y. Yamamura, S. Kotani, I. Azuma, A. Koda, and T. Shiba, eds., Excerpta Medica, Amsterdam (1982).

17. H. Friedman, Immunosuppression by murine leukemia viruses, in: "Viruses and Immunity," H. Koprowski, ed., Academic Press, New York (1978).

18. H. Friedman, Cellular immunity and Friend leukemia virus infection, in: "Virus Tumorigenesis and Immunogenesis," W. S. Ceglowski and H. Friedman, eds., Academic Press, New York (1972).

19. H. Friedman and H. Goldner, Relationship between immunologic maturity and viral oncogenesis in hamsters, J. Nat. Cancer Inst. 44:809 (1970).

20. H. Friedman and S. Specter, Virus induced immunomodulation, in: "Advances in Immunopharmacology," J. Hadden, L. Chedid, P. Mullen, and F. Spreafico, eds., Pergamon Press, New York (1981).

21. H. Friedman and S. Specter, Virus induced immunomodulation in: "Immunopharmacology," L. Chedid and J. Hadden, eds., Pergamon Press, London (1980).

22. H. Friedman, S. Specter, and M. Bendinelli, Viruses and the immune response, in: "Bacterial and Viral Inhibition and Modulation of Host Defenses," G. Falconi, ed., Academic Press, London (1984).

23. H. Friedman, S. Specter, C. Butler, and M. Bendinelli, Friend leukemia virus induced immunosuppression: reversal by bacterial products and activated macrophages, in: "Advanced Comp Leukemia," D. S. Yohn and V. R. Blakeslee, eds., Elsevier Biomedical, New York (1982).

24. J. Holland, K. Spindler, F. Horodyski, E. Grabau, S. Nichol, and S. Van de Pol, Rapid evolution of RNA genomes, Science 215:1577 (1982).

25. E. Israel, B. Beiss, and M. A. Wainberg, Viral abrogation of lymphocyte mitogenesis: induction of a soluble factor inhibitory to cellular proliferation, Immunol. 40:77 (1980).

26. J. R. Kateley, I. Kamo, G. Kaplan, and H. Friedman, Suppressive effect of leukemia virus-infected lymphoid cells on in vitro immunization of normal splenocytes, J. Nat. Cancer Inst. 53:1371 (1974).

27. M. M. Katz, A. White, and A. L. Goldstein, Lymphocyte populations of AKR/J mice. II. Effect of leukemogenesis on migration patterns, response to PHA, and expression of theta antigen, J. Immunol. 111:1519 (1973).

28. I. Kamo, J. Kateley, G. Kaplan, and H. Friedman, Immunosuppression in vitro induced by leukemia virus infected splenocytes, Proc. Soc. Exp. Biol. Med. 148:383 (1975).

29. G. C. Koo, W. S. Ceglowski, M. Higgins, and H. Friedman, Immunosuppression by leukemia viruses. VI. Ultrastructure of individual antibody-forming cells in the spleens of Friend leukemia virus-infected mice, J. Immunol. 106:815 (1971).

30. G. C. Koo, W. S. Ceglowski, and H. Friedman, Immunosuppression by leukemia viruses. V. Ultrastructural studies of antibody-forming spleens of mice infected with Friend leukemia virus, J. Immunol. 106:815 (1971).

31. J. M. Mansfield (ed.), "Parasitic Diseases," Vol. I, Marcel Dekker, Inc., New York (1981).

32. R. F. Mortensen, W. S. Ceglowski, and H. Friedman, Susceptibility and resistance to Friend virus: effect on production of migration-inhibition factor, J. Nat. Cancer Inst. 52:499 (1974).

33. M. R. Proffitt, Virus-lymphocyte interactions: implications for disease, in: "Virus-Lymphocyte Interactions - Implications for Disease," M. R. Proffitt, ed., Elsevier/North Holland, Amsterdam (1979).

34. J. H. Schwab, Suppression of the immune response by microorganisms, Bacteriological Reviews 39:121 (1975).

35. S. Specter and H. Friedman, Viruses and the immune response, Pharmacol. and Therapeutics A2:595 (1978).

36. A. Toniolo, D. Matteucci, M. P. Pistillo, Z. Gori, and M. Bendinelli, Early replication of Friend leukemia viruses in spleen macrophages, J. Gen. Virol. 49:203 (1980).

37. W. H. Wainwright, R. W. Veltri, and P. M. Sprinkle, Abrogation of cell-mediated immunity by a serum blocking factor isolated from patients with infectious mononucleosis, J. Infec. Dis. 140:22 (1979).

38. D. Westmoreland, A lymphoblastoid response of human fetal lymphocytes to ultraviolet-irradiated herpes simplex virus, J. Gen. Virol. 47:151 (1980).

39. E. F. Wheelock and S. T. Toy, Participation of lymphocytes in viral infections, Adv. in Immunol. 16:123 (1973).

40. J. F. Woodruff and J. J. Woodruff, The effect of viral infections on the function of the immune system, in: "Viral Immunology and Immunopathology, A. L. Notkins, ed., Academic Press, New York (1975).

II. SPECIFIC VIRAL INFECTIONS AND IMMUNITY

EPSTEIN-BARR VIRUS (EBV) AND IMMUNODEFICIENCIES

Werner Henle and Gertrude Henle

The Joseph Stokes, Jr. Research Institute
The Children's Hospital of Pennsylvania
Philadelphia, Pennsylvania 19104

Primary EBV infections induce either infectious mononucleosis or silent seroconversions (1). In both instances, a persistent latent viral carrier becomes established. Both arms of the immune system are engaged in the primary as well as the persistent EBV infection; B-lymphocytes are an early target of EBV and form the habitat of the persisting viral genome; T-lympho-cytes serve to subdue the primary infection and to control the persistent carrier state. It is not surprising, therefore, that immunodeficiencies influence, for better or worse, the interactions of the virus with its host. Study of EBV infections in immunologically compromised individuals should provide pertinent information on the immune mechanism(s) normally responsible for control of the virus. In turn, the EBV-specific serology may serve as another parameter in the assessment of immunocompetence (2).

In this discussion, we shall present examples of EBV-specific antibody responses to primary EBV infections and following activation of the ensuing persistent viral carrier state in patients with genetic iatrogenic or dis-ease-induced immune defects. Antibodies of the immune globulin classes G, M, or A to EB viral capsid antigen (VCA) and to the diffuse (D) or restricted (R) components of the early antigen (EA) complex were determined by indirect immunofluorescence (3) and antibodies to the EBV-associated nuclear antigen (EBNA) by anti-complement immunofluorescence (4). A current primary EBV infection is characterized by elevated titers of IgM and IgG antibodies to VCA and absence as yet of antibodies to EBNA which emerge only several weeks to months after onset of illness (5). Most acute IM patients also show transient anti-D responses while in late convalescence low levels of anti-R may appear. In silent seroconversions only anti-R may transiently arise (6). The differential appearance of antibodies to VCA, D and R, on one hand, and to EBNA, on the other, denotes that the corresponding antigens are derived from separate sets of cells under different circumstances (5). A recent primary EBV infection is identified by low or no longer detectable levels of IgM anti-VCA and not yet or barely measurable levels of anti-EBNA. After long past primary EBV infections usually only IgG anti-VCA and anti-EBNA remain detectable, mostly at moderate titers but occasionally low levels of anti-R, very rarely anti-D, may also be found if the anti-VCA titers are relatively high.

Depending upon the type of immune defect primary EBV infections may be mild or silent, as one may surmise from absence of information to the contrary in the histories of seropositive patients, be unusually severe and often fatal as in the X-linked lymphoproliferative (XLP) syndrome in which male family members succumb to fulminant IM in the absence of EBV-specific antibody responses or develop life-threatening complications (7-9). IM itself may possible be on rare occasions a cause of defective immune responses in male as well as female patients without previously known immunodysfunction. We have followed several such patients with truly "chronic IM" who acquired various severe complications of the disease in the course of several years and developed excessively high IgG antibody titers to VCA and D (up to 1:40,960 and 1:10,240, respectively) and more moderate titers of IgA antibodies to these antigens, whereas the anti-EBNA titers remained within the normal range (10,14). Complaints of IM patients of persistent fatigue, intermittently recurrent fever and lymphadenopathy undoubtedly have a clinical basis but the antibody spectra and titers of such patients often fall within, or only slightly above the normal range. However, antibodies to EBNA may be of low titer or absent in some of these patients.

Turning to genetic immune defects, the accelerated lymphoproliferative phase of the Chediak-Higashi syndrome (CHS) seems to depend upon a prior EBV infection (12). This autosomal recessive syndrome is characterized by partial albinism, CNS abnormalities, recurrent bacterial infections due to dysfunction of phagocytic cells which carry abnormal giant lysosomes, a reduction in natural killer (NK) cell activity and a high incidence of lymphoproliferative malignancies. None of ten as yet seronegative CHS patients studied by us had entered the accelerated phase, including two patients who surprisingly have survived to adulthood (unpublished). Five of these seronegative patients subsequently seroconverted with only mild or no signs of IM. While their EBV-specific antibody responses conformed initially to expectation, the IgG anti-VCA titers failed to decline, as expected during late convalescence from IM, but rather increased. Antibodies to R emerged and reached titers equal to or exceeding the anti-VCA titers, a pattern frequently observed in EBV-associated Burkitt's lymphoma (13). These changes occurred concomitant with the development of the accelerated, lymphoproliferative phase of the CHS. Antibodies to EBNA also emerged but the titers did not exceed the normal range.

We had the opportunity to study primary EBV infections also in several organ allograft recipients who in part had received antithymocyte globulin (ATG) and/or Cyclosporin A (CyA) in addition to routine immunosuppression. Four primary EBV infections were observed in renal allograft recipients at Massachusetts General Hospital in the wake of the transplant operation which was combined with cytomegalovirus (CMV) infection in two cases (14; unpublished). They took a mild course but evoked unusual EBV-specific antibody responses. While production of IgG antibodies to VCA followed the normal pattern, no or only a low level of IgM antibodies to VCA were detected, no anti-D emerged, and anti-R and anti-EBNA became measurable at low titers more than four months later (unpublished). In another patient, studied in collaboration with Dr. Hanto and associates (15), a mild primary EBV infection long after, and therefore unrelated to the transplant operation, was followed within 15 weeks by the development of a polyclonal B-cell lymphoma which harbored EB viral DNA in amounts equivalent to multiple genomes per cell. This patient had a normal IgM anti-VCA response but retained high IgG anti-VCA and anti-D titers throughout the observation period.

Two cardiac allograft recipients studied in collaboration with Dr. Bieber and his associates (16) developed mild signs of IM seven to twelve weeks after the transplant which was followed nine weeks later in one of the patients by a polyclonal EBV-positive B-cell lymphoma which responded

transiently to acyclovir treatment. Both patients had received ATG and
CyA. The EBV-specific antibody responses were very similar but also unusual
for primary EBV infections. They revealed passively transferred IgG antibodies to VCA and EBNA immediately after the transplant procedure which
decayed according to a half life of about four weeks. Active antibody production became evident after the passive antibodies had reached low or non-
detectable levels. However, no significant levels of IgM antibodies to VCA
and to heterophil antigen emerged as observed also in the renal allograft-
associated primary EBV infections. No antibodies to EA components became
detectable in the lymphoma patient, whereas anti-R appeared during late
convalescence in the other patient.

Lack of a proper IgM anti-VCA response was observed again in a seronegative patient 80 days after receiving bone marrow from a donor who likewise was seronegative. The patient therefore became infected probably by
the transfusion of blood products (17). It seems evident from these observations that passively transmitted antibodies, even if not measurable in the
recipient, can retard the infectious process initiated by EBV and interfere
with proper antibody responses, a suggestion which deserves further study.
It is also conceivable, however, that lymphocytes from donated blood and
blood products establish residence and propagate in immunosuppressed patients
and continue to maintain the viral carrier state in the new environment.

ACTIVATION OF PERSISTENT EBV INFECTIONS IN IMMUNODEFICIENCIES

Normally, a stable equilibrium exists in viral carriers between EBV
and host defenses as deduced from nearly constant anti-VCA and anti-EBNA
titers over decades. The equilibrium fails to materialize or becomes upset
in some genetic or acquired immunodeficiencies.

Patients with ataxia-telangiectasia (A-T), an autosomal recessive
primary immunodeficiency characterized by progressive ataxia, oculocutaneous
telangiectasia and recurrent sinopulmonary infections, have among others,
T-cell deficiencies of varying degrees of severity. They withstand, however,
primary EBV infections without apparent difficulty but show subsequently an
overrepresentation of elevated anti-VCA and anti-R titers yet often no or
only low levels of antibodies to EBNA (18-20). Low anti-EBNA titers correlated with severe T-cell dysfunction (18,20). A-T patients are at an increased risk of developing malignancies, among them B-cell lymphomas (21).
One of these was found recently to harbor multiple EBV genomes per cell
(22). However, this patient's EBV-specific antibody titers did not distinguish him from other A-T patients. The severe T-cell deficiency indicated
by the absence of antibodies to EBNA probably facilitated emergence of the
tumor.

ATG and CyA activate the persistent EB viral carrier state in allograft
recipients within a few weeks as evident from four-fold or greater rises in
anti-VCA titers, the emergence of low titers of anti-R, and increased oropharyngeal excretion of EBV (11,16,22-25). Also, antibodies to other viruses
harbored by the patient increase in titer (24). In two cardiac allograft
recipients who received ATG and CyA diffuse, polyclonal B-cell lymphomas
were detected 11 and 15 weeks after the transplant which contained EB viral
DNA and EBNA-positive cells (16). However, other patients who also received
ATG and CyA did not develop B-cell lymphomas even though they had shown
EBV-specific antibody responses comparable to those of the lymphoma patients.
Seropositive bone marrow recipients also show substantial rises in antibodies
to VCA and R or D within a four month period after the graft (17). None of
the patients in this study developed lymphomas.

As to disease-related immunosuppression, juvenile patients with Hodgkin's disease (HD), had at diagnosis anti-VCA titers within the normal range,

but an enhanced incidence of anti-R and low anti-EBNA titers (26). The ratio between the geometric mean titers (GMT) of anti-VCA and anti-EBNA was nine instead of the normally observed two to four. In the course of treatment and continuing thereafter the anti-VCA but not anti-EBNA titers increased substantially so that the ratio between the two GMTs rose ultimately to 17.

In approximately 1% of adult patients with HD or non-Hodgkin lymphomas (NHL) the anti-VCA titers were found to climb to excess ($\geq$1:5120) accompanied by very high titers of either anti-D or anti-R, whereas anti-EBNA titers remained within the normal range (27,28). While these patients were in remission, various types and degrees of immune defects were detected, referable to EBV-specific T-cell but not NK cell activities.

Patients with the acquired immunodeficiency syndrome (AIDS) have shown, in our experience, an overrepresentation of elevated anti-VCA and anti-EA titers (Anti-R or anti-D) which did not appear to exceed the elevations seen in other immunodeficiency states. The AIDS patients had, with rare exceptions, anti-EBNA titers which the normal range suggesting that the subset of T-cells responsible for release of EBNA from EBV-transformed B-lymphocytes was functioning. Only an occasional AIDS patient was found to have excessively high anti-VCA and anti-R or anti-D titers. A number of AIDS patients have developed Burkitt's lymphomas which were monoclonal, showed the characteristic translocation between chromosome 8 and chromosome 14 or 22, and harbored EBV genomes as evident from expression of EBNA in the tumor cells (29). The EBV-specific antibody patterns recorded for these patients did not distinguish them from AIDS patients without lymphomas. Also, the antibody patterns in sera from lymphoma-bearing AIDS patients which we were able to examine in our laboratory did not reflect the presence of the tumors.

CONCLUDING REMARKS

The various examples discussed reflect the profound influence exerted by immunodeficiencies on EB virus-specific antibody responses in primary and/or persistent EBV infections. Some defects may cause similar and others rather distinct changes in the EBV-specific antibody patterns. One can visualize how given defects may affect antibody production. A deficiency or dysfunction of B-lymphocytes readily explains reduced or lacking antibody responses as observed in the XLP syndrome or in hypo- or agammaglobulinemias. A deficiency or dysfunction of suppressor/cytotoxic T-lymphocytes may account for excessively high antibody titers because antibody production is not shut off, as seen in rare cases of chronic IM or the occasional HD and NHL patient. A deficiency or dysfunction of natural killer (NK) cells and the probably identical cells responsible for antibody-dependent cellular cyto-toxicity (ADCC) will permit viral replication to go to completion within productively infected B-cells which normally would be destroyed by NK cell or the ADCC reaction as soon as viral antigens are inserted in the cell membrane; i.e., greater amounts of antigen become available for enhanced antibody stimulation, as apparent, for instance, in CHS patients. A deficiency or dysfunction of virus-specific killer T-lymphocytes will allow EBV-transformed B-lymphocytes to survive and divide to increased numbers with two possible effects: too little EBNA is released for continued antibody production, as evident from the absence of anti-EBNA in many A-T patients; and an increased number, though not necessarily percentage, of EBV genome carrying B-lymphocytes may become spontaneously induced to replicate virus, yielding increased quantities of antigens with consequently enhanced antibody production, as also seen in A-T patients. It is likely that in many conditions several defects occur simultaneously which indeed is expected to be the case in therapeutic immunosuppression of allograft recipients.

ACKNOWLEDGMENTS

The work done by the authors was supported by research grant CA 33324 from the National Institutes of Health, U.S. Public Health Service.

REFERENCES

1. G. Henle and W. Henle, The virus as the etiologic agent of infectious mononucleosis, in: "The Epstein-Barr Virus," M. A. Epstein and B. G. Achong, eds., Springer-Verlag, Berlin, Heidelberg and New York (1979).
2. W. Henle and G. Henle, Epstein-Barr virus-specific serology in immuno-logically compromised individuals, Cancer Res., 41:4222 (1981).
3. W. Henle, G. Henle, and C. A. Horwitz, Epstein-Barr virus-specific diagnostic tests in infectious mononucleosis, Human Pathol. 5:551 (1974).
4. B. M. Reedman and G. Klein, Cellular localization of an Epstein-Barr virus (EBV)-associated complement-fixing antigen in producer and non-producer lymphoblastoid cell lines, Int. J. Cancer 11:499 (1973).
5. G. Henle, W. Henle, and C. A. Horwitz, Antibodies to Epstein-Barr virus-associated nuclear antigen in infectious mononucleosis, J. Infect. Dis. 130:231 (1974).
6. R. J. Biggar, G. Henle, J. Böcker, E. T. Lennette, G. Fleisher, and W. Henle, Primary Epstein-Barr virus infections in African infants. II. Clinical and serological observations during seroconversion, Int. J. Cancer 22:244 (1978).
7. R. Bar, C. J. DeLor, K. P. Clausen, P. Hurtubise, W. Henle, and J. Hewetson, Fatal infectious mononucleosis in a family, New Eng. J. Med. 290:363 (1974).
8. D. T. Purtilo, C. K. Cassel, Y. P. S. Yang, R. Harver, S. R. Stevenson, B. H. Landing, and G. F. Vawter, X-linked recessive progressive combined variable immunodeficiency (Duncan's disease), Lancet 1:935 (1975).
9. D. T. Purtilo, K. Sakamoto, A. Saemundsen, J. L. Sullivan, A.-C. Synnerholm, M. Anvret, J. Pritchard, C. Sloper, C. Sieff, J. Pincott, I. Packman, K. Rich, F. Cruzi, J. A. Cornet, R. Collins, N. Barnes, J. Knight, B. Sandstedt, and G. Klein, Documentation of Epstein-Barr virus infection in immunodeficient patients with life-threatening lymphoproliferative diseases by clinical, virological, and immuno-pathological studies, Cancer 41:4226 (1981).
10. E. M. Edson, L. K. Cohen, W. Henle, and J. L. Strominger, An unusual high-titer human anti-Epstein-Barr virus (EBV) serum and its use in the study of EBV-specific proteins synthesized in vitro and in vivo, J. Immunol. 130:919 (1983).
11. R. T. Schooley, D. I. Arbit, W. Henle, and M. S. Hirsch, T-lymphocyte subset interactions in the cell-mediated immune response to Epstein-Barr virus (submitted for publication).
12. F. Merino, G. O. Klein, W. Henle, P. Ramirez-Dugue, M. Forsgren, and C. Amesty, Elevated antibody titers to Epstein-Barr virus and low natural killer cell activity in patients with Chediak-Higashi syndrome, Clin. Immunol and Immunopathol. 27:326 (1983).
13. W. Henle and G. Henle, Antibodies to the R component of EBV-induced early antigens in Burkitt's lymphoma may exceed in titer antibodies to EB viral capsid antigen, J. Nat. Cancer Inst. 58:785 (1977).
14. R. T. Schooley, M. S. Hirsch, R. B. Colvin, A. B. Cosimi, N. E. Tolkoff-Rubin, R. T. McCluskey, R. C. Burton, P. S. Russell, J. T. Herrin, F. A. Delmonico, J. V. Giorgi, W. Henle, and R. H. Rubin, Association of herpesgroup virus infections with T-lymphocytes subset alterations, glomerulopathy, and opportunistic infections following renal transplantation, New Eng. J. Med., 308:307 (1983).

15. D. W. Hanto, K. J. Gajl-Pecsalska, G. Frizzera, D. C. Arthur, H. H. Balfour, K. McClain, R. L. Simmons, and J. S. Najarian, Epstein-Barr virus-induced polyclonal and monoclonal B-cell lymphoproliferative diseases occurring after renal transplantation, Ann. Surg. 198:356 (1983).

16. C. P. Bieber, R. I. Heberling, S. W. Jamieson, P. E. Oyer, M. Cleary, R. Warnke, A. Saemundsen, G. Klein, W. Henle, and E. B. Stinson, Lymphoma in cardiac transplant recipients associated with cyclosporin A, prednisone and antithymocytic globulin (ATG), in: Immune Deficiency and Cancer: Epstein-Barr Virus and Lymphoproliferative Malignancies, D. T. Purtilo, ed., Plenum Press, New York (1984).

17. B. Lange, W. Henle, J. D. Meyers, L. C. Yang, C. August, P. Koch, A. Arbeter, and G. Henle, Epstein-Barr virus related serology in marrow transplant recipients, Int. J. Cancer 26:151 (1980).

18. A. I. Berkel, W. Henle, G. Henle, G. Klein, F. Ersoy, and O. Sanal, Epstein-Barr virus related antibody patterns in Ataxia-Telangiectasia, Clin. Exp. Immunol. 35:196 (1979).

19. J. Joncas, N. Lapointe, F. Gervais, M. Leyfritz, and A. Wills, Unusual prevalence of antibodies to Epstein-Barr virus early antigen in ataxia-telangiectasia, Lancet 1:1160 (1977).

20. E. Vilmer, G. M. Lenoir, J. L. Virelizier, C. Griscelli, Epstein-Barr virus serology in immunodeficiencies: an attempt to correlate with immune abnormalities in Wiscott-Aldrich and Chediak-Higashi syndromes and ataxia-telangiectasia, Clin. and Exper. Immunol. 55:249 (1984).

21. J.H. Kersey, B. D. Spector, and R. A. Good, Primary immunodeficiency diseases and cancer: the immunodeficiency-cancer registry, Int. J. Cancer 12:333 (1973).

22. A. K. Saemundsen, A. I. Berkel, W. Henle, G. Henle, M. Anvret, P. Sanal, F. Ersoy, M. Caglar, and G. Klein, Epstein-Barr virus carrying lymphoma in an ataxia-telangiectasia patient, Br. Med. J. 282:425 (1981).

23. R. S. Chang, J. P. Lewis, R. D. Reynold, M. J. Sullivan, and J. Neuman, Oropharyngeal excretion of Epstein-Barr virus by patients with lymphoproliferative disorders and renal homografts, Ann. Int. Med. 88:34 (1978).

24. S. H. Cheeseman, W. Henle, W. Rubin, N. E. Tolkoff-Rubin, A. B. Cosimi, K. Cantell, J. T. Herrin, P. H. Black, P. H. Russel, and M. S. Hirsch, Epstein-Barr virus infection in renal transplant recipients: effect of antithymocyte globulin and interferon, Ann. Int. Med. 93:39 (1980).

25. B. Strauch, L. Andrews, N. Siegel, and C. Miller, Oropharyngeal excretion of Epstein-Barr virus by renal transplant recipients and other patients treated with immunosuppressant drugs, Lancet 1:234 (1974).

26. B. Lange, A. Arbeter, J. Hewetson, and W. Henle, Longitudinal study of Epstein-Barr virus antibody titers and excretion in pediatric patients with Hodgkin's disease, Int. J. Cancer 22:521 (1978).

27. M. G. Mascucci, R. Szigeti, I. Ernberg, M. Bjorkholm, H. Mellstedt, G. Henle, W. Henle, G. Pearson, G. Masucci, E. Svedmyr, B. Johansson, G. Klein, Cell mediated immune reactions in three patients with malignant lymphoproliferative disease in remission and abnormally high EBV-antibody titers, Cancer Res. 41:4292 (1981).

28. G. Masucci, H. Mellstedt, M. G. Masucci, R. Szigeti, I. Ernberg, M. Bjorkholm, K. Tsukuda, G. Henle, W. Henle, G. Pearson, G. Holm, P. Biberfeld, B. Johansson, and G. Klein, Immunological characterization of Hodgkin's and Non-Hodgkin's lymphoma patients with high antibody titers against Epstein-Barr virus associated antigens, Cancer Res. 44:1288 (1984).

29. J. L. Ziegler, W. Drew, R. C. Miner, L. Mintz, E. Rosenbaum, J. Gershow, E. T. Lennett, J. Greenspan, E. Shillitoe, J. Beckstead, C. Casavant, and K. Yamamoto, Outbreak of Burkitt's-like lymphoma in homosexual men, Lancet 2:631 (1982).

DEPRESSIVE EFFECT OF EPSTEIN-BARR VIRUS TRANSFORMED CELL FRACTIONS

ON RESPONSIVENESS OF HUMAN LEUKOCYTES TO MITOGENS

Jian-Lin Zhang, Lee Hsu, Steven Specter, Herman Friedman,
Meihan Nonoyama, and Andor Szentivanyi

University of South Florida College of Medicine
Tampa, Florida and Showa University Institute for
Biomedicine in Florida, St. Petersburg, Florida

INTRODUCTION

Epstein-Barr virus (EBV) has been readily demonstrated to infect human
B lymphocytes from tonsils or peripheral blood in vitro and impart to these
cells the ability to proliferate indefinitely (1-4). EBV is considered an
etiologic agent for infectious mononucleosis worldwide as well as Burkitt's
lymphoma in equitorial Africa and nasopharyngeal carcinoma in China. While
the molecular biology of such transformation of B lymphocytes is not yet
completely understood, it has been determined that the EBV genome is integrated into the transformed cells (3). Patients with Burkitt's lymphoma
and other EBV associated diseases demonstrate altered immune competence;
however, there is little information available concerning the role of the
virus in precipitation of these effects (5). In this regard, Werkmeister
et al. reported that Daudi cells, which are an EBV transformed cell line,
release into their culture fluid a substance capable of inhibiting phytohemagglutinin induced mitogenesis of lymphocytes (6).

Studies in this laboratory indicated that a continuous cell line transformed by EBV markedly depressed the blastogenic responsiveness of normal
human peripheral blood leukocytes (PBL) stimulated in vitro by plant mitogens
(unpublished observations). Suppression was related both to tumor cell
number and time of addition of tumor cells to PBL. These results suggest
that EBV transformed cells are immunosuppressive and that this could be due
to the presence of infectious virus or its genome. However, an additional
lymphoblastoid tumor cell line from a Burkitt's lymphoma patient, but EBV
negative, had a similar immunodepressive activity. Thus the role of the
virus in this suppression is unclear. It is possible that any B lymphoblastoid cells with an appropriate stimulus may produce suppressive activity.
In this chapter we present studies on the suppressive activity associated
with cell-free preparations from two B lymphoblastoid cell lines.

EXPERIMENTAL METHODS AND PROCEDURES

Cell Lines

The two cell lines used for this study were as follows: 1) B95-8
cells initially induced by EBV transformation of marmoset lymphocytes in

Table 1. Suppressive Effects of Cell-Free Preparations from Lymphoblastoid Cells on Blastogenic Responses of Peripheral Blood Leukocytes Stimulated In Vitro with Conconavalin A

Addition to Cultures[a]	No Added Cells (Controls)	Con A Induced Blastogenesis[b]					
		B95-8 Cells			BJAB Cells		
		CPM	SI	Percent of Control	CPM	SI	Percent of Control
None	415±36	32,100±2680	77.3	100	32,100±2640	77.3	100
Sonicate 1:2	265±32	965± 48	3.6	3.0	840± 59	3.2	2.6
1:20	380±19	1,840± 210	4.8	5.7	23,600±1840	61.1	73.5
1:200	366±41	27,850± 870	85.7	86.7	31,560±2400	87.8	98.3
Supernatant 1:2	430±27	730± 48	1.7	2.3	4,710±1560	10.9	14.6
1:20	324±22	20,500±1760	83.1	63.9	25,600±3258	78.8	79.8
1:200	310±39	28,250±3150	91.1	88.0	24,500±1970	79.0	76.3

[a] Indicated dilution of 0.1 ml of a cell-free preparation from 10^6 tumor cells added to cultures of 10^6 peripheral blood leukocytes from normal individuals.

[b] Average response for 3-4 cultures per group 72 hr after in vitro stimulation with 5 μg Con A.

vitro that are known to shed the virus; and 2) BJAB cells, derived from a Burkitt's lymphoma patient but which do not shed EBV and give no evidence of the presence of the viral genome (3,4). Both cell lines were maintained as suspensions at a concentration of 10^6 viable nucleated cells/ml RPMI 1640 medium, and frozen at -70°C until used. For each experiment an aliquot of a cell suspension was thawed and then the cells were cultured at 37°C in medium containing 10% fetal bovine serum and antibiotics. The cells were then subcultured every four days.

Cell-free Preparations

Suspensions of 10^6 viable nucleated cells were sonicated by six pulses of 30 seconds each with a Raytheon sonicator. Cellular debris was removed by centrifugation at 15000 x g for 10 min at 4°C and the supernatant obtained. In addition, cell-free culture supernatant fluids were obtained from individual 48 hr cultures by centrifugation at 1500 x g for 30 min at 4°C. Sonicates or supernatants were stored at -70°C until used. For inactivation experiments, cell-free preparations were treated by boiling at 100°C for 10 min or exposed to ultraviolet light for 20 min at a distance of 15 cm at 25°C. In other experiments the cell-free preparations were centrifuged at 100,000 x g for 1 hr at 4°C and the resulting supernatant and pellet utilized.

Blastogenic Assays

Peripheral blood leukocytes were obtained from normal volunteers, both male and female, aged 20 to 50. Suspensions of mononuclear cells were prepared by standard Ficoll-Hypaque gradient separation (7). For blastogenic tests 10^5 viable nucleated leukocytes in 0.1 ml medium were placed in individual wells of 96 well flat bottom microtiter plates. The cells were stimulated by addition of 0.1 ml of a 5 μg concentration of concanavalin A (Con A), pokeweed mitogen (PWM), or phytohemagglutinin (PHA). Graded dilutions of a cell-free preparation were then added to appropriate wells. All plates were incubated for 72 hr at 37°C in a humidified atmosphere of 95% air and 5% CO_2. Each culture was pulsed for the final 18 hr with 0.5 μCI ^{3}H-thymidine (Schwartz Biochemical, Portland, ME). The amount of radioactivity taken up into the cellular DNA was determined by collecting the cells on glass fiber filter paper using a Brandel cell harvester. Filter discs were placed in a counting vial with 3 ml Econofluor cocktail (New England Nuclear, Boston, MA). Vials were then counted using a Packard spectrometer, Model 3380 (7,8).

EXPERIMENTAL RESULTS

Previous studies had shown that both the B95-8 and BJAB lymphoblastoid cell lines suppressed the responsiveness of normal human peripheral blood leukocytes to Con A, PWM or PHA using as few as 10^5 tumor cells treated with mitocycin C so they would not replicate (unpublished observations). Such cells inhibited 90% or more the expected blastogenic responsiveness of the normal peripheral blood leukocytes. As shown in Table 1, cell-free preparations from these cell lines also markedly suppressed the Con A blastogenic response of normal peripheral blood leukocytes. For these experiments graded dilutions of cell-free preparations from 10^6 cells of both of the tumor cell lines were added at the time of culture initiation. A 1:2 or 1:20 dilution of the cell-free sonicate from B95-8 cells suppressed 95% or more the blastogenic response of the peripheral blood leukocytes. The 1:200 dilution showed no significant suppression. In contrast, only the 1:2 dilution of the supernatant from cultures of the B95-8 cells was suppressive; higher dilutions had much less or no effect on the blastogenic response. Sonicates and the supernatant from BJAB were only suppressive at a 1:2 dilution.

Inhibition of blastogenic responsiveness to the mitogens PWM and PHA occurred when cell-free sonicates and culture supernatants from either B95-8 or BJAB cells were added to cultures of normal peripheral blood leukocytes (Tables 2 and 3). However, cell-free supernatant from B95-8 at a dilution of 1:2 up to 1:200 inhibited the blastogenic responses to PHA mitogens by > 83%. BJAB preparations at a dilution of 1:2, caused only less than 70% suppression while greater dilution resulted in loss of suppressive activity. Sonicates from B95-8 cells were less active than supernatants, while sonicates from BJAB were more active than culture supernatant. PWM responses were suppressed to the same degree by sonicates and supernatants of both cell lines.

The time of addition of either cell-free sonicate to the leukocyte cultures markedly affected the level of suppression. Significant suppression occurred only when the cell-free preparations were added (Table 4) on the day of culture initiation and stimulation with mitogen. Slight suppression occurred when the cell-free sonicates were added one day after culture initiation and stimulation. No suppression was evident when they were added on day +2 at the time of pulsing with thymidine nor day +3 when the cultures were being tested for thymidine uptake.

Studies to characterize the suppressive factor(s) in the cell-free preparations were performed using various inactivation procedures. As is apparent in Table 5, boiling the cell-free sonicates for 10 min markedly inactivated suppressive activity for Con A responses. Boiling for 20 min or longer completely diminished the suppressive activity (data not shown). Similarly, exposure of the sonicate to UV light for 20 min markedly reduced suppressive activity. Finally, after centrifugation of the cell-free sonicate at 100,000 x g for 1 hr. diminution of the suppressive activity of the supernatants was evident with the greatest loss of activity occurring with the B95-8 as compared to BJAB preparations. The pellets obtained by centrifugation of the B95-8 sonicates, after resuspension to the original volume, had moderate suppressive activity (data not shown). This was not evident with the BJAB pellets. Treatment of the sonicates with trypsin (20 μg for 30 min at 25°C) markedly diminished the suppressive activity of sonicates from both cell lines, but similar treatment with RNase or DNase failed to affect the suppressive activity (data not shown).

DISCUSSION AND CONCLUSIONS

The results of this study show that cell-free preparations from lympho-blastoid cells derived either from EBV transformed lymphocytes or from a Burkitt's lymphoma patient can affect the blastogenic responsiveness of normal human leukocytes. Various transformed cell lines have been estab-lished from patients infected with EBV or with lymphomas associated with this virus. However, from the results of the present study it appears that EBV itself is probably not the direct mediator of suppression, mainly because similar suppressive effects were observed with cell-free preparations from a lymphoblastoid line, BJAB, which does not shed EBV and give no evidence of carrying the EBV genome (6).

Although it is not clear what subcellular component(s), if any, are responsible for the suppressive effects induced by either of the two cell lines, it seems unlikely that a nonspecific factor such as "cold" thymidine could account for the effects noted. Heating the cell-free preparations for as little at 10 min at 100°C markedly diminished the suppressive effects. Addition of cell-free preparations to cultures of human peripheral blood leukocytes after a delay of two or three days, or immediately before or after pulsing with thymidine, also failed to affect the uptake of thymidine, indicating that competition with cold thymidine or some other inhibitor of

Table 2. Effect of Cell-Free Sonicate or Culture Supernatant from Lymphoblastoid Cells on Blastogenic Response of Peripheral Blood Leukocytes Stimulated In Vitro with PHA

Addition to Cultures[a]	Mitogen Stimulation[b]					
	B95-8 Cells			BJAB Cells		
	No Mitogen (Control)	CPM	SI	No Mitogen (Control)	CPM	SI
None	214±27	42,249±2,861	148.8	214±27	42,249±2,861	148.8
Sonicate 1:2	346±41	3,512± 197	10.3	275±22	8,460± 498	30.9
1:20	314±22	14,260±1,630	45.3	360±47	15,210± 976	42.3
1:200	360±29	37,980±2,791	105.5	312±21	45,468±2,131	145.7
Supernatant 1:2	410±56	1,456± 59	3.6	320±46	13,643±1,950	42.6
1:20	378±19	3,150± 298	8.3	297±17	46,227±3,105	155.7
1:200	340±31	5,870± 431	17.3	276±30	45,964±2,968	166.6

[a]Indicated concentration of cell-free clarified sonicate or supernatant from 10^6 B95-8 or BJAB cells cultured for 4 days in vitro added to cultures of 10^6 peripheral blood leukocytes from normal individuals

[b]Average response of 3-4 cultures per group 72 hr after in vitro stimulation with 5 µg of indicated mitogen and addition of 0.1 ml of indicated cell-free preparation.

53

Table 3. Effect of Cell-free Sonicate or Culture Supernatant from Lymphoblastoid Cells on Blastogenic Response of Peripheral Blood Leukocytes Stimulated In Vitro with PWM

| Addition to Cultures[a] | Mitogen Stimulation[b] | | | | | |
| | B95-8 Cells | | | BJAB Cells | | |
	No Mitogen (Control)	CPM	SI	No Mitogen (Control)	CPM	SI
None	214±27	6,051±134	21.3	214±27	6,051±134	21.3
Sonicate 1:2	346±41	1,459±128	4.3	275±22	1,875±215	6.8
1:20	314±22	3,098±268	9.9	360±47	4,056±314	11.3
1:200	360±29	7,160±486	19.9	312±21	5,264±292	16.9
Supernatant 1:2	410±56	1,591±261	3.9	320±46	2,156±168	6.7
1:20	378±19	2,185±383	5.8	297±17	3,958±235	13.3
1:200	340±31	5,210±297	15.3	276±30	5,765±380	20.9

[a]Indicated concentration of cell-free clarified sonicate or supernatant from 10^6 B95-8 or BJAB cells cultured for 4 days in vitro added to cultures of 10^6 peripheral blood leukocytes from normal individuals.

[b]Average response of 3-4 cultures per group 72 hours after in vitro stimulation with 5 µg of indicated mitogen and addition of 0.1 ml of indicated cell-free preparation.

Table 4. Blastogenic Response of Normal Human Blood Leukocytes to a Con A or PHA After Incubation with Cell-free Sonicate from B95-8 Cells

Time of Addition to Cultures[a]	No Mitogen (Control)	Blastogenic Response[b]			
		Con A		PHA	
		CPM	SI	CPM	SI
None (Control)	324	27,610±4,871	85.2	48,210±3,865	148.8
Day 0	410	1,970± 168	4.8	2,636± 192	6.4
+1	392	28,650± 972	73.1	37,158±2,473	94.8
+2	340	34,710±1,870	102.1	52,643±4,318	154.8
+3	312	32,935±2,136	105.6	50,760±3,861	162.7

[a]Cultures of 10^6 normal blood leukocytes incubated with 0.1 ml of a 1:2 dilution of cell-free sonicate from B95-8 cells at indicated time after culture initiation.

[b]Average CPM ± SD and SI for 3-4 cultures 72 hr after culture initiation and stimulation with 5 μg Con A or PHA.

Table 5. Effect of Heat, UV Light, or Centrifugation on the Inhibitory Activity of
Cell-free Sonicates from Lymphoblastoid Cells on the Blastogenic
Response of Human Blood Leukocytes Stimulated In Vitro.

Addition to Cultures[a]	In Vitro Treatment[b]	No Mitogen (Control)	Blastogenic Response[c] Con A	
			CPM	SI
None (Control)	--	420±27	38,680±2,706	92.1
B95-8 Sonicate	None	567±43	1,970± 382	3.5
	Heat (100°C)	386±47	31,436± 279	81.6
	UV Irradiation	481±38	32,735± 470	68.1
	Centrifugation	530±65	29,365± 312	55.4
BJAB Sonicate	None	531±31	3,072± 270	5.9
	Heat (100°C)	360±27	27,458± 416	76.3
	UV Irradiation	448±53	39,721± 305	88.9
	Centrifugation	526±22	19,964± 276	37.6

[a] Cultures of 10^6 normal human peripheral blood leukocytes treated in vitro with 0.1 ml of a 1:2 dilution of cell-free sonicate from 10^6 B95-8 or BJAB cells on day of culture initiation.

[b] Cell-free sonicate treated as indicated prior to addition to leukocyte cultures.

[c] Average CPM ± SD and SI from 3-4 cultures per group 72 hr after in vitro stimulation with 5 µg Con A and incubation with treated sonicates.

thymidine incorporation was not responsible for the effects noted. It is
more likely that a factor already present in the transformed cell lines or
synthesized by the cells during culture directly affected the blastogenic
responsiveness of normal leukocytes.

It seems important to note that extensive studies in experimental animals infected with retroviruses such as leukemogenic RNA viruses have shown
that not only infected or transformed cells suppress blastogenic responsiveness of normal syngeneic lymphoid cells in vitro, but also purified tumor
viruses as well as virus associated factors (5). Thus, it is possible that
EBV itself may activate cells to synthesize and/or release a factor responsible for suppression of normal immunocompetent cells. This factor could be
present as a normal constituent or product of healthy lymphoid cells in
relatively small amounts but is expressed in greater quantity in rapidly
dividing lymphoblastoid cells, including those derived from Burkitt's lymphoma patients without evidence of direct EBV infection.

It is now widely recognized that cells constituting the immune response
system are under direct and continuous control by a wide variety of immunoregulatory molecules. Not only are lymphokines, including IL-1 and IL-2
and interferons, important in enhancing or suppressing immune responses in
vivo and in vitro, but also many other factors, including small molecular
weight substances. In this latter category, accounting only for those
effector molecules, where the cell-type has been identified, the spectrum
of effector-storing, synthesizing, or transporting cells, includes the
neutrophil leukocyte (leukotrienes, eosinophil chemotactic factor of anaphylaxis, kinin-generating substances, histamine-releasers, and a neutrophil
inhibitory factor), the basophilic leukocyte (histamine, leukotrienes, the
eosinophilic and neutrophil chemotactic factors, and a platelet activating
factor), the murine basophilic leucocyte (histamine, leukotrienes, serotonin,
the eosinophilic chemotactic and platelet activating factors), the eosinophilic leucocyte (some histamine and leuktrienes as well as the platelet activating factor), the tissue mast cell (all effector molecules listed so far),
the murine tissue mast cell (in addition to all effectors present in mast
cells across species lines, serotonin), the "chromaffin positive" mast cell
(dopamine in suncinants; in other mammals norepinephrine), the enterochromaffin cell (serotonin), the chromaffin cell (catecholamines), the platelet
(depending on species: histamine, serotonin, catecholamines, and prostaglandins), the neurosecretory cell (all the previously mentioned biogenic
amines together with acetylcholine, and prostaglandins), and the nerve cell
[potentially all amine effectors, prostaglandins, and kinins (9,10)]. Many,
if not most of these effector molecules realize their immunoregulatory potential through their influence on the adenylate cyclase--cyclic AMP system of
the various cells that participate in the organization of the immune response
(11,12,13).

Studies from a number of laboratories in recent years have shown that
such factors, when present in increased concentrations, may adversely affect
lymphoproliferative responsiveness to antigens and mitogens. It has long
been known that suppressive factors are also released by a wide variety of
tumors, both in vivo and in vitro. Thus it seems likely from the present
study that lymphoblastoid cells induced by EBV, similar to other oncogenic
viruses, may result in production of immunomodulating mediators by the tumor
cell. However, it is also evident from this study that lymphoblastoid cells
free of EBV but derived from a patient with Burkitt's lymphoma, which is
widely regarded to be associated with EBV infection, may also release a
similar suppressive factor. Further characterization experiments are necessary to identify and isolate the specific suppressive factor(s) noted in
these studies and to determine whether these are similar or different from
those that have already been investigated (5). Also, the inhibitory effects
of the lymphoblastoid cell extracts on responsiveness of normal human leuko-

cytes to antigens which specifically stimulate B lymphocytes, as compared to those that stimulate T lymphocytes, should also be undertaken. Regardless of the mechanisms involved, it appears clear from these studies that cell-free preparations and culture supernatants from two distinct lymphoblastoid cell lines can depress the blastogenic responsiveness of normal human leukocytes in vitro to three distinct mitogens.

REFERENCES

1. J. G. Stevens, Herpetic latency and reactivation, in: "Oncogenic Herpesviruses," F. Rapp, ed., CRC Press, Boca Raton, FL (1980).
2. G. de-The, Epidemiology of Epstein-Barr virus and associated diseases in man, in: "The Herpesviruses," B. Roizman, ed., Plenum Press, New York (1983).
3. J. E. Robinson and G. Miller, Biology of lymphoid cells transformed by Epstein-Barr virus, in: "The Herpesviruses," B. Roizman, ed., Plenum Press, New York (1983).
4. W. Henle and G. Henle, Immunology of Epstein-Barr virus, in: "The Herpesviruses," B. Roizman, ed., Plenum Press, New York (1983).
5. S. Specter and H. Friedman, Viruses and the immune response, Pharm. Ther. 2:595 (1978).
6. J. Werkmeister, R. Zbroja, W. McCarthy, and P. Hersey, Detection of an inhibitor of cell division in cultures of tumor cells with immuno-suppressive activity in vitro, Clin. Exp. Immunol. 40:168 (1980).
7. J. S. Garvey, N. E. Cremer, and D. H. Sussdorf, "Methods in Immunology," W. A. Benjamin, Inc., Reading, PA (1977).
8. F. Vanky and J. Stjernsward, Lymphocyte stimulation test for detection of tumor specific reactivity in humans, in: "In Vitro Methods in Cell Mediated and Tumor Immunity," B. Bloom and J. R. David, eds., Academic Press, New York (1976).
9. A. Szentivanyi and J. Szentivanyi, Cellular and molecular foundations of immunity, immunololgic inflammation and hypersensitivity. Component parts and their relation to neurohumoral control mechanisms, in: "Sodeman's Pathologic Physiology - Mechanisms of Disease," Seventh Edition, W. A. Sodeman and T. M. Sodeman, eds., W. B. Saunders Company, Philadelphia and London (1985a).
10. A. Szentivanyi and J. Szentivanyi, The pathophysiology of immunologic and related diseases, in: "Sodeman's Pathologic Physiology - Mechanisms of Disease," Seventh Edition, W. A. Sodeman and T. M. Sodeman, eds., W. B. Saunders Company, Philadelphia and London (1985b).
11. A. Szentivanyi, E. Middleton, J. F. Williams, and H. Friedman, Effect of microbial agents on the immune network and associated pharmaco-logic reactivities, in: "Allergy: Principles and Practice," Second Edition, E. Middleton, C. E. Reed, and E. F. Ellis, eds., The C. V. Mosby Company, St. Louis (1983).
12. A. Szentivanyi, J. J. Krzanowski. and J. B. Polson, The autonomic nervous system and altered effector responses, in: "Allergy: Principles and Practice," Third Edition, E. Middleton, C. E. Reed, and E. F. Ellis, The C. V. Mosby Company, St. Louis, in press (1986a).
13. J. Szentivanyi, A. Szentivanyi, J. F. Williams, and H. Friedman, Virus associated immune and pharmacologic mechanisms in disorders of respiratory and cutaneous atopy, in this volume (1986b).

CYTOMEGALOVIRUS INFECTION AND THE IMMUNE SYSTEM

Mary Ann South, David A. Fuccillo, and
John L. Sever

National Institute for Neurologic and Communicative
Disorders and Stroke, National Institutes of Health
and Microbiological Associates
Bethesda, Maryland

INTRODUCTION

The interaction of human cytomegalovirus (CMV) with the immune system offers an unusual display of findings. CMV infection produces changes in the immune network which can result in depression of immune function. These clinical and immunological effects of CMV infection in various types of hosts are discussed here and are summarized in the accompanying table. In patients with immune deficiencies, especially of the cellular immune response, there is an environment conducive to serious CMV infections. In these cases, CMV functions as an opportunistic infectious agent. The double interaction offers a system for study of both the virus and immune system, and makes CMV prevention and treatment a high priority for clinical research efforts.

CONGENITAL CMV INFECTION

Infection with CMV is the most common of the congenital infections. At least 1% of all infants are infected in utero with this virus; in some studies the frequency is as high as 2.5% (1). Almost all of these infants are asymptomatic at birth, but evidence of damage can be demonstrated eventually in more than 10% of them. This damage can include hearing loss, brain damage with consequent mental retardation and/or neurologic deficit, chorioretinitis, and inguinal hernia. The occurrence of hearing loss (about 15% in one study) (2), cannot be predicted from the initial symptomatology, being found in almost equal frequency in children who were asymptomatic and those who were symptomatic at birth. Both brain and eye damage have been found to correspond roughly to the severity of the infectious syndrome in the neonate, so that severe disease affecting these systems is rare in the asymptomatically infected children.

Severe CMV infection which is symptomatic in the newborn period occurs in 1/15,000 births, or roughly 1% of all infants congenitally infected with CMV. These infants can develop a symptom complex, called cytomegalic inclusion disease (CID), which indicates disseminated CMV infection. Symptoms discernible at birth include hepatosplenomegaly, thrombocytopenia, anemia, lymphadenopathy, jaundice, central nervous system depression, respiratory distress due to interstitial pneumonia, microcephaly, cerebral calcifications, and skin rash of two types. These are petechiae due to the thrombocytopenia, and areas of extramedullary hematopoiesis presenting as "blueberry muffin" spots, which is due to the intrauterine anemia. These are the same presenting symptoms which may occur in other congenital infections.

Soon after the intrauterine infection occurs, there is polyclonal B cell activation, with precocious anatomic and functional development of the antigen-driven component of the B cell system. Immune recognition of CMV antigen can begin at 24-48 weeks gestation. After this period, the fetus can mount an immune response which includes a specific antibody response to the infecting virus. Cellular immunity has not been studied in the abortus with CMV, but in later life it is generally intact. Lymphocyte proliferation is normal for non-specific mitogens and in mixed lymphocyte reaction (3), but in response to CMV antigens is poor (4-6), especially when the congenitally infected person is less than one year of age (7).

Most infants with congenital CMV infection do not demonstrate immunologic abnormalities. If they ever had such abnormalities they may have already passed through them by the time they are born. Thus Montgomery et al. (3) found normal responses for proliferation to phytohemagglutinin, pokeweed mitogen, and in mixed lymphocyte culture in 11 infants in the first week of life. There was a positive response in all six of the infants tested for CMI by delayed hypersensitivity skin response after sensi-sensitization with keyhole limpet hemocyanin. Humoral immunity is also generally intact, with at least 90% of congenitally infected infants having CMV-IgM antibody even at the time of birth.

Variations of this intact immunity have been noted. Abnormalities in the T cell subsets have been found by two groups. We have observed (8) an infant with reversed T-helper/T-suppressor (T_H/T_S) ratio, due to a decreased number of T-helper cells, which persisted throughout his first year of life. He also had a lack of CMV-IgM and a delay in production of CMV-IgG antibody. Despite these immunologic abnormalities, this infant has not experienced opportunistic infections, resembling in this regard other infants with congenital CMV. Pass et al. (9) found four of 48 congenitally infected children to have reversed T_H/T_S ratios also due to a decrease in the T-helper cell fraction. Three of these four were infants less than one year of age, but 27 other infants had normal ratios. The mean number of T-helper cells was significantly lower in the symptomatic infants than in asymptomatic infants or older children.

PERINATALLY ACQUIRED CMV INFECTION

CMV can be acquired during birth from an infected cervix, shortly after birth from infected colostrum or milk, or from another infected infant in the newborn nursery. Premature or otherwise ill infants are most susceptible to infection in this period, and are especially prone to develop serious disease due to transfusion related CMV infection (10). These infants can develop a syndrome which in many respects resembles CID. Mortality is high and is due mostly to respiratory complications. In these infants there has not been a systematic search for immune abnormalities such as the T cell subset imbalance sometimes found in congenital infection.

ACQUIRED CMV INFECTION

Between 30 and 60 percent of normal adults are seropositive for CMV. One peak of infection occurs before age two, and is usually asymptomatic. Another peak occurs in early adulthood. Transmission is by intimate contact. These infections may be asymptomatic, cause a flu-like illness, or rarely produce an infectious mononucleosis syndrome. This syndrome can produce quite severe symptoms, especially if the infection is contracted from a direct intravenous inoculation as in blood transfusions. There are no other known predisposing factors to the development of this syndrome in the immunologically normal host.

The normal immune response to CMV infection includes an antibody response by one month with a peak about two months after onset of illness. The lymphocyte proliferative response lags behind the antibody, with onset at about two months and peak three months or more following development of symptoms (11). This timing of the development of specific immunity to CMV might be regarded as a delayed response due to the virus' direct effect on the immune system.

Transfusion acquired CMV infection was first described as a complication of open-heart surgery, and was called "post-perfusion syndrome." Symptomatically it is an infectious mononucleosis-like syndrome, and often is accompanied by pneumonia and other severe manifestations in the compromised host (10). It can follow any transfusion of infected blood products.

T cell subsets have been analyzed in CMV mononucleosis syndrome. There is a reversed T_H/T_S ratio, due to an increase in the T suppressor cell fraction. This reversed ratio occurs in infectious mononucleosis syndrome due to either CMV or EBV, but in CMV the reversal lasts longer (up to ten months) (12) than in EBV (about two months) (13). The lymphocyte proliferative response can be temporarily decreased (14), more markedly in transfusion-acquired than in community-acquired infection (15,16).

CMV INFECTION IN THE IMMUNOLOGICALLY COMPROMISED HOST

CMV infection has not presented as a clinical problem in patients with humoral immune deficiency states, but patients with compromise of cell-mediated immunity (CMI) are susceptible to severe and fatal disease with CMV infection, as with most other viruses (Table 1).

Primary Immune Deficiencies

Primary deficiencies of CMI are seen in the genetically determined immune deficient states such as severe combined immune deficiency and Di George syndrome. Since these patients have no T cell response at all, they do not exhibit the same symptoms or pathology that occurs in those with secondary and less complete CMI deficiency. In these patients, CMV most commonly causes an indolent lower respiratory tract infection, often in combination with another opportunist such as Pneumocystis carinii. The effect of CMV on the rudimentary immune systems of these patients has not been studied.

Secondary Deficiency of CMI Due to Drug Suppression

Patients with secondary deficiency of CMI due to drug suppression include those maintained on immunosuppressive drugs for cancer chemotherapy, organ transplantation, or treatment of a collagen-vascular or autoimmune disease. Patients who are on immunosuppressive drugs have variable suppression of the T cell system depending on the drugs being used. There is no increase in incidence or severity of CMV infection in patients who are treated only with corticosteroids alone. However, in patients who have received an organ transplant the graft usually cannot be maintained with corticosteroids alone. The T cell system is the primary target for immunosuppressive therapy and therefore the drug regimens used will uniformly depress CMI. The suppression must be maintained for the lifetime of the

Table 1. Effects of CMV Infection on Clinical Symptomatology and T Cells
in the Immunologically Compromised Host

CMV Infection	Clinical Effect	Effect on T Cells
Congenital	1% severely ill (CID) and permanently damaged; 10% milder delayed damage.	Helper T cells decreased (found in a few infants).
Perinatally Acquired	May cause CID with high mortality in prematures and transfusion related cases.	Unknown.
Acquired in Adulthood	Infectious mononucleosis syndrome in a few. Serious disease when acquired from transfusion.	Suppressor T cells increased; proliferative responses decreased for a short time.
In primary immuno-deficiency	Augmentation of symptoms from other infectious agents.	Unknown.
In patients immunosuppressed by drugs	Serious multisystem disease.	Helper T cells decreased, suppressor T cells increased.
In bone marrow transplant recipients	Interstitial pneumonia, other multisystem disease.	Helper T cells decreased, suppressor T cells increased.
In AIDS patients	Interstitial pneumonia, other multisystem disease.	Helper T cells decreased.

graft; this places the organ transplant recipient at risk for a long period
of time. Better suppressive regimens are being devised; for example,
cyclosporin (17) seems to produce a more selective depression and the complications of CMV infection are proportionately decreased.

The source of infection in transplant patients can be from reactivation
of a pre-existent CMV infection, from transplanted organs, or from blood
transfusions, as well as the usual routes. The infection can result in
severe symptomatology, most commonly involving the lungs, liver, or central
nervous system, and may contribute to the severity of the primary illness
or may be fatal.

In drug-suppressed patients, CMV produces the same immunologic findings
as in the normal host with CMV mononucleosis, involving the residual T
cells (18).

Bone Marrow Transplant Recipients

Patients who receive bone marrow transplants are even more thoroughly
suppressed than the organ transplant recipients, since their pre-transplant

conditioning must aim to destroy not only T cells but the more resistant NK cells, requiring more stringent cytotoxic treatment by drugs or irradiation than is used in any other situation. There is a very high frequency of severe CMV pneumonia in those recipients who already have CMV, receive marrow from a CMV positive donor, or contract CMV during the course of the transplant. In addition graft-versus-host reactions are aggravated by CMV infection.

During reconstitution of the lymphoid system after marrow transplant, there is often a T cell subset abnormality similar to that found in CMV mononucleosis. Verdonck and DeGast (19) have analyzed patients who received autologous marrow, and therefore have no graft rejection nor graft-versus-host disease to complicate interpretation of the data. Those who had CMV infec- tion had reconstitution of the T cell system at a slower rate than the un- infected recipients. The T_H/T_S ratio was constantly reversed and function- ally there was an excess of T suppressor activity in CMV infected but not in uninfected recipients. This study definitely incriminated CMV as the cause of these common findings in transplant recipients.

Acquired Immune Deficiency Syndrome (AIDS)

Almost 5,000 adults and more than 50 infants have been reported to the U. S. Centers for Disease Control as AIDS patients (20). In adult AIDS, CMV infection is almost universal. Detels et al. (21) found 96% of 89 homosexually active men seropositive for CMV; 100% were seropositive for at least one of the herpes group viruses. The symptoms of CMV infection in the AIDS patient are similar to that found in other patients with secondary immunodeficiency. CMV gastroenteritis is a newly described condition in AIDS (22,23). CMV retinitis is common in this group as in other immunocompromised patients (24).

AIDS patients classically have a reversal of T_H/T_S ratio (25). They usually have a multiplicity of infections in addition to the AIDS agent, so that it is difficult to determine which factor is causing this particular immunologic abnormality. Infant AIDS, however, represents a less complicated infectious situation. A study (26) of 13 patients diagnosed as having infant AIDS found two of them with normal T_H/T_S ratios, and these two children had no evidence of CMV or other herpes group virus infection. These two cases suggest that CMV or other herpes viruses, rather than the AIDS agent, may be primarily responsible for the reversal of the T_H/T_S ratio.

TREATMENT AND PREVENTION OF CMV INFECTION

Treatment

Treatment of established CMV infection has been attempted using anti-viral drugs and immune factor therapy. In general, there is no treatment which is effective in curing the viral infection. Several treatments, however, can suppress viral excretion and so may be of value in selected clinical situations. Anti-viral drugs definitely effective in CMV suppression include cytosine arabinoside (ARA-C) and adenine arabinoside (ARA-A, Vidarabine) (27). ARA-A is chosen for anti-viral treatment because it is less cytotoxic than ARA-C, but even so it is used only in selected clinical circumstances. For example, ARA-A is unacceptable for CMV treatment in bone marrow transplant patients because of its toxicity to the newly en-grafted immature cells. Acyclovir is less toxic than ARA-A but also has less anti-CMV effect (28).

Immune factors which have been used to treat CMV include immune serum globulin, transfer factor, and interferon. Immune serum globulin, containing specific CMV-IgG antibody in high titer, has been of possible value in decreasing viral excretion (29). This is especially true for the forms of immunoglobulin which can be given intravenously, so that very large doses of neutralizing antibody can reach infected sites. The IV forms are doubly valuable in thrombocytopenic patients to whom intramuscular injections cannot be given. A hyperimmune anti-CMV IV preparation shows greatest promise of effectiveness for treatment of high risk groups (30).

Transfer factor has been reported to be of value in the treatment of CMV retinitis (31). It has not been tried on a large scale, and there are no controlled studies comparing CMV immune transfer factor to that made from donors who are CMV seronegative. Studies in other disease models have suggested that a major clinical effect of transfer factor is in a nonspecific enhancement of the immune response. Transfer factor is now being fractionated and the fractions active in this nonspecific enhancement are being analyzed (32).

Interferon (33) has been used successfully to decrease CMV excretion and symptomatology in renal transplant patients.

Prevention

CMV seronegative persons in high risk groups should be protected from CMV infection in every possible way (34). All transfusions should be from seronegative donors. In preparation for transplantation, consideration should be given to the CMV serologic status of both recipient and possible donors. In hospital situations where high risk patients may be exposed, it is wise to isolate known infected patients such as infants with congenital CMV. Outside the hospital, however, it is not necessary to isolate these individuals, since this infection is not airborne and there is no danger of transmission through casual contact. Although the risk is very small, seronegative pregnant women as well as persons in other high risk groups should avoid infants and others who are known to be excreting CMV.

Prevention of CMV disease by vaccine is a possibility in the near future. Two candidate live virus vaccines are now in clinical trials. One is derived from Towne strain and the other from AD-169. Attempts are also being made to isolate subunits lacking viral DNA which will be effective in producing protective immunity to CMV without the possibility of continued latent infection with the vaccine virus (27).

CONCLUSION

Over the past 20 years CMV has been established as a causative agent of congenital infection with long term morbidity. In addition, the importance of CMV as a pathogen has been recognized in the adult host with a primary or secondary immunodeficient state. In these cases, CMV may be involved as an opportunistic infection. Transfusion acquired CMV has become a clinical problem as the frequency of transfusion has increased, particularly during recently developed and highly complex medical and surgical procedures. Thus, a great deal of effort is being directed toward treatment and prevention of this infection.

REFERENCES

1. S. Stagno, R. F. Pass, M. E. Dworsky, and C. A. Alford, Congenital and perinatal cytomegalovirus infections, Seminars in Perinatology 7:31 (1983).
2. S. Stagno, D. W. Reynolds, C. S. Amos, A. J. Dahle, F. P. McCollister, I. Mohindra, R. Ermocilla, and C. A. Alford, Auditory and visual

defects resulting from symptomatic and subclinical congenital cytomegaloviral and toxoplasma infections, Pediatrics 59:669 (1977).

3. J. R. Montgomery, E. O. Mason, Jr., A. P. Williamson, M. M. Desmond, and M. A. South, Prospective study of congenital cytomegalovirus infection, Southern Medical J. 73:590 (1980).

4. R. C. Gehrz, S. C. Marker, S. O. Knorr, J. M. Kalis, and H. H. Balfour, Jr., Specific cell-mediated immune defect in active cytomegalovirus infection of young children and their mothers, Lancet 2:844 (1977).

5. D. W. Reynolds, P. H. Dean, R. F. Pass, and C. A. Alford, Specific cell-mediated immunity in children with congenital and neonatal cytomegalovirus infection and their mothers, J. Infect. Dis. 140:493 (1979).

6. S. E. Starr, M. D. Tolpin, H. M. Friedman, K. Paucker, and S. A. Plotkin, Impaired cellular immunity to cytomegalovirus in congenitally infected children and their mothers, J. Infect. Dis. 140:500 (1979).

7. R. F. Pass, M. E. Dworsky, R. J. Whitley, A. M. August, S. Stagno, and C. A. Alford, Specific lymphocyte blastogenic responses in children with cytomegalovirus and herpes simplex virus infections acquired early in infancy, Infect. Immun. 34:166 (1981).

8. M. A. South, W. Rodriguez, D. Fuccillo, L. Nerurkar, A. Yachie, and J. L. Sever, Immunologic findings in a case of congenital CMV compared to infants with AIDS, Chapter 6 in this book.

9. R. F. Pass, M. A. Roper, and A. M. August, T lymphocyte subpopulations in congenital cytomegalovirus infection, Infect. and Immun. 41:1380 (1983).

10. S. P. Adler, Transfusion-associated cytomegalovirus infections, Reviews Infect. Dis. 5:977 (1983).

11. M. Ho, Cytomegalovirus: biology and infection, in: "Current Topics in Infectious Disease," W. B. Greenough, III and T. C. Merigan, eds., Plenum Publishing, New York (1982).

12. W. P. Carney, R. H. Rubin, R. A. Hoffman, W. P. Hansen, K. Healey, and M. S. Hirsch, Analysis of T lymphocyte subsets in cytomegalovirus mononucleosis, J. Immunol. 126:2114 (1981).

13. E. L. Reinharz, C. O'Brien, P. Rosenthal, and S. F. Schlossman, The cellular basis for viral induced immunodeficiency: analysis by monoclonal antibodies, J. Immunol. 125:1269 (1980).

14. C. R. Rinaldo, M. J. Levin, W. P. Carney, P. H. Black, and M. S. Hirsch, Interactions of lymphocytes with cytomegalovirus, in: "Virus Lymphocyte Interactions: Implications for Disease," M. R. Proffit, ed., Elsevier North-Holland, Amsterdam (1979).

15. C. R. Rinaldo, W. P. Carney, B. S. Richter, P. H. Black, and M. S. Hirsch, Mechanisms of immunosuppression in cytomegaloviral mononucleosis, J. Infect. Dis. 141:488 (1980).

16. M. J. Levin, C. R. Rinaldo, Jr., P. L. Leary, J. A. Zaia, and M. S. Hirsch, Immune response to herpesvirus antigens in adults with acute cytomegalovirus mononucleosis, J. Infect. Dis. 140:851 (1979).

17. J. S. Dummer, A. Hardy, A. Poorsattar, and M. Ho, Early infections in kidney, heart, and liver transplant recipients on cyclosporin, Transplantation 36:259 (1983).

18. R. T. Schooley, M. S. Hirsch, R. B. Colvin, A. B. Cosimi, N. E. Tolkoff-Rubin, R. T. McCluskey, R. C. Burton, P. S. Russell, J. T. Herrin, F. I. Delmonico, J. V. Giorgi, W. Henle, and R. H. Rubin, Association of herpesvirus infections with T-lymphocyte-subset alterations, glomerulopathy, and opportunistic infections after renal transplantation, N. Eng. J. Med. 308:307 (1983).

19. L. F. Verdonck and G. C. DeGast, Is cytomegalovirus infection a major cause of T-cell alterations after (autologous) bone marrow transplantation? Lancet 1:932 (1984).

20. Update: Acquired Immunodeficiency Syndrome (AIDS) - United States, Morbidity and Mortality Weekly Report 33:337 (1984).

21. R. Detels, B. R. Visscher, J. L. Fahey, K. Schwartz, R. S. Greene, D. L. Madden, J. L. Sever, and M. S. Gottlieb, The relation of cytomegalovirus and Epstein-Barr virus antibodies to T-cell subsets in homosexually active men, JAMA 251:1719 (1984).

22. S. L. Gertler, J. Pressman, P. Price, S. Brozinsky, and K. Miyai, Gastrointestinal cytomegalovirus infection in a homosexual man with severe acquired immunodeficiency syndrome, Gastroenter. 85:1403 (1983).

23. A. B. Knapp, D. A. Horst, G. Eliopoulos, H. F. Gramm, L. W. Gaber, K. R. Falchuk, Z. M. Falchuk, and C. Trey, Widespread cytomegalovirus gastroenterocolitis in a patient with acquired immunodeficiency syndrome, Gastroenter. 85:1399 (1983).

24. A. H. Friedman, J. Orellana, W. R. Freeman, M. H. Luntz, M. B. Starr, M. L. Tapper, I. Spigland, H. Rotterdam, R. M. Tejada, S. Braunhut, D. Mildvan, and U. Mathur, Cytomegalovirus retinitis: a manifestation of the acquired immune deficiency syndrome (AIDS), Brit. J. Ophthal. 67:372 (1983).

25. J. L. Fahey, H. Prince, M. Weaver, J. Groopman, B. Visscher, K. Schwartz, and R. Detels, Quantitative changes in T helper or T suppressor/cytotoxic lymphocyte subsets that distinguish acquired immune deficiency syndrome from other immune subset disorders, Amer. J. Med. 76:95 (1984).

26. G. B. Scott, B. E. Buck, J. G. Leterman, F. L. Bloom, and W. P. Parks, Acquired immunodeficiency syndrome in infants, New Eng. J. Med. 310:76 (1984).

27. S. A. Plotkin, S. Michaelson, C. A. Alford, S. E. Starr, P. D. Parkman, J. S. Pagano, and F. Rapp, The pathogenesis and prevention of human cytomegalovirus infection, Pediatr. Infect. Dis. 3:67 (1984).

28. J. D. Meyers, J. C. Wade, R. W. McGuffin, S. C. Springmeyer, and E. D. Thomas, The use of acyclovir for cytomegalovirus infections in the immunocompromised host, J. Antimicrobial Chemotherapy 12:181 (1983).

29. J. D. Meyers, J. Leszcynski, J. A. Zaia, N. Flournoy, B. Newton, D. R. Snydman, G. G. Wright, M. J. Levin, and E. D. Thomas, Prevention of cytomegalovirus infection by cytomegalovirus immune globulin after marrow transplantation, Ann. Int. Med. 98:442 (1983).

30. R. M. Condie and R. J. O'Reilly, Prevention of cytomegalovirus infection by prophylaxis with an intravenous hyperimmune native unmodified cytomegalovirus globulin, Am. J. Med. 36:134 (1984).

31. M. W. Rytel, T. M. Aaberg, T. H. Dee, and L. R. Heim, Therapy of cytomegalovirus retinitis with transfer factor, Cell. Immunol. 19:8 (1975).

32. A.A. Gottlieb, J. L. Farmer, M. Falum, C. Kardinal, and A. Levine, Partial immunoreconstitution of acquired immunodeficiency syndrome (AIDS) patients with an immunomodulator derived from human leukocyte dialysates

33. M. S. Hirsch, R. T. Schooley, A. B. Cosimi, P.S. Russell, F. L. Delmonico, N. E. Tolkoff-Rubin, J. T. Herrin, K. Cantell, M. Farrell, T. R. Rota, and R. H. Rubin, Effects of interferon-alpha on cytomegalovirus reactivation syndromes in renal-transplant recipients, New Eng. J. Med. 308:1489 (1983).

34. A. S. Yeager, F. C. Grumet, E. B. Hafleigh, A. M. Arvin, J. S. Bradley, and C. G. Prober, Prevention of transfusion acquired cytomegalovirus infections in newborn infants, J. Pediatr. 98:281 (1981).

IMMUNOLOGIC FINDINGS IN A CASE OF CONGENITAL CMV

COMPARED TO INFANTS WITH AIDS

Mary Ann South, William Rodriguez, David Fuccillo,
Lata Nerurkar, Akihiro Yachie, and John L. Sever

National Institute for Neurologic and Communicative
Disorders and Stroke, and National Cancer Institute
National Institutes of Health, Bethesda, MD
Children's Hospital National Medical Center and
George Washington University, Washington, D.C.

INTRODUCTION

Infections with viruses of the herpes group, particularly cytomegalovirus (CMV), have been associated with a transient reversal of T-helper/-
T-suppressor (T_H/T_S) ratio. This reversal has been reported with CMV mononucleosis, immunosuppressed patients with CMV infection, and a few cases of
congenital CMV. In none of these reports has the reversed T_H/T_S ratio been
causally associated with other immune abnormalities. The reversed ratio is
also a frequent finding in acquired immune deficiency syndrome (AIDS), and
it is unclear as to what causal relationships may exist among the CMV infection of AIDS patients, the AIDS agent, the reversed T_H/T_S ratio, the other
immune defects of AIDS, and the susceptibility to opportunistic infections
experienced by AIDS patients. We have studied a child with congenital CMV
throughout the first year of life who exhibited a persistently reversed
T_H/T_S ratio, a lack of antibody to CMV in the IgM class, a delay in CMV-IgG
antibody formation, and an unusually prolonged high titer of CMV excretion
in his urine. In spite of these immunologic changes, he has not experienced
opportunistic infections. This case study helps to clarify some of the
above relationships.

CASE REPORT

The patient was a male child delivered of a 14-year old Hispanic mother,
who had immigrated ten years earlier from El Salvador. She was not an IV
drug user or a prostitute, and she had no abnormal physical findings. Medical history during her pregnancy was unremarkable except for a flu-like
illness at four months gestation. The neonate was small for gestational
age, jaundiced, and had hepatosplenomegaly, a rash resembling "blueberry
muffin" spots, and central nervous system depression. Laboratory studies
revealed thrombocytopenia, anemia (but no leukopenia), hypergammaglobulinemia, and brain calcifications.

The immunologic and virologic findings in the newborn period and at
sequential followup for the first year of life are presented in Table 1 and
Figure 1. CMV was cultured from urine at a titer of more than 10^7 $TCID_{50}$/ml,

and also from buffy coat, throat swab, and cerebrospinal fluid at the age of two weeks. His T cell subsets were measured at this time, using the OKT series of monoclonal antibodies in which T_4 is related to helper and T_8 to suppressor function. There was a marked decrease of T_4 positive cells with a normal number of T_8 positive cells, producing a reversed T_4/T_8 ratio of 0.8. The mother's T_4 and T_8 cell numbers were normal with a ratio of 1.5, although she was still excreting CMV in urine at a titer of $10^4 TCID_{50}$/ml. The indirect ELISA CMV-IgG antibody titer was 1:8192 for both mother and newborn baby. The baby's ELISA CMV-IgM was negative although his total serum IgM was 70 mg/dl.

On followup exam, the patients, CMV-IgG titer decreased to undetectable levels by four months of age; the other findings persisted unchanged. At four and five months of age his T cells proliferated normally in response to PHA, Con A, and PWM. His B cells secreted immunoglobulins normally, and his T cells were not unusually suppressive and were able to supply help to normal B cells in secreting immunoglobulins. All these functions were comparable to an age matched control. At eight months of age, his CMV-IgG rose to 1:10,140. Despite this IgG antibody, the CMV shedding continued at the same high level, and the CMV-IgM remained negative. The T helpers remained low, producing a continuously reversed ratio which never rose above 0.8. The anemia and thrombocytopenia had corrected and he was never lymphopenic. All these findings persisted through one year of age. During this year he had only three transient infections, none of which were opportunistic.

DISCUSSION

This patient with congenital CMV infection presents several unusual findings. First, his clinical symptoms were unusually severe. Of all infants congenitally infected with CMV, only 5% have typical cytomegalic inclusion disease (1). This patient had every aspect of that disease in particularly severe form, suggesting that he may have been infected very early in gestation. Indeed, the mother had a history of a flu-like illness

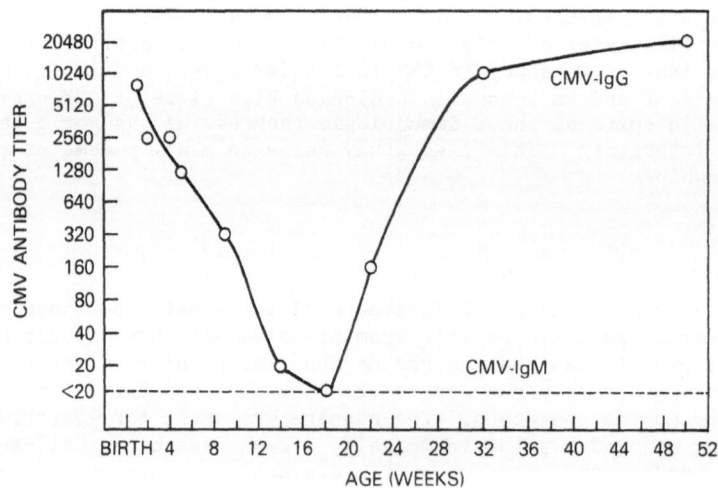

Fig. 1. The patient's CMV antibody measured by indirect ELISA. CMV antibody in the IgM class (broken line) remained undetectable. CMV antibody (maternally derived) in the IgG class (solid line) dropped to undetectable levels by 18 weeks of age, before climbing to high levels again at 8 months.

Table 1. Measurements of T-Cell Subsets and Urinary Excretion of CMV in the Newborn Period and at Sequential Follow-up for the First Year of Life

| | Patient | | | | | | Normal | | |
| | Age | | | | | | | | |
	2 wk.	4 wk.	14 wk.	22 wk.	32 wk.	50 wk.	Adult	Newborn	20 wk.
T_3 (total T)%	27	24	36	43	26	53	71	43	43
T_4 (helper)%	11	12	13	19	2	15	48	32	24
T_8 (suppressor)%	14	18	22	24	22	38	22	12	16
T_4/T_8 Ratio	0.83	0.66	0.60	0.80	0.08	0.40	2.13	2.96	1.51
Virus in Urine	+	$10^{7.3}$	$10^{7.4}$	$10^{6.5}$	$10^{7.5}$	$10^{6.5}$			

The patient's T cell subsets measured by cytofluorographic method utilizing OKT series of monoclonal antibodies. Normals are mean values of adult daily controls in the same laboratory, 8 cord blood specimens and a normal infant two weeks younger than the patient, measured at 20 weeks of age. Viral cultures were performed with human foreskin fibroblast cells (Flow 7000).

at four months of gestation. She may have experienced her primary CMV and transmitted it to her fetus at that time. Second, urinary excretion of CMV continued at about 10^7 $TCID_{50}$/ml throughout the first year of life, whereas most infants with congenital CMV will have decreased their viral titer in urine to about 10^4 $TCID_{50}$/ml by one year of age (1). Third, there was never a CMV-IgM antibody response, while 90% of infants with congenital CMV infection have CMV-IgM antibody even in cord blood (1). There was a delay in initiation of the CMV-IgG antibody response. Infants with congenital CMV regularly begin to make CMV-IgG either in utero or directly after birth, so that as the maternally derived antibody decays, the infant's own IgG antibody replaces it, keeping the titer at a nearly steady level through the first few months of life. In contrast, our patient's maternally derived antibody had completely disappeared before he had his own CMV-IgG detectable by ELISA. And fourth, the T_H/T_S ratio was reversed due to a decrease in the number of helper cells, and remained so during his entire first year of life.

The reversal of this patient's T_H/T_S ratio is not in itself completely unexpected. Adult patients with CMV mononucleosis (2) also have a reversed T_H/T_S ratio, but the reversal is due to an augmentation of T_S cell numbers. AIDS patients, who typically have the T_H/T_S ratio reversed (3), have decreased helper cells, just as found in our patient. Other infants and children with congenital CMV have been reported by Pass et al. (4) to have a reversal of the T_H/T_S ratio. These patients were of various ages when they were studied. The younger symptomatic infants were most likely to have low or reversed T_H/T_S ratios. A reduced number of helper cells contributed to the lowered ratio rather than an increased number of suppressor cells. These findings are consistent with those in our patient. As with our patient, none of the individuals with either CMV mononucleosis or congenital CMV have been reported to have the opportunistic infections which the AIDS patients experience.

Table 2 summarizes the T cell subset findings in CMV mononucleosis, congenital CMV, and AIDS, and compares the susceptibility to opportunistic infection in these conditions. Congenital CMV is like CMV mononucleosis in the lack of susceptibility to opportunistic infections, but is more like AIDS in its T cell subset relationships. In trying to understand this apparent inconsistency, a study of infant AIDS provides a most instructive comparison. Scott et al. (5) reported a detailed study of 14 infant AIDS cases in Miami. Two of these infants had normal T_H/T_S ratios. These two had no infection with any viruses of the herpes group, e.g. CMV, Epstein-Barr virus, herpes simplex types 1 and 2, and varicella-zoster. However, they both had opportunistic infections consisting of Pneumocystis carinii pneumonia and candidiasis. In contrast, adults are virtually never seronegative for all the herpes viruses, and the adult AIDS patients often have active infection with more than one member of this viral group.

Comparison of these four groups of individuals (Table 2) suggests that the T cell subset abnormality is not responsible for the susceptibility to opportunistic infections in AIDS. Further, the comparison of AIDS, infant AIDS, and CMV infections suggests that the CMV, rather than the AIDS agent, may actually be responsible for the T cell subset abnormality. The effect of the CMV (or other herpes virus group) infection may be different in the mature intact T cell system of the CMV mononucleosis patients than in a compromised T cell system. Either immaturity, as in fetal T_H cells or infection with the AIDS retrovirus, which is known to grow in the T_H cell fraction (6), could be responsible for such a compromise in the T cells. In the patient already thus compromised, a superimposed herpes group infection could destroy T_H cells, whereas in the normal and mature patient the effect would be only an increase in the T_S cell numbers as compensation for the polyclonal activation of the B cells with resultant hypergammaglobulinemia. In this respect the immature fetal T cells would be analogous

Table 2. Conditions with Abnormal T Cell Subsets Producing Reversed T_H/T_S Ratios

Condition	Usual Findings		
	T_H	T_S	Opportunistic Infections
Congenital CMV	Low	Normal	No
CMV Mononucleosis	Normal	High	No
Adult AIDS	Low	Normal	Yes
Infant AIDS			
with CMV	Low	Normal	Yes
without CMV	Normal	Normal	Yes
Bone Marrow Transplant			
with CMV	Low	High	Yes
without CMV	Normal	Normal	Yes

to the newly differentiated T cells of transplant recipients (Table 2). Verdonck and DeGast (7) compared recipients with and without CMV. The CMV infected recipients had a slow reconstitution of their T cells with a constantly reversed T_H/T_S ratio, and a slow recovery of the specific immune responses.

Perhaps our patient's similarity to the bone marrow transplant recipients can explain his continued high viral excretion and his abnormally delayed IgG-CMV antibody response as well as his prolonged decrease of the T_H cell fraction. If our patient become infected at four months gestation, he had CMV antigen present before the specific immune responsiveness for CMV normally develops. The lymphoid cell system, although present, had not matured. Thus, he would be in a situation exactly like the marrow recipients who already have CMV infection when engraftment occurs and lymphoid reconstitution begins. If this was true, our patient could be expected to react just as he did.

It is a reasonable assumption that our patient does not have AIDS in addition to his congenital CMV reversal and delayed CMV antibody response. His mother was not in any high risk group for AIDS, and still has no symptoms. He has not subsequently been exposed to anyone in a high risk group. He did have blood transfusions in the first month of his life, but they were taken from regular blood donors who were carefully screened and followed up and who have remained asymptomatic. Our patient had symptomatic CMV infection and the reversed T_H/T_S ratio from birth, and even at 12 months of age had no opportunistic infection. In contrast, as reported by Shannon et al. (8), an infant apparently acquired both CMV and AIDS from transfusions as a neonate. This patient developed opportunistic infections (Pneumocystis and Candida) at ten months of age. He had a normal T_4/T_8 ratio at four months of age, but by five and one-half months had a ratio of 0.8 with progressive decrease until last studied at 16 months. Further, in the Miami study (5) 8/14 patients had clinically apparent AIDS in the first three months of life, and all were symptomatic by eight months of age. Thus it appears that the incubation period for infant AIDS, whether acquired from the mother or via transfusion, is shorter than the year during which we have studied our patient.

SUMMARY AND CONCLUSIONS

We have studied a child with congenital CMV longitudinally and have found the T-helper/T-suppressor ratio reversed, no CMV-IgM antibody, and high urinary excretion of CMV at 10^7 $TCID_{50}$/ml, all persisting through his first year of life. There was a delay in appearance of CMV-IgG antibody until five months of age.

The analysis of this infant's findings and comparison with CMV mononucleosis, AIDS in both infants and adults, and bone marrow transplant recipients, draws us to two conclusions. First, CMV infection can produce T_H/T_S ratio reversal, both in congenital and acquired forms of the disease. This reversal is due to an increase in the T-suppressor fraction in the intact adult, but is more related to a decrease in T-helpers in newborns and other immunologically compromised individuals. Second, the reversal of T_H/T_S ratio, whether due to decrease of helper cells or increase of suppressor cells, does not cause susceptibility to opportunistic infections.

REFERENCES

1. S. Stagno, R. F. Pass, M. E. Dworsky, and C. Alford, Congenital and Perinatal Cytomegalovirus Infections, Seminars in Perinatology 7:31 (1983).
2. W. P. Carney, R. H. Rubin, R. A. Hoffman, W. P. Hansen, K. Healey, and M. S. Hirsch, Analysis of T lymphocyte subsets in cytomegalovirus, J. Immunol. 126:2114 (1981).
3. J. L. Fahey, H. Prince, M. Weaver, J. Groopman, B. Visscher, K. Schwartz, and R. Detels, Quantitative changes in T helper or T suppressor/cytotoxic lymphocyte subsets that distinguish acquired immune deficiency syndrome from other immune subset disorders, Am. J. Med. 76:95 (1984).
4. R. F. Pass, M. A. Roper, and A. M. August, T lymphocyte subpopulations in congenital cytomegalovirus infection, Inf. Imm. 41:1380 (1983).
5. G. B. Scott, B. E. Buck, J. G. Leterman, F. L. Bloom, and W. P. Parks, Acquired immunodeficiency syndrome in infants, New Eng. J. Med. 310:76 (1984).
6. M. Popovic, M. G. Sarngadharan, E. Read, and R. C. Gallo, Detection, isolation, and continuous production of cytopathic retroviruses (HTLV-III) from patients with AIDS and pre-AIDS, Science 224:497 (1984).
7. L. F. Verdonck and G. C. DeGast, Is cytomegalovirus infection a major cause of T cell alterations after (autologous) bone-marrow transplantation? Lancet 1:932 (1984).
8. K. Shannon, E. Ball, R. L. Wasserman, F. K. Murphy, J. Ludy, and G. R. Buchanan, Transfusion-associated cytomegalovirus infection and acquired immune deficiency syndrome in an infant, J. Pediatr. 103:859 (1983).

HERPES SIMPLEX VIRUS AND IMMUNITY

Steven Specter

Department of Medical Microbiology and Immunology
University of South Florida College of Medicine
Tampa, Florida

INTRODUCTION

The interactions between herpes simplex virus (HSV) and the host immune system have been extensively investigated both in man and experimental animals. HSV may serve in these interactions as, (1) an antigen to stimulate specific immune responses to the virus, (2) an immune suppressive agent, initiating both specific and non-specific depression of immune reactivity, and (3) a non-specific stimulant of host defense responses. Each role for HSV will be examined and the mechanism(s) responsible for each will be discussed.

IMMUNITY TO HSV

Host defense against HSV begins with natural resistance involving both macrophages and natural killer cells (1-3). This subject is dealt with elsewhere in this volume and will not be discussed in this chapter (see chapters by C. Lopez and S. Mogensen).

Primary infection with HSV, leads to production of anti-HSV antibodies, development of anti-HSV cellular immunity and generally resolves with recovery from infection. The humoral immune response includes development of both type specific antibodies and immunoglobulins which cross-react between HSV type 1 and HSV type 2. Contrary to many other virus infections antibody is not associated with prevention of subsequent clinical disease due to this virus. Recurrent disease may occur in up to 50% of individuals who have measurable antibodies to HSV. Virus has the ability to remain latent within host ganglion cells. Thus the virus is protected from the neutralizing effects of antibody. Primary HSV1 induced infection may manifest itself as a subclinical infection, mild stomatitis, or severe systemic disease. The factors affecting the course of acute primary infection, both immunologic and non-immunologic, are not understood (4).

In addition to the development of antibodies, there is a very prominent cellular immune response to HSV. Several investigators have suggested that T lymphocytes contribute to the establishment and maintenance of latency and reactivation of HSV from latency (5-11). It has not been clearly delineated how HSV reactivation occurs in the presence of a healthy T-lymphocyte responsiveness in an individual who harbors latent HSV. It is possible

Table 1. Herpes Simplex Virus Induced Suppression of PHA Stimulated
Human Lymphocytes

		PHA	100a	PHA + HSV 10	1
HSV Seropositive[c]	S.I.[b]	25.6±5.0	4.0±0.6	9.3±1.3	13.7±2.0
	%	-	(16)	(36)	(54)
HSV Seronegative[d]	S.I.	25.8±4.2	5.7±2.6	10.5±3.2	16.0±3.5
	%	-	(22)	(41)	(62)

a Multiplicity of infection
b Stimulation index = cpm ^{3}H-thymidine with PHA/cpm ^{3}H-thymidine in
   control
c Anti-HSV CF titer ≥1:16; n=44
d Anti-HSV CF titer <1:Ø8; n=16
e Percent versus PHA alone ± S.E.

that when T cell activity is reduced yielding a lower level of immunity HSV
recrudescences. This will be discussed in greater detail below.

MODULATION OF IMMUNITY BY HSV

    The ability of viruses to alter immune responses is a widely recognized
phenomenon dating back to the observation in the early 1900's by Von Pirquet
that individuals infected with measles virus had depressed anti-tuberculin
responses (12). However, the ability of herpes simplex viruses to negatively
affect a variety of immune reactions was not documented until the 1970's
(12-17). The changes noted in both specific immune function and non-specific
or polyclonal reactivity vary greatly depending upon the system utilized.

    Kleinerman et al. (16) demonstrated that monocyte chemotaxis of human
peripheral blood leukocytes (PBL) is severely depressed in the presence of
live HSV, whereas UV inactivated virus has no effect. The authors were not
able to associate this with any cytotoxic effect of the virus on the PBL
(16). Centifanto et al. demonstrated that patients with a history of ocular
or labial recurrent HSV, while in the quiescent phase, did not demonstrate
inhibition of migration of peripheral blood leukocytes, thus expressing
deficient leukocyte inhibitory factor (LIF) activity in the presence of UV
inactivated HSV-1 (18). Plaeger-Marshall and Smith demonstrated that live,
but not heat inactivated, HSV-1 could inhibit blastogenesis by PBL from HSV
seropositive and seronegative individuals. This inhibition was observed in
responses to various antigens and mitogens. Inhibition by HSV was unaltered
by removal of monocytes from the assay (17).

    Conversely, several investigators have reported that either live or
inactivated HSV may enhance blastogenic responses to specific antigen (19-24)
while some investigators suggest that there is no effect of HSV on blastogenic or migration inhibition assays (17,20,25). It is difficult to pinpoint
the cause(s) for the diverse nature of these results. The most consistent
data are those indicating that inactivated HSV serves as a good antigen for
stimulating immune lymphocytes to incorporate ^{3}H-thymidine and that live
HSV may be immunosuppressive.

Table 2. Herpes Simplex Virus Induced Reversal of Migration
Inhibition due to the Presence of Streptokinase-Strepto-
dornase[a]

| | SK-SD | SK-SD + HSV | | |
		1[b]	10	100
		HSV Seropositive (n=44)		
Percent migration[c]	28±4	43±5	82±4	84±4
% Positive for M.I.[d]	93	84	41	34
		HSV Seronegative (n=16)		
Percent migration	31±8	39±7	55±8	56±8
% Positive for M.I.	88	88	63	69

a Patient peripheral blood leukocytes were incubated in the presence
   or absence of antigen in RPMI 1640 with 10% fetal bovine serum.
   Cells were in 20 μl agarose droplets in flat bottom 96-well micro-
   liter plates. Cells were allowed to migrate out of the droplets
   for 48 hours and then the diameter of migration measured. Average
   migration for control wells without antigen were considered 100%
   migration.
b Multiplicity of infection
c Percentage migration as compared to controls without SK-SD ± S.E.
d Percentage of those cultures with <80% migration vs. controls. A
   lower percentage of positive cultures is indicative of the immunosuppressive activity of HSV.

Studies performed by the author that examined HSV and immune responsiveness yielded results similar to those reported in the literature. Live HSV
strongly depressed CMI responses in human peripheral blood lymphocytes (PBL)
as measured by phytohemagglutinin (PHA) blastogenesis (Table 1) and migration
inhibition (Table 2). However, murine spleen cell blastogenic responses to
PHA in the presence of HSV were unaffected (Table 3). Mouse spleen cells
did show apparent suppression when antibody responses in vitro were tested
to sheep erythrocytes (Table 4). In studies using both seropositive and
seronegative individuals blastogenic responses were not demonstrable to HSV
using live virus (data not shown).

MECHANISM(S) OF HSV IMMUNOSUPPRESSION IN A LATENT HSV MODEL

Aurelian and co-workers have studied the relationship between herpes
simplex virus and cellular immune function (5,7,10). A recent report by
Iwasaka et al. has elucidated, at least in part, some of the mechanisms by
which HSV can suppress immune responsiveness (7). Their studies indicate
that recurrent HSV in the guinea pig can be examined in three phases; recrudescence (0-7 days post recurrence), convalescence (8-14d) and quiescence
(>15d or no disease). If ^{3}H-thymidine incorporation by lymphoid cells from
these HSV infected animals is examined five days after addition of UV inactivated HSV one finds the poorest responses in guinea pigs with recrudescence,
slightly increased responses in convalescence and strong responses in those

animals that were in quiescence or were HSV seropositive and had no evidence of recurrent disease. Spleen cells or PBL from guinea pigs with recrudescent HSV were capable of inhibiting ^{3}H-thymidine responses to HSV antigen in HSV immune animals, indicating the presence of suppressor cells in the animals with active infection. No such cells could be found in PBL from guinea pigs during convalescence or quiescence. These cells were demonstrated to produce three soluble factors with molecular weights of 5-30,000, 50-60,000 and 110-160,000, each capable of suppressing blastogenic responses to UV inactivated HSV. However, the mechanisms of the suppression by the three factors is not identical, since the smaller fraction was also capable of inhibiting concanavalin A (Con A) responses. The two larger fractions had no effect on Con-A responses.

Thus, HSV induces immunosuppressive factors produced by leukocytes which have both specific and non-specific activity during the recrudescent phase but not in convalescence or quiescence. The crucial observation which is lacking is to determine whether these factors are generated before establishing clinical disease so that they actually contribute to initiation of recrudescence or whether they are produced afterward and are the result of recrudescence. Thus, there is still uncertainty as to whether depressed immunoresponsiveness results in the ability of HSV to recur clinically or whether suppression is an after effect of recurrence.

The authors hypothesize two levels of control for recurrent disease. The first level results in increased virus shedding from persistently infected cells, but does not necessarily result in clinical disease, because an anamnestic response precludes spread of the virus. However, if immunity to HSV is generated slowly or is depressed (for whatever reason) then these specific suppressor substances may function at a second level favoring continued virus replication and clinical disease. This hypothesis remains to be tested.

While these data offer strong evidence that HSV can induce depressed immune responsiveness, it is apparent that such reduced responsiveness is not a consistent finding. Even in the studies reported by Iwasaka et al. four of seven animals exhibited strong blastogenic responses to HSV during recrudescence (7). Thus, HSV appears to exhibit a selective immunosup-

Table 3. PHA Induced Murine Lymphocyte Stimulation in the Presence and Absence of Herpes Simplex Virus

	MOI[a]	cpm[b]	Stimulation Index
Control		3415	–
HSV	100	3811	1.1
PHA		13870	4.1
PHA + HSV	100	13268	3.9

[a] Multiplicity of infection
[b] Average cmp for 12 cultures per group ± S.E. Cells were incubated with PHA for 48 hrs. then pulsed with ^{3}H-thymidine for an additional 18 hrs. Cells were collected on glass fiber filter paper, placed in 5 ml fluor and counted in a liquid scintillation counter.

Table 4. Herpes Simplex Virus Induced Suppression of Antibody
Plaque Forming Cells to Sheep Erythrocytes

	MOI[a]	PFC/10^6 spleen cells[b]	% of control
Control	-	234 ± 26	-
HSV	100	115 ± 46	49
	10	211 ± 35	90
	1	206 ± 52	88

[a] Multiplicity of infection
[b] Average 9-12 cultures per group of in vitro lymphocyte
cultures for anti-sheep PRC plaque forming cells ± S.E.

pression, based on the numerous studies cited here. What factors enable
HSV to express its immune depressive activity is presently unclear.

IMMUNOSTIMULATORY EFFECTS OF HSV

Several reports have indicated that inactivated HSV serves as a good
antigen for stimulation of lymphocyte blastogenesis in HSV immune individuals
(11,14,15). This is a direct reaction to antigen. Hersh and co-workers
(personal communication) have studied the ability of heat- inactivated HSV
to modulate natural killer (NK) cell activity. Killing of K562 target cells
in the presence or absence of the inactived HSV was evaluated. In normal
individuals and AIDS patients enhanced natural killer cell activity against
K562 cells was observed. This stimulated NK function may have been associated with the ability of HSV to stimulate interferon production since interferon was produced in cultures of HSV infected cells. However, interferon
levels in NK cell cultures were not measured.

Mochizuki et al. demonstrated enhanced antibody formation to TNP in
mice infected with HSV, indicating a polyclonal B cell activation by HSV
(25).

CONCLUSIONS

The interactions between HSV and the host immune system are variable;
they may include specific immunity to the virus, a generalized immune enhancement or immunosuppression. The circumstances determining which responses
will be generated in a particular infection are poorly understood. Recently,
factors which might affect this outcome have been described and may explain
the mechanism(s) by which HSV alters immunoresponsiveness. With regard to
suppression, HSV has been demonstrated to induce specific and non-specific
suppressor factors (7) and depress production of lymphokines (10). Enhanced
NK cell activity may be attributable to interferon induction by HSV.

The search continues for identification of other factors which will
determine how and why HSV re-establishes in local sites in the face of host
immunity to the virus. Whether immune depression precedes recrudescence or
vice versa is the critical question to be answered. Based on the observations cited herein, it seems evident that once established, HSV can sustain

immune suppression but only for a short time. Most studies suggest that relatively high numbers of virus particles are required for immune suppression. Thus, the data suggest that non-immunologic host factors, e.g. hormones may be responsible for the initial immune depression which allows HSV to escape host immunity and recrudesce. These factors may only need to have a small negative effect on immune regulation in favor of HSV reactivation. Once established, the virus may locally maintain the infection to cause clinical disease until systemic immunity is mobilized. These interactions between HSV and the immune system may be so unpredictable because of a delicate balance involving immune and non-immune factors which are required to limit HSV replication during latency. Determination of the nature of these factors and how they affect the expression of HSV infection may ultimately lead to the ability to control and possibly prevent recurrent HSV infection.

REFERENCES

1. C. Ching and C. Lopez, Natural killing of herpes simplex virus type-1 infected target cells: normal human responses and influence of antiviral antibody, Infect. Immun. 26:49 (1979).
2. H. Friedman and S. Specter, Immunotherapy and immunoregulation, in: "Chemotherapy of Viral Infections," P. E. Cane and L. A. Caliguiri, eds., Springer-Verlag, Berlin (1982).
3. S. C. Mogensen, Role of macrophages in natural resistance to virus infections, Microbiol. Rev. 43:1 (1979).
4. S. L. Shore and P. M. Feorino, Immunology of primary herpes virus infections in humans, in: "The Human Herpesviruses," A. J. Nahmias, W. R. Dowdle, and R. F. Schinzai, eds., Elsevier/North Holland, Amsterdam (1981).
5. L. Aurelian, J. F. Sheridan, A. D. Donneberg, E. Chaikof, and S. Nigida, Cellular and humoral immunity in herpes virus infections, in: "Microbiology-1981," D. Schlessinger, ed., American Society for Microbiology, Washington, D.C. (1981).
6. T. J. Hill, Mechanisms involved in recurrent herpes simplex, in: "The Human Herpesviruses," A. J. Nahmias, W. R. Dowdle, and R. F. Schinazi, eds., Elsevier/North Holland, Amsterdam (1981).
7. T. Iwasaka, J. F. Sheridan, and L. Aurelian, Immunity to herpes simplex virus type 2: recurrent lesions are associated with the induction of suppressor cells and soluble suppressor factors, Infection and Immunity 42:955 (1983).
8. H. Openshaw, T. Sekizawa, C. Wohlenberg, and A. L. Notkins, The role of immunity in latency and reactivation of herpes simplex viruses, in: "The Human Herpesviruses," A. J. Nahmias, W. R. Dowdle, and R. F. Schinazi, eds., Elsevier/North Holland, Amsterdam (1981).
9. H. Openshaw, L. V. Shavrina Asher, C. Wohlenberg, and A. L. Notkins, The role of immunity in latency and reactivation of herpes simples viruses, in: "The Human Herpesviruses," A. J. Nahmias, W. R. Dowdle, and R. F. Schinazi, eds., Elsevier/North Holland, Amsterdam (1981).
10. J. F. Sheridan, A. D. Donnenberg, and L. Aurelian, Immunity to herpes simplex virus type 2. IV. Impaired lymphokine production correlates with a perturbation in the balance of T lymphocyte subsets, J. Immunol. 129:326 (1982).
11. E. J. Shillitoe, J. M. A. Wilton, and T. Lehner, Sequential changes in cell-mediated immune responses to herpes simplex virus after recurrent herpetic infection in humans, Infect. Immun. 18:130 (1977).
12. S. Specter and H. Friedman, Viruses and the immune response, Pharmac. Ther. A. 2:595 (1978).
13. R. Cappel, C. Henry, and L. Thiry, Experimental Immunosuppression induced by herpes simplex virus, Arch. Virol. 49:67 (1975).

14. I. I. El Araby, M.A. Chernesky, W. E. Rawls, and P. B. Dent, Depressed herpes simplex virus-induced lymphocyte blastogenesis in individuals with severe recurrent herpes infections, Clin. Immunol. Immunopathol. 9:253 (1978).

15. H. Kirchner, M. Schwenteck, H. Northoff, and E. Schopf, Devective in vitro lymphoproliferative responses to herpes simplex virus in patients with frequently recurring herpes infections during the disease-free interval, Clin. Immunol. Immunopathol. 11:267 (1978).

16. E. S. Kleinerman, R. Snyderman, and C. A. Daniels, Depression of human monocyte chemotaxis by herpes simplex and influenza viruses, J. Immunol. 120:641 (1978).

17. S. Plaeger-Marshall and J. W. Smith, Inhibition of mitogen and antigen-induced lymphocyte blastogenesis by herpes simplex virus, J. Infect. Dis. 138:506 (1978).

18. Y. M. Centifanto, Z. S. Zam, J. I. McNeill, and H. E. Kaufman, Leukocyte migration inhibitory factor in HSV infections, Invest. Ophthalmol. Visual Sci. 17:863 (1978).

19. H. Kirchner, G. Darai, H. M. Hirt, K. Keyssner, and K. Munk, In vitro mitogenic stimulation of murine spleen cells by herpes simplex virus, J. Immunol. 120:641 (1978).

20. P. S. Morahan, M. D. Breining, and M. B. George, Immune responses to vaginal or systemic infection of Balb/c mice with herpes simplex virus type 2, J. Immun. 119:2030 (1977).

21. G. L. Rosenberg, P. A. Farber, and A. L. Notkins, In vitro stimulation of sensitized lymphocytes by herpes simplex virus and vaccinia virus, Proc. Nat. Acad. Sci. 69:756 (1972).

22. M. Scriba, Stimulation of peripheral blood lymphocytes by herpes simplex virus in vitro, Infect. Immun. 10:430 (1974).

23. E. J. Shillitoe, J. M. A. Wilton, and T. Lehner, Sequential changes in T and B lymphocyte responses to herpes simplex virus in man, Scand. J. Immunol. 7:357 (1978).

24. R. W. Steele, M. M. Vincent, S. A. Hensen, D. A. Fuccillo, I. A. Chapa, and L. Canales, Cellular immune responses to herpes simplex virus type 1 in recurrent herpes labialis: in vitro blastogenesis and cytotoxicity to infected cell lines, J. Infect. Dis. 131:528 (1975).

25. D. Mochizuki, S. Hedrick, J. Watson, and D. T. Kingsbury, The interaaction of herpes simplex virus with murine lymphocytes. I. Mitogenic properties of herpes simplex virus, J. Exp. Med. 146:1500 (1977).

HEPATITIS B VIRUS, IRON AND IRON-BINDING PROTEINS

Baruch S. Blumberg

Institute for Cancer Research
Fox Chase Cancer Center
Philadelphia, Pennsylvania

INTRODUCTION

Contemporary discussions of immunity in man usually center on various forms of cellular and humoral response. However, bacteria, fungi, protozoa and tumor cells need iron for their growth. A response of the mammalian host to infection and possibly also to the growth of tumor cells is to deny to the invading agent and replicating cells the iron present in the host. Weinberg (1) has prepared a comprehensive analysis of the relation of iron and iron-binding proteins to what has been referred to as "nutritional immunity." Additional references will be found in his paper.

The purpose of the present review is not to marshal the evidence to support or reject the argument that serum and storage iron levels are important in the control of infection and tumor growth; Weinberg's paper (1) is, in part, intended to do that. It is presented, rather, as a compilation of observational and experimental data that may be useful in understanding a series of observations related to hepatitis B virus (HBV), iron and iron-binding proteins that have been made over the past ten years.

Several mechanisms affect the relation between host iron and invading agent. The host can mobilize iron-binding materials at or near the site of infection to withhold humoral and tissue iron and prevent its utilization by the bacteria. The first of these materials to be discovered was conalbumin, a powerful binder of iron and a major constituent of egg white. Lactoferrin, an iron-binding protein originally found in milk, is also present in tears, nasal exudate, saliva, mucus, bile and seminal fluid; it accounts for much of the antibacterial action of these secretions. The specific granules of polymorphonuclear neutrophilic leucocytes contain large amounts of lactoferrin which has a profound effect on their ability to counteract infection by depriving microorganisms of iron.

Transferrin is the major iron-binding protein of serum. Its current name focuses attention on its role in transporting iron, but its original name, siderophilin (2), emphasized its ability to bind iron and its subsequent effect on infection. The probability of infection may increase if transferrin levels are lowered, as is the case in protein malnutrition (i.e. kwashiorkor) or when iron saturation is increased, allowing invading bacteria to remove host iron more readily.

Ferritin is the major iron binding protein of cells and is found in large amounts in the liver, spleen and bone marrow (3). Its function is to store iron which can then be made available for the synthesis of hemoglobin and other iron-containing proteins. Men have up to about two grams of storage iron. Women, during the childbearing period, may have little storage iron; the levels usually increase after menopause. Ferritin is also present in serum, and, in an otherwise normal individual, the serum levels reflect the total iron stores of the body. This relation, however, may not be seen with inflammation, infection and malignancy where increased serum ferritin levels can be independent of iron stores.

Crystalline ferritin has been isolated from liver and spleen. It consists of a protein shell (apoferritin) which covers a core made up of a maximum of 4000 atoms of iron. Apoferritin has a molecular weight of about 450,000 and is composed of 24 subunits; two classes of subunits, 19,000 (L) and 21,000 (H) can be distinguished (4). Ferritin from different sources may be made up of different ratios of the subunits. The ratio of subunits is related to the isoelectric points (pI) of the ferritin molecule and the rate of iron uptake. Investigators have found that ferritin from certain tumors has acidic pI, with a higher H/L ratio of subunits and lowered iron content.

A second general mechanism which the body uses to respond to infection and to the presence of cancer cells is to withhold iron. The intestinal absorption of iron is decreased and iron is shifted to the tissue compartment (e.g. liver, bone marrow) where it binds to ferritin and is stored. Extremely low levels of iron may require treatment in order to allow the immune system to function, but excess therapy with iron during infection can be detrimental.

A major mechanism for denying iron is to block the release of iron contained in macrophages, which have acquired the metal from decaying erythrocytes. The increased amount of iron remaining in the macrophages then stimulates the production of ferritin whose levels may then rise in tissue and in the blood. In malignancies, a ferritin which does not bind iron well may also be produced in large quantities. A key regulator of the iron metabolism in the cell is the hormone leukocytic endogenous mediator (LEM, also termed interleukin-1) which is released by monocytes activated by infection or immune responses.

At the site of infections, large quantities of iron could become available to the invading bacteria due to the breakdown of red blood cells. However, the hemoglobin-binding protein haptoglobin is increased under these circumstances, and the resultant hemoglobin-haptoglobin complex is taken up by the reticuloendothelial system and cleared by it.

An additional, important mechanism for the control of iron during infection is the fever response. The temperature elevation decreases the ability of the iron-binding proteins (siderophores) of the gram-negative bacteria to take up host iron. There is a competition between the binding proteins of the invading organism and those of the host for the available iron. Many of the protective effects described favor the retention of the iron by the host and its denial to the invading organism.

Weinberg (1) has described a variety of mechanisms by which alterations in iron levels and binding can improve the response to infection, that is the enhancement of "nutritional immunity," and counter-measures which diminish the effect. Moderate restrictions of iron may enhance immunity, but severe restrictions can be detrimental; there appears to be an optimal level of available iron which is most advantageous to the host. In an actual clinical situation it may be difficult to know exactly what this is. A variety of observations in re-feeding camps for victims of famine in Africa showed that sudden improvements in nutrition with augmented iron intake could actually increase the frequency and severity of infections including tuberculosis, brucellosis and malaria.

Various bacterial endotoxins and cell wall extracts can decrease available iron and enhance host protection. There are a large series of observations and experiments that indicate that acute and chronic infections as well as therapeutic injections of cell wall components can have an antineoplastic effect. Pearl (5) found that, in a survey of autopsies, bodies that had evidence of active tuberculosis had much lower incidence of concurrent cancer than did the bodies which did not have such infection. A popular form of cancer therapy for many years has been the use of non-viable extracts of bacterial products (Streptococcus pyogenes and Serratia marcescens) in an attempt to cause tumor regressions (see review by Nauts (6)). This form of therapy has not gained wide acceptance, but there is experimental evidence to support the clinical impressions. These bacterial extracts can result in a hypoferremia which might decrease tumor growth.

There is experimental evidence that some iron chelators can serve to combat infection or decrease carcinogenesis while others actually make the iron available to microorganisms and tumor cells and enhance their growth. The addition of excess amounts of iron can enhance infection or tumor growth. Patients with inherited or acquired hemochromatosis have an increased susceptibility to infection as well as to tumor generation and growth. Ingestion of alcohol increases iron levels. African males who consume large quantities of home brewed alcoholic beverages develop siderosis, and this may be related to an increased frequency of cancer of the liver in these individuals.

Pathological organisms and tumor cells may have siderophores which act to bind the iron made available to them by the host. The amount and affinities of these siderophores vary from organism to organism and, presumably, in various tumor cells.

This short review of the effects of iron and iron-binding proteins on microorganisms and tumor cells will, it is hoped, provide a background to consider a series of studies on the relation of iron and iron-binding proteins to HBV. We will review our work in this field and then suggest how phenomena related to iron may explain some curious observations that have been made on the behavior of HBV. Possible uses of this information in therapy and prevention will also be discussed.

Serum Iron Levels in Carrier and Non-carrier Patients with Down's Syndrome

Our introduction to the iron problem came as part of the original investigation of the nature of the "Australia antigen" (Au, HBsAg). Au was contained in a precipitin band found in an immunodiffusion reaction between the serum of an Australian aborigine and a much transfused patient with hemophilia. We were testing the hypothesis that Au was located on a hepatitis virus (7).

One test of the hypothesis was based on an extensive study of patients with Down's syndrome, many of whom had Au in their blood. We postulated that the patients with Au (who had no obvious symptoms of clinical hepatitis) would have chemical evidence of mild liver dysfunction that was more abnormal than the equivalent measurements in the Down's syndrome patients who did not have Au (8). We measured "liver chemistries" including SGPT (now ALT), SGPT, cephalin flocculation, thymol turbidity, BSP, total protein, and serum albumin, all of which showed that the patients with Au were more abnormal than those without it. There was no significant differences in bilirubin, prothrombin time and alkaline phosphatase. Since serum iron levels were known to be elevated in patients with acute hepatitis, its measurement was included in the studies.

Some time in 1973, our colleague Dr. Alton I. Sutnick brought to our attention an article published by a group of Dutch investigators which reported a curious observation on patients with end stage kidney disease undergoing renal dialysis treatment (9). A group of 11 patients had developed anicteric hepatitis in all but one case associated with HBsAg. They experienced a spontaneous rise in hemoglobin levels and required fewer transfusions than a "control" group of patients who did not have hepatitis B.

At that time we could not study patients on renal dialysis, but we had extensive information on hepatitis in Down's syndrome patients. Sutnick et al. (10) then devised and executed a comparison study of 20 patients with Down's syndrome who had HBsAg in their serum and an additional 20 who did not have the antigen. Measurements were made of serum iron and related factors as well as SGPT as an indication of liver dysfunction.

We found, as predicted from the Dutch observation, that the serum iron, hemoglobin, and hematocrit were significantly higher in the HBsAg(+) patients than in those who were HBsAg(-). The total iron binding capacity (essentially a measurement of the binding capacity of the serum transferrin that is not already occupied by iron) was also higher in the hepatitis group. In a series of correlation studies we found that the elevation of iron was not correlated with elevations of the SGPT and, therefore, the elevation of the serum iron in the HBsAg(+) patients could not be accounted for by the breakdown of liver cells alone but was in some way a function of the presence of the virus itself. It also suggested the possibility that the carrier state was advantageous to the patients in that it allowed them to maintain higher levels of serum iron, hemoglobin and hematocrit. We also predicted that there would be similar findings in renal dialysis patients which would then explain the Dutch observations.

Iron Levels and Host Response to HBV Infection

The iron project remained dormant but not forgotten until mid-1978 when our attention was focused on nutritional problems. We, and other workers in the field, had by this time concluded a large body of studies testing the hypothesis that persistent infection with the HBV is necessary for the development of primary cancer of the liver (11,12). It became apparent that HBV was required for the development of PHC, but that other factors were also involved. We wanted to understand as much as possible about pathogenesis in order to affect the course of disease in people who had already become carriers of HBV.

In humans, nearly all iron is derived from eating, therefore it can be considered nutritional. Iron had the further advantage of being manipulatable, that is, if we learned that it was involved in the pathogenesis of chronic liver disease and primary cancer of the liver, it was conceivable that iron levels could be altered to favorably affect outcome.

Our second study included a group of 201 patients receiving renal dialysis, including 39 carriers of HBV, 76 with anti-HBs, and 86 without evidence of HBV infection (13). There were 113 males and 88 females. We first tested the hypothesis derived from the Down's syndrome study and confirmed that serum iron was higher in carriers of HBV than in non-carriers.

We confirmed other observations made in the first study (Table 1). The percent iron saturation and SGPT were also higher in the carriers than in those with anti-HBs, but this difference was only significant in the males. Ironically, we did not find any difference between the carriers and the others in respect to hemoglobin, hematocrit or red blood cell count which had been expected from the original Dutch studies and from the Down's syndrome study.

Table 1. Mean Values for Groups of Renal Dialysis Patients

	SI, mg/dl			TIBC, mg/dl			% Iron saturation			SGPT, international units/liter		
	Male	Female	Total	Male	Female	Total	Male	Female	Total	Male	Female	Total
HBsAg(+)	114	214	145 **	278	305	285	42.4 **	46.5	43.6 **	28.1 **	20.8 **	25.8 **
Anti-HB(+)	95	107	102	304	284	294	29.6	36.3	33.0	11.5 ***	6.2 ***	10.8 ***
No evidence of infection	103	95	99	283	281	282	34.6	33.4	34.1	14.8	21.4	17.2
Total	103	117		288	286		34.9	36.4		16.9	15.9	

	RBC, 10^6 cells/mm^3			HB, g/dl			Hematocrit, %		
	Male	Female	Total	Male	Female	Total	Male	Female	Total
HBsAg(+)	2.6	2.2	2.5	6.8	6.7	6.8	22.4	21.8	22.2
Anti-HBs(+)	2.6 *	2.3	2.5	7.1 **	6.3	6.7	23.5 *	20.8	22.1
No evidence of infection	2.4	2.3	2.3	6.7	6.4	6.6	21.9	20.8	21.5
Total	2.5 **	2.3		6.9 *	6.4		22.6 *	20.0	

Differences were assessed by the Mann-Whitney test. % iron saturation = serum iron (SI)/total iron-binding capacity (TIBC). RBC = red blood cells. * is p = 0.05; ** is p = 0.01; *** is p = 0.001.

After completing the analysis of single factors we did a logistic regression analysis to determine the interactions between the variable serum iron, sex, SGPT levels and HBV status (HBsAg, anti-HBs or no response) considered together (Table 2). This was an inductive analysis, that is, the data were analyzed without any preset hypothesis to re-test and complement the original deductive analysis.

We found that interactions of the variables taken two at a time could account for the distribution of the data, and it was not necessary to consider three-way or high order interactions. The inductive study confirmed the original observations: carriers had higher serum iron levels than non-carriers, carriers had higher SGPT levels than non-carriers, and the HBV response was sex related, that is, males were more likely to become carriers and females to develop anti-HBs (14,15). We also found that there were independent interactions between serum iron and SGPT and between HBV response and SGPT, that is, the elevation of iron could be associated with liver cell breakdown but that it also was elevated as a consequence of the carrier state independent of any significant liver cell damage (as measured by SGPT elevation).

We had confirmed, in large part, our original observation that serum iron was raised as a consequence of the HBV carrier state independent of liver cell breakdown. This was found to be true despite the possible masking effects in dialysis patients, or iron therapy, the anemia of chronic renal disease and the decrease in iron absorption due to the use of aluminum hydroxide. A series of questions was raised by these findings.

(1) We suggested that these studies should be repeated in other populations, including non-hospitalized populations in regions of the world with high frequencies of carriers. Our first studies had been done in patient groups known to have immunological and other abnormalities, and we wanted to know if these iron differences had an impact at the population level.

(2) Were the raised iron levels a consequence of the infection with HBV or did they precede them and make the putative carriers more prone to chronic infection with HBV?

Table 2. Distribution of Data According to HBV Response, SGPT Level, Serum Iron Level, and Sex. Renal Dialysis Patients.

	Low iron		Middle iron		High iron	
	Male	Female	Male	Female	Male	Female
Low SGPT (≤ 15 international units/liter)						
HBsAg(+)	3	2	6	2	5	3
Anti-HBs(+)	12	11	11	14	6	11
No evidence of infection	19	9	10	9	6	3
High SGPT (>15 international units/liter)						
HBsAg(+)	1	0	1	1	11	4
Anti-HBs(+)	4	0	1	0	2	3
No evidence of infection	1	3	4	3	8	9

(3) Were HBV carriers more likely to become infected with bacteria as a consequence of their raised iron levels?

(4) We had recently found that incubations of HBV with certain species and strains of Pseudomonas resulted in a loss of HBsAg antigenicity (16). We questioned if this were in some way related to the HBV-iron interaction.

(5) Millman et al. (17) found that transferrin was firmly bound to HBsAG. We suggested that the binding of iron via transferrin to the virus and the liver cell transferrin receptor might facilitate the entry of HBV into cells and thereby promote its infectivity.

(6) We made the hypothesis that increased iron stores might increase the possibility of the development of primary hepatocellular carcinoma in carriers, that is, that iron is involved in the pathogenesis of the cancer and that alterations in iron or iron storage could be used to favorably alter the outcome.

Most of these hypotheses were tested during the next several years, and the consequences of these studies will now be discussed.

Serum Iron Levels in Non-hospitalized Asymptomatic Carriers

In 1977 we had collected sera from members of the community living in the village complex of Tip in an area of central Senegal about 200 kilometers east of Dakar as part of an extensive study of primary cancer of the liver and HBV (18). From this collection we selected 193 sera for the iron study, including 40 carriers, 59 with anti-HBs and 94 who had no evidence of infection. Measurements similar to those completed on the Down's syndrome and renal dialysis patients were undertaken, with the exception that the SGPT determinations were performed on sera that had been stored frozen for about three months. The enzyme loses its activity under these conditions and, although the values could be used for comparison within the Tip population, they could not be compared directly to the earlier studies.

The results were, in general, similar to those of the first two studies (Table 3). The iron levels overall were lower in the Tip study, probably a reflection of the low iron intake of the population. Serum iron levels were higher in the carriers than in the non-carriers. We did an inductive analysis of the data including the variables serum iron, sex, SGPT levels and HBV status similar to that done in the renal dialysis study. Again, only two factor interactions were required to model the distribution. Two of the interactions found in the dialysis study were confirmed. (1) The serum iron was increased in carriers independent of SGPT elevation and (2) the SGPT was increased in the carriers compared to the other HBV responses. Two additional interactions were also observed: between SGPT and sex and between serum iron and sex. The latter was particularly interesting; the serum iron differences between those who were HBsAg(+) and those HBsAg(-) was greatest for the females.

The elevation in serum iron in carriers seen in the two patient groups had now been confirmed in a non-hospitalized population group. It raised again the possibility of advantage to the carriers who could retain more iron, particularly under conditions such as those in Africa with a low dietary intake of the element. This was seen particularly in the females who, in any case, would most benefit from increased iron retention during the period they were losing blood regularly through menstruation. This concept of advantage to the carrier state was consistent with the notion advanced in some of our earliest studies that the carrier trait behaves as a genetic polymorphism.

Table 3. Mean Serum Iron Levels (mg/dl) in Down's Syndrome Patients, Renal Dialysis Patients and Non-hospitalized People from Tip, Senegal.

| | Down's Syndrome | | | Renal Dialysis | | | Tip, Senegal | | |
	Male	Female	Total	Male	Female	Total	Male	Female	Total
HBsAg(+)	164	–	164	114	214	145	77	81	79
HBsAg(−)	84	–	84	98	100	100	75	58	65
N	40		40	103	117	220	81	112	193

In each case, the serum iron is higher in carriers (HBsAg(+)) than in non-carriers (HBsAg(−)). N = number of people tested. Females were not tested in the Down's syndrome study. The HBsAg(−) values for the renal dialysis patients are approximate.

Serum Iron Levels Before and After Infection

In an effort to control the spread of HBV, we had, since 1972, been monitoring a group of renal dialysis patients in the Philadelphia area. Specimens of blood were collected two times a month and tested for HBV. At the time our surveillance of this group began, HBV was extremely common in such units and there was a very high probability that patients would become infected, some to remain carriers and others to rid themselves of the infection and develop anti-HBs. (An important consequence of this surveillance program was the complete control of HBV infection. Hepatitis due to HBV is now rare in the dialysis unit we served as well as in most others where the epidemiologic measures were used.)

Two groups of patients were identified; 1) those who, after infection became carriers and, 2) those who became transiently infected. Serum iron levels and other measurements were made on both of these groups one month before, at the time of the and 6-12 months after infection (19). In the patients destined to become carriers, serum iron levels were not elevated before the infection but arose immediately after infection and remained high in the late follow-up period. In the transients, the serum iron levels were not elevated prior to the infection, rose at the time of infection, but decreased in the follow-up period (Table 4). Hence, our question had been answered: the iron in the carrier state was not elevated prior to exposure to HBV but remained elevated after infection.

A distinction, however, could be made between the putative carriers and the transients. Among the carriers, if iron levels had decreased between the first and second time periods, then all of these individuals had increases during the post-conversion period, and if there was a decrease in the post-conversion period there would have been an increase in the pre-conversion period. The carriers never had decreasing iron levels in both time periods, whereas the transients often did. There appeared to be differences in binding and/or storage proteins between the carriers and the transients, and these were investigated in subsequent studies.

In the discussion of this chapter we reaffirmed the hypothesis that bacterial infection and death might be more common in the carriers compared to non-carriers at certain times in their lives. We also suggested that

Table 4. Mean Iron Levels in Carriers and Transients Before (sample 1),
          Immediately After (sample 2), and 6-12 Months After (sample 3)
          Seroconversion.

HBV status	Mean iron levels, µg/dl		
	Sample 1	Sample 2	Sample 3
Carrier	97.7	115.3	119.6
Transient	100.7	115.8	101.4

For carriers, the mean iron levels before seroconversion were significantly
less than the other two values (p <0.05).

the relation between HBV and the sex ratio of offspring and overall fertility
that we had observed during the course of several large studies (20,21)
might also be linked to the iron levels, possibly through the intermediary
of the bacterial infection.

        We elaborated further on the iron-PHC hypothesis. Edmondson and Steiner
had, in 1954 (22), found that in cases of PHC there is little or no iron
present in the malignantly transformed liver cells but that large quantities
of iron may be present in the cells surrounding the cancer which do not
appear to be transformed. Similarly, whole HBV virus, surface and core
antigen can be found in the surrounding cells but are much less frequent in
the cancer cells. Fernandez-Pol (23) had shown experimentally that removal
of iron (using a chelating agent prepared from a plant substance) decreases
the growth of live tumors in tissue culture. We postulated that the HBV-
infected liver cells surrounding the malignant cells would supply iron to
the cancer cells which did not have a sufficient amount and thereby
encourage or stimulate their growth. Carriers with elevated storage iron
and iron-binding proteins (e.g. ferritin) would be at greater risk of
developing PHC than other carriers. We had, in effect, made a model to
explain a portion of the pathogenetic mechanism, and various direct and
indirect studies have been designed to test it. We will return to this
matter later.

        In all these comparisons of carriers and non-carriers, the differences
in serum iron levels, ferritin and transferrin measurements are small; most
measurements fall into what is usually considered to be normal limits.
However, these differences exist for many years, and in some cases decades,
and could, over a long period of time, have a profound effect on the pathogenesis of a chronic disease.

        McGlynn et al. (24) have reported a curious finding which could be
explained by the interactions of microorganisms and host iron. They found
that, among a group of southeast Asians living in Philadelphia, HBV carriers
who were tuberculin (PPD) positive were much less likely to also be HBeAg(+)
than those negative for PPD and had lower levels of ALT elevation than carriers who were HBeAg(-). This suggests that either the presence of the
Mycobacterium or the ability to immunologically react to it (or both) inhib-
its the replication of HBV and its ability to kill infected liver cells.
This is reminiscent of the findings of Pearl and those reviewed by Nauts
(see above). It could be associated, in part, with the ability of Mycobacterium to effect the binding and metabolism of iron, and this notion can be
tested directly.

Lustbader et al. (25) studied the role of serum ferritin as a predictor of host response to HBV infection. Our attention was, in part, focused on ferritin as a consequence of the extensive studies reported on ferritin and prognosis in neuroblastoma in children. Hann and her colleagues (26,27) found that elevated levels of ferritin predicted a poor outcome in patients with advanced neuroblastoma. In addition, the studies reviewed above (19) suggested that iron binding proteins were likely to distinguish between those who, after infection, were likely to become carriers from those who would develop anti-HBs. We predicted that individuals fated to be carriers would have higher ferritin levels before infection, than those who were to become transiently infected.

Three factors were already known that could be used to predict the development of the carrier state in an infected individual.

(1) Sex. Males were more likely to become carriers than females, and females were more likely to be only transiently infected and then develop anti-HBs.

(2) Age. Younger people (but over the age of about three months) were more likely to become carriers than adults.

(3) Geography. Certain populations were more likely to become carriers than others.

The ferritin study design was similar to that already described for the iron study. Dialysis patients who had at least one serum sample positive for HBsAg were selected. Two other criteria had to be satisfied for inclusion in the study: (1) the serum sample collected two months prior to the first detection of HBsAg had to be negative for both HBsAg and anti-HBs, and (2) a serum sample had to be obtained 12 months after the positive serum. Two possible outcomes, persistent infection or transient infection and five variables: sex, serum iron, serum ferritin, transferrin, and ALT (formerly SGPT) were considered. Data obtained on the serum sample collected prior to the positive sample were to be used to predict the outcomes (persistent or transient infection).

A difference in the direction was predicted in the sera collected before infection occurred in the mean log serum ferritin values of transiently and persistently infected individuals (Table 5). Persistently infected individuals had higher ferritin values than the transients. The difference was significant in females ($p < .001$) but not in males ($p = .11$). All the variables were then considered together in a stepwise linear discriminant analysis to determine the best combinations to predict outcome. As expected, sex was the most significant variable. Log serum ferritin was also significant ($p \ .05$). The best model to describe the predictive capacities of the variables was

$$y = 0.412 - 1.931\ S + 1.257\ F$$

where $S = 1$ for males, $S = 2$ for females, and F is the log (base 10) of serum ferritin concentration. The value of y predicts if the infected person will become transiently or chronically infected. Values of y greater than 0 predicted that the subject would develop a persistent infection, and values of y less than 0 that the subject would develop a transient infection.

Hence, the development of this quantitative formula allowed one to predict if a person would become a carrier or only transiently infected based on their sex and serum ferritin value. It also unexpectedly allowed

Table 5. Serum Ferritin as a Predictor of Host Response to HBV Infection

Classification	N	Serum iron (μg/dl)	Transferrin (mg/dl)	F	ALT	S
			Males			
Persistent	23	85.0±32.7	309± 86.9	1.98±0.62	8.83± 3.97	1
Transient	8	87.3±31.4	313±110	1.60±0.37	10.9 ± 6.45	1
			Females			
Persistent	6	132 ±63.6	310± 95.6	2.42±0.57	10.7 ±10.3	2
Transient	17	98.6±46.4	313± 98.1	1.64±0.51	7.24± 6.48	2
			All Patients			
Persistent	29	94.7±44.0	303± 87.0	2.07±0.63	9.21± 5.66	1.21
Transient	25	95.0±41.8	313± 99.7	1.62±0.46	8.40± 6.54	1.68

Data collected two months before HBsAg was found in the serum of patients undergoing hemodialysis treatment. F, log serum ferritin (serum ferritin was measured in nanograms per milliliter); ALT, alanylaminotransferase, measured in Karmen units (14); S, arbitrary value of 1 for males and 2 for females. Results are given as means ± standard deviations. Only the difference in F values for females was significant at the .05 level. The classification of infection as persistent or transient was made one year after HBsAg was first detected.

predictions of the ability of an infected individual to muster an antibody response to the surface antigen of the virus (anti-HBs) after becoming rid of HBsAg. This is described in the original paper; briefly, the analysis indicated that low levels of ferritin predisposed to the development of anti-HBs.

Does ferritin also have a role in determining if individuals vaccinated against HBV will or will not develop anti-HBs? In the field trials about 95% of vaccinated individuals develop antibody. The frequency is very much lower in dialysis patients. There is little known about why some inoculees do not develop antibody, and the possible role of ferritin in this process can be tested directly. It seems unlikely that the process would be the same as natural infection since killed vaccine is used and viability in liver cells is unlikely to be an issue in determining antibody production.

These findings made an important contribution to the pathogenetic model for primary hepatocellular carcinoma we were developing. Birgegard (28) had reported that the increased levels of ferritin seen during acute viral infections were the consequence of increased synthesis of ferritin. The model recommended by Lustbader et al. (25) postulates that the cells with an increased propensity to ferritin production are also more likely to become infected with HBV and to provide a suitable environment for replication. Infection with HBV, in turn, stimulates the production of even more ferritin in a positive feedback mechanism. This accounts for the increased levels of ferritin seen prior to infection and the even higher levels after infection has become persistent.

Iron, HBV, Death, and Disease

In the mid-1960's, the late Albert Damon conceived and executed a study of populations living in the Solomon Islands, some of which had only recently come into contact with western civilization and its medical baggage. Although the studies concentrated on hypertension and cardiovascular disease, unusually comprehensive medical and serological studies were also done. Near-total village populations of several Solomon Island communities were surveyed and followed up in subsequent years. The existence of this data base allowed a study of the long term mortality effects of HBV infection and also the interaction between HBV, iron binding protein levels and mortality. Accurate data or cause of death was not available in the Solomon Islands study, and only the end point of death was used in the analysis.

Early in the study of HBsAg we completed a cross sectional analysis of 1802 people resident on the island of Cebu in the central Philippines (29). The frequency of carriers was found to decrease with age. We offered three possible explanations: (1) There is a higher mortality in the carriers of HBsAg; (2) there is a decrease in the titer of HBsAg with increasing age; (3) both of these mechanisms are operating. There is considerable evidence that the titer of HBsAg does decrease with age, and the Solomon Islands population allowed us to examine the first explanation.

Details of this analysis are given in the original publication (30), and only general conclusions will be given here. Information on the HBV status was obtained from sera collected between 1966-1970, at the initiation of the surveys, and the mortality of individuals was obtained on revisits to the islands up to 1980. We compared HBV status at the initiation of the survey with the subsequent mortality experience. In both males and females, children (15 and under) with high titer anti-HBs are at decreased risk of death compared to children with no evidence of infection (chi-squared = 10.4, 1 d.f., p <0.05). In the breakdown of the data by the different village communities the strongest association of anti-HBs with decreased mortality is seen in the communities with the highest infection rates for HBV. This suggests that the protective effect is primarily against HBV itself, although it may also protect against death from other causes.

Beasley and his colleagues in Taiwan have been following prospectively a group of male government workers with a high incidence of HBV infection. They found that HBsAg carriers had a much higher mortality risk (about three times greater than non-carriers) and that the risk was almost all attributable to death from PHC. Taken overall, the Solomon Islands study did not show any excess risk of death among the carriers. However, the Solomon Islands population is very much younger than that studied by Beasley, who selected, initially, workers 40-59 years of age.

To compare this Solomon Islands study with the Taiwan study, an analysis was done only of males who were aged 40-59 at the beginning of the study. There were 11 deaths among 31 HBsAg carriers compared to 20 deaths among 90 men who were not carriers, a relative risk of 1.8. These numbers are small, but they suggest that the excess mortality associated with HBsAg carriers does not occur until later in life and that the protective effect of the anti-HBs acts primarily earlier in life. This is compatible with the known pathogenesis of HBV in which the effects of chronic liver disease, cirrhosis and PHC are associated with long term exposure to HBV. Mortality in the young may be associated with acute events, including HBV infection, but also probably other childhood diseases.

Iron Binding Proteins, HBV and Mortality in the Solomon Islands

It is widely recognized that insufficient iron intake may result in iron deficiency anemia which is associated with the impairment of the immune response and increased susceptibility to infection. Since the end of the second World War, nutritional programs for the fortification of foods to increase iron intake have been instituted in some countries. This has been done in the expectation that they could, at a population level, decrease the frequency of anemia and enchance resistance to infections, among other beneficial effects. Crosby (31) has objected to these programs warning against the dangers of excess iron in members of the population who have hemochromatosis and other possible forms of toxicity.

As already discussed, excess amounts of iron may also increase the susceptibility to bacterial (and probably other) infections, and there are several clinical and epidemiologic studies which support this notion (see Weinberg (1)). The possible danger of excess iron was already perceived in 1868 by Trousseau, a professor of clinical medicine in Paris, who warned against excessive iron therapy because of the fear that it would induce clinical episodes of tuberculosis (32). Iron overload and a consequent increased susceptibility can occur in humans, as Weinberg point out, by (1) increased intake of iron from exogenous sources; (2) destruction of liver cells in which iron is stored bound to ferritin; (3) hemolysis which occurs in malaria, leukemias, lymphomas and hemoglobinopathies; and (4) decreased synthesis of iron binding protein (transferrin) as a result of poor nutrition, as in kwashiorkor.

In the Solomon Islands, infection has been a major cause of death. We tested the hypothesis that individuals who died during the observation period would be more likely to have increased iron stores at the time of entry than those who had survived (33). In normal people, serum ferritin levels are directly and transferrin levels indirectly related to body iron stores. Specifically, two hypotheses were tested: (1) the 1966-70 serum ferritin levels of people who had died by 1978 (group D) were higher than those of a control group who had survived to 1978 (group A); and (2) the serum transferrin levels in group D were lower than those in group A. A total of 156 deaths had occurred in the population of 2500. Each death was compared with a live control matched for age, sex, subpopulation group and HBV serology (HBsAg(+), anti-HBs, no response). There was sufficient serum available to constitute 105 pairs to test the transferrin hypothesis, and 94 pairs the ferritin hypothesis.

The differences were in the direction predicted for both transferrin and ferritin (Table 6), and the results were significant at the 0.05 level by a parametric test, non-parametric test, or both. An analysis of possible confounding factors (i.e. nutritional status, existing illness at the time the sera were collected, or the years at which the death occurred) indicated that these could not account for the differences observed. There was, however, an interaction with HBV status; the differences in ferritin were most striking in the HBsAg(+) carriers.

In order to study the joint effects of ferritin, transferrin and HBV on mortality, a conditional logistic regression model was applied to the data. The conclusions supported the findings from the single variable analysis, that is, that lower transferrin and higher ferritin (hence, probably higher iron stores) were associated with increased mortality and, in addition, showed that the effect was most evident in HBsAg carriers rather than in the other HBV response groups. The HBV interaction was seen only in females in this analysis. There was also an interaction with hemoglobin; individuals with lower hemoglobin levels at the beginning of the study had a greater probability of death. This combination of low hemoglobin and high iron stores is seen in chronic infections and chronic illness of various kinds.

These findings were taken to support the hypothesis that increased iron, particularly in HBsAg carriers predisposed to death, which by inference would have included many deaths from infection. We concluded the paper by stating that we did not think that the results warranted any change in nutritional practice, but we hoped that it would stimulate additional studies to learn if iron supplementation could, in some circumstances, be harmful to certain members of the population.

Neutrophil Function, HBV and Liver Cell Injury

Recent studies by Vierucci et al. (34) suggest an additional model which could reinforce this process. They studied neutrophil function in a group of nine children with chronic active hepatitis due to HBV and compared them to an equal number of controls. The patient observations were then reinforced by in vitro studies in which isolated neutrophil function was studied with and without the addition of (1) serum containing HBV; (2) isolated HBsAg; and (3) isolated HBcAg. They found profound alterations in the neutrophils of the patients compared to controls and in the neutrophils treated with the HBV preparations. There was an increase in oxidative metabolism in the resting cells of HBsAg carriers demonstrated by an increase in the production of superoxide anion generating activity and an increase in NBT reduction in unstimulated cells. The superoxide formation was reduced after the cells of the carriers were stimulated with zymosan. There was also a reduced capacity of the cells of the HBsAg carriers to kill ingested bacteria after 60 minutes of incubation. The decreased bactericidal activity was shown by studies on phagocytosis and killing of E. coli and Candida albicans. There was one effect seen in vitro but not in vivo, a decrease in chemotaxis. They reasoned that, in the intact host, some compensatory mechanism existed which overcame the direct effects of HBV on the cells.

The most significant effect of the HBV infection was the induction of the respiratory burst in the neutrophils, apparently as a consequence of

Table 6. Comparison of 1966–1970 Serum Ferritin and Transferrin Levels of Solomon Islanders Dead by 1978 (Group D) and Alive in 1978 (Group A).

	Ferritin	Transferrin
No. of pairs	94	105
Group D		
Mean	62.6 ng/ml	242.4 mg/dl
Range	2.2–290 ng/ml	109–394 mg/dl
SEM*	5.4	5.5
Group A		
Mean	51.6 ng/ml	269.4 mg/dl
Range	1.9–408 ng/ml	120–460 mg/dl
SEM*	5.5	5.6
Mean difference	11.0	−27.0
t statistic	1.5	3.2
One-tailed p value	0.07	0.001
Wilcoxon rank test	1728.5	1563.0
One-tailed p value	0.03	0.001

*SEM = standard error of the mean

the presence of the virus or of an antigen-antibody complex with HBV. Similar effects have been seen with virus-antibody complexes with influenza virus and syncytial virus. Presumably, the production of the oxygen radicals could aid host defense by destruction of the virus. It could be due to either increased production or decreased detoxification because of some inadequacy of enzymes such as superoxide dismutase or catalase. In due course, it might also adversely affect the phagocytic activity of the neutrophil.

In addition to the effects on invading organisms and on the neutrophils themselves, the oxygen radicals may also cause inflammation and tissue damage. They have been found to induce peroxidation in lysosomal membranes, depolymerize hyaluronate, affect myoblasts and activate platelet function. It has been suggested that high iron levels in synovial fluid in patients with rheumatoid arthritis can catalyze the formation of free radicals and cause damage to joint tissue (35). The combination of high iron levels and HBV in liver tissue may, therefore, cause severe cellular damage through the intermediary of the oxygen radicals.

A Model for Iron, Iron Binding Proteins and HBV Infection

It is now possible to construct a model based on the observations on iron and HBV in an attempt to explain in part the pathogenesis of HBV infection and disease and to recommend procedures that could affect their course.

Some individuals infected with HBV will have liver cells that contain relatively large amounts of ferritin or an augmented ability to generate the protein, and this could be under genetic control. Within a single liver, cells will be heterogeneous in respect to their ferritin content and potential to generate it. Cells with higher amounts of ferritin or the capacity to synthesize it would be more likely to become infected with HBV. This in turn would produce further increased amounts of ferritin. Infection with HBV would increase the iron content of the liver cells, and when this exceeds the binding capabilities of the ferritin, free iron levels would increase in the cell (as already suggested, the excess iron could come from the released storage iron in the liver cells which are killed by the infecting HBV, from macrophages and other inflammatory cells, from the iron accumulation associated with alcohol intake, and probably by other mechanisms). This would stimulate the production of oxygen radicals with consequent damage to the liver cells. Cell death would be followed by regeneration and scarring, leading to the pathological picture of advanced liver disease and cirrhosis.

The increased probability of HBV infection of the cells containing the high ferritin and iron levels may be a consequence of the large number of transferrin binding sites (transferrin receptors) on the surface of these cells. This notion is based on the testable hypothesis that HBV-cell attachment and entry points are the same as or related to the transferrin binding sites through which iron enters the cell.

Additional tissue destruction could result from the effects of HBV and iron on the phagocytic cells as proposed by Vierucci et al. (34). It would also diminish the host's ability to resist bacterial and other infections, as discussed above, and add to their mortality risks.

Iron, Iron Binding Proteins, HBV and the Development of PHC

The model can be extended to explain the relation of iron and iron binding proteins to HBV and PHC.

An important feature of the pathology of PHC is the absence of stainable iron in the neoplastic cells of the tumor; high levels of stainable iron may be seen in the non-malignant cells which surround them (22). Tumor cells contain a form of ferritin, acidic ferritin, which, according to some studies (3), does not bind iron well, while the non-tumor cells contain ferritin with strong iron binding characteristics (basic ferritin). In addition, the malignantly transformed cells, those with little or no iron, do not contain large quantities of or, in many cases, any whole HBV or its components. The surrounding non-malignant cells, those with large amounts of storage iron, may contain whole virus, HBsAg, and HBcAg. All cells, including tumor cells, require iron to grow and divide. The model suggests that the iron-containing cells, infected with replicating HBV, can supply the iron to be malignant cells and thereby stimulate their growth and division. This suggests a possible mechanisms for inhibiting the growth of the tumor by, in some way, inhibiting the transport of iron from the infected iron-containing cells to the malignant cells or by decreasing the overall supply of iron.

London and Blumberg (12,36) have proposed a model for the development of PHC in individuals who are carriers of HBV. They postulate the existence of two kinds of liver cells. The R cells are less differentiated cells common in the fetus but rare in the mature liver. When infected with HBV, the R cells may integrate the HBV-DNA into their own, but the virus does not replicate in the cells. The S cells are more fully differentiated cells which, when infected with HBV, may or may not undergo integration, but the virus can replicate in the cell.

The less differentiated R cells can divide to form either (1) two S cells during the process of differentiation; (2) an S cell and an R cell when destroyed liver cells are being replaced; (3) two R cells in the early fetus or at other times when the liver is growing at a rapid rate. The fully differentiated S cell, on the other hand, does not divide very readily and, if it does, can produce only other S cells. When an S cell is infected, replication of the virus will ensue and, in due course, the cell will die as a consequence of the immune responses of the host, the oxygen radical mechanisms already described, and other processes. Hence, the S cells are at a selective disadvantage compared to the R cells. The death of the S cells will stimulate the division of the R cells until a point is reached when uncontrolled division occurs with the production of two R cells each time an R cell divides. This may occur after the HBV-DNA becomes integrated into the R cell DNA, thus controlling its division. When the R cell mass becomes sufficiently large, it is perceived by the patient and recognized as clinical cancer.

It is possible to relate the London-Blumberg R/S developmental model for PHC to the iron-HBV model already described. The less differentiated R cells would be the equivalent of the malignant cells which contain little or no stainable iron. Whole virus and parts of the virus would be absent from these cells, although integration may have occurred. The S cells would correspond to the cells with the basic ferritin and large amounts of stored iron which are readily invaded by HBV and in which viral replication occurs. They are killed by the oxygen radicals and other processes as a consequence of the long HBV infection. The death of the S cells stimulates the division of the R cells. The continuous process of death, scarring, cell division and the increase of the R cell component over time results in the pathological and clinical picture of chronic liver disease, cirrhosis and primary cancer of the liver.

Altering Pathogenesis

This model recommends an approach to "therapy" which is different from that usually used in cancer treatment. Most cancer treatments are directed to the killing of as many cancer cells as possible. Since normal cells,

96

particularly developing and dividing cells, are similar to cancer cells, they will also be killed in the process, thus limiting the aggressiveness and extent of therapy.

It is now known that carriers of HBV (at least in some geographical regions) are at a very high risk of developing PHC, and it may, in due course, be possible to identify those at greatest risk. Hence, measures should be developed to slow down the pathological process to allow the carrier to remain asymptomatic until he or she can live out a normal life span. We have referred to this (37) as "prevention by delay." Several possibilities recommend themselves that could be applied to the carriers before symptoms develop and before uncontrolled division (of the R cells) commences.

Can the replication of the virus be decreased by inhibiting the amount of iron (and/or ferritin) available to the host? Does HBV enter the cells in the same place or in the same manner as iron? Is there some measure that can be used to competitively inhibit this entry? Is the polymerized albumin binding site (38) such a location? Can replication of HBV be inhibited by inactivating its polymerase in a manner which is not also detrimental to the host?

It is hoped that as these models are tested and developed, practical intervention measures to prevent the development of disease in carriers can be discovered and implemented.

ACKNOWLEDGMENTS

This work was supported by USPHS grants CA-06551, RR-05539 and CA-06927 from the National Cancer Institute and by an appropriation from the Commonwealth of Pennsylvania.

REFERENCES

1. E. D. Weinberg, Iron withholding: a defense against infection and neoplasia, Physiological Reviews 64:65 (1984).
2. A. L. Schade and L. Caroline, An iron-binding component in human blood plasma, Science 104:340 (1946).
3. M. Worwood, Ferritin in human tissues and serum, Clinics in Hematology 11:275 (1982).
4. J. W. Drysdale, T. G. Adelman, P. Arosio, D. Casarcale, P. Fitzpatrick, J. T. Hazard, and M. Yokota, Human isoferritins in normal and disease states, Seminars in Hematology 14:71 (1977).
5. R. Pearl, Cancer and tuberculosis, Am. J. Hyg. 9:97 (1929).
6. H. C. Nauts, The apparently beneficial effects of bacterial infection on host resistance to cancer: end results in 435 cases, Cancer Res. Inst. Monograph 8:1 (1958).
7. B. S. Blumberg, B. J. S. Gerstley, D. A. Hungerford, W. T. London, and A. I. Sutnick, A serum antigen (Australia antigen) in Down's syndrome, leukemia and hepatitis, Ann. Int. Med. 66:924 (1967).
8. A. I. Sutnick, W. T. London, B. S. Blumberg, and B. J. S. Gerstley, Persistent anicteric hepatitis with Australia antigen in patients with Down's syndrome, Am. J. Clin. Path. 57:2 (1972).
9. A. J. Kolk-Vegter, E. Bosch, and A. M. Leeuwen, Influence of serum hepatitis on haemoglobin level in patients on regular haemodialysis, Lancet 1:526 (1971).
10. A. I. Sutnick, B. S. Blumberg, and E. Lustbader, Elevated serum iron levels and persistent Australia antigen (HBsAg), Ann. Int. Med. 81:855 (1974).

11. B. S. Blumberg, B. Larouze, W. T. London, B. Werner, J. E. Hesser, I. Millman, G. Saimot, and M. Payet, The relation of infection with the hepatitis B agent to primary hepatic carcinoma, Am. J. Pathol. 81:669 (1975).

12. W. T. London and B. S. Blumberg, Hepatitis B and related viruses in chronic hepatitis, cirrhosis and hepatocellular carcinoma in man and animals in: "Chronic Active Liver Disease," S. Cohen and R. D. Soloway, eds., Churchill Livingstone, New York (1982).

13. C. Felton, E. D. Lustbader, C. Merten, and B. S. Blumberg, Serum iron levels and response to hepatitis B virus, Proc. Natl. Acad. Sci. USA 76:2438 (1979).

14. A. Vierucci, W. T. London, B. S. Blumberg, A. I. Sutnick and F. Ragazzini, Australia antigen and antibody in transfused children with thalassemia, Arch. Dis. Childhood 47:760 (1972).

15. W. T. London and J. S. Drew, Sex differences in response to hepatitis B infection among patients receiving chronic dialysis treatment, Proc. Natl. Acad. Sci. USA 74:2561 (1977).

16. S. Mazzur, J. Corbett, and B. S. Blumberg, Loss of immunologic reactivities of Australia antigen after incubation with bacteria, Proc. Soc. Exp. Biol. Med. 142:327 (1973).

17. I. Millman, H. Hutanen, F. Merino, M. E. Bayer, and B. S. Blumberg, Australia antigen: physical and chemical properties, Res. Commun. Chem. Path. Pharm. 2:667 (1971).

18. E. Feret, B. S. Blumberg, P. Whitford, and E. Lustbader, Serum iron levels and the response to infection with hepatitis B virus in the population of Tip, Senegal, West Africa, in preparation (1984).

19. B. S. Blumberg, E. D. Lustbader, and P. L. Whitford, Changes in serum iron levels due to infection with hepatitis B virus, Proc. Natl. Acad. Sci. USA 78:3222 (1981).

20. J. S. Drew, W. T. London, E. D. Lustbader, J. E. Hesser, and B. S. Blumberg, Hepatitis B virus and sex ratio of offspring, Science 201:687 (1978).

21. J. Drew, W. T. London, B. S. Blumberg, and S. Serjeantson, Hepatitis B virus and sex ratio on Kar Kar Island, Human Biology 54:123 (1982).

22. H. A. Edmondson and P. E. Steiner, Primary carcinoma of the liver, Cancer 7:462 (1954).

23. J. A. Fernandez-Pol, Iron: possible cause of the G_1 arrest induced in NRK cells by picolinic acid, Biochem. Biophys. Res. Commun. 78:136 (1977).

24. K. A. McGlynn, E. D. Lustbader, and W. T. London, Tuberculin skin test reactivity and hepatitis B e antigen status, in preparation (1984).

25. E. D. Lustbader, H. L. Hann, and B. S. Blumberg, Serum ferritin as a predictor of host response to hepatitis B virus infection, Science 220:423 (1983).

26. H. L. Hann, A. E. Evans, I. J. Cohen, and J. E. Leitmeyer, Biologic differences between neuroblastoma stages IV-S and IV. Measurement of serum ferritin and E-rosette inhibition in 30 children, N. Engl. J. Med. 305:425 (1981).

27. H. L. Hann, A. E. Evans, S. E. Siegel, H. Sather, D. Hammond, and R. Seeger, Serum ferritin levels as a guide to prognosis in patients with stage IV neuroblastoma, Proc. Am. Soc. Clin. Oncol. 2:72 (Abstract #C-282) (1983).

28. G. Birgegard, The source of serumferritin during infection. Studies with concanavalin A-Sepharose absorption, Clin. Sci. 59:385 (1980).

29. B. S. Blumberg, L. Melartin, R. A. Guinto, and B. Werner, Family studies of human serum isoantigen system (Australia antigen), Am. J. Human Genet. 18:594 (1966).

30. R. G. Stevens and B. S. Blumberg, Hepatitis B in the Solomon Islands, in: "Health Effects of Westernization: Biomedical Survey in the Solomon Islands," J. Rhoads, W. Howells, and J. Friedlaender, eds., Oxford University Press, in press (1984).

31. W. H. Crosby, Editorial: Fortification of food with carbonyl iron, Am. J. Clin. Nutr. 31:572 (1978).

32. A. Trousseau, True and false chlorosis, in: "Lectures on Clinical Medicine," Vol. 5, Lindsay and Blakiston, Philadelphia (1872).

33. R. G. Stevens, S. Kuvibidila, M. Kapps, J. Friedlaender, and B. S. Blumberg, Iron-binding proteins, hepatitis B virus, and mortality in the Solomon Islands, Am. J. Epidemiol. 118:550 (1983).

34. A. Vierucci, M. de Martino, E. Graziani, M. E. Rossi, W. T. London, and B. S. Blumberg, A mechanism for liver cell injury in viral hepatitis: effects of hepatitis B virus on neutrophil function in vitro and in children with chronic active hepatitis, Pediatric Res. 17:814 (1983).

35. D. R. Blake, N. D. Hall, P. A. Bacon, P. A. Dieppe, B. Halliwell, and J. M. C. Gutteridge, The importance of iron in rheumatoid disease, Lancet 2:1142 (1981).

36. B. S. Blumberg and W. T. London, Hepatitis B virus: pathogenesis and prevention of primary cancer of the liver, Cancer 50:2657 (1982).

37. B. S. Blumberg and W. T. London, Hepatitis B virus pathogenesis and prevention of primary cancer of the liver, in: "Accomplishments in Cancer Research 1981, General Motors Cancer Research Foundation," J. G. Fortner and J. E. Rhoads, eds., J. B. Lippincott Company, Philadelphia (1983).

38. S. G. Franklin, I. Millman, and B. S. Blumberg, Hepatitis B surface antigen and polymerized albumin binding activity in sheep serum, Proc. Natl. Acad. Sci. USA 81:564 (1984).

THE IMMUNE SYSTEM IN EXPERIMENTAL COXSACKIEVIRUS-B3 INFECTION

A. Toniolo, D. Matteucci, F. Basolo, and M. Bendinelli

Institutes of Microbiology, Hygiene and Pathological
Anatomy and Histology, University of Pisa, Pisa, Italy

In humans, members of the Coxsackievirus B group (CBV) produce a variety of clinical diseases, including epidemic pleurodynia, meningitis, encephalitis, pericarditis, myocarditis, and pancreatitis. With the possible exception of a few reported cases of anemia, lymphopenia, and thrombocytopenia especially in infants (1,2) and two cases of association between neonatal CBV-1 infection and Pneumocystis carinii pneumonia (3), these viruses are not regarded as common causes of damage to the hematopoietic and the immune systems. To our knowledge, however, studies on the immunologic functions of patients with clinical CBV infections are lacking.

We have previously shown that immunodeficiency is a primary consequence of CBV infection of adult mice (4,5). In particular, types 3, 4 and 6 reduce the antibody response to poliovirus and to heterologous red blood cells (RBC), whereas CBV-3 also suppresses the generation of cell-mediated responses. As shown in Table 1, adult mice immunized in vivo or in vitro with several different antigens have quite low responses to sheep and horse RBC, as well as to TNP conjugated to RBC. In addition, the development of contact sensitivity to oxazolone and to picryl chloride is impaired in these mice. In general, those immune responses which are dependent on the collaboration of both B and T cells are reduced by about 50% in the early phase of infection; in contrast, the response to "pure" T-independent antigens (TNP-Ficoll, for instance) is relatively unaffected. We first investigated whether this powerful suppression of immunological functions was due to an impairment of the proliferative capability of spleen lymphocytes. As shown in Table 1, the response to Con-A and to PWM was of the same level in infected as in normal mice. whereas the response to LPS--a B cell activator--was unexpectedly enhanced. Whatever the causes for the enhanced B cell proliferation, these experiments indicate that infection does not prevent lymphocyte division. Evidence from in vitro experiments showed that CBV-3-induced immunodeficiency is due in part to malfunction of spleen macrophages. In fact, when normal macrophages were substituted for by infected macrophages in a Mishell-Dutton system, the plasma cell generation in response to RBC was strongly reduced. In contrast, spleen cell cultures from infected mice, if deprived of endogenous macrophages and supplemented with equivalent numbers of normal adherent cells, developed near-normal responses. This may be taken as evidence that the antigen-presenting cells are functionally altered during infection. Accordingly, electron microscopy of infected spleens showed non-specific structural changes of macrophages, but failed to detect intracellular viral particles. Although

Table 1. Immune Reactivity of CBV-3-infected BALB/c Mice.

Stimulus	Response (% of control)
SRBC[1]	47
Poliovirus[1]	48
Oxazolone[1]	55
SRBC	34
TNP-HRBC	26
TNP-Ficoll	92
Con-A	98
PWM	108
E. coli LPS	157

[1] In vivo immunization; other data refer to in vitro
assays. See references 4 and 5 for details.

different approaches were attempted, we were unable to demonstrate that
CBV-3 can infect spleen macrophages in vivo. However, since minute amounts
of viral infectivity could have escaped detection even by the sensitive
infectious center assay, it remains unclear whether the observed alterations
reflect the direct effect of virus on these cells or, alternatively, are a
consequence of the enhanced phagocytic functions seen in infected animals.
In addition to macrophage alterations, experiments in vitro have shown that
CBV-3 infection activates non-specific T suppressor cells in a high proportion of mice; this has been confirmed by the rise of Lyt $1^-,2^+$ T lymphocytes
in the spleen during the first eight days of infection. Though it is difficult to quantify the immunodepressive role of these cells, they certainly
contribute to the observed immunodeficiency.

In the course of these studies we noticed that infected mice underwent
a dramatic reduction of both weight and cellularity of lymphoid organs. In
particular, the weight of thymus, spleen, and lymph nodes decreased very
rapidly during infection, so that approximately eight days post-infection
all the animals had atrophic organs (Table 2). The heart, liver, and total
body weights also tend to fall, but at a reduced rate as compared to lymphoid
organs. During the first ten days of infection, although the numbers of
nucleated cells in these organs were progressively reduced, cell viability
remained unchanged; this is in agreement with the unimpaired proliferative
ability of lymphocytes.

Histologic studies showed that the main lesion in the thymus is represented by the early retraction of epithelial-reticular cells, followed by
the loss of both cortical and medullary lymphocytes. Necrosis or inflammatory changes were not observed in infected lymphoid organs, which, eventually
became fibrotic and atrophic. Approximately ten days post-infection, the
thymus virtually disappeared; similar events occurred in the spleen and
lymph nodes, where B- and T-dependent areas appeared equally affected. No
lesions suggestive of direct viral cytopathology could be detected by optical
or electron microscopy. Ten days after infection, the spleen weight was
reduced by about two-thirds and a massive degree of fibrosis was evident.
As shown by immunofluorescence and by complement-dependent cytotoxicity,
although the total counts of nucleated cells in the spleen were falling in
the course of infection, the relative proportions of B and T cells remained

Table 2. Weight of Lymphoid Organs During CBV-3
Infection of BALB/c Mice.

| Day | Mean Weight (% of control)[1] | | | |
	Thymus	Spleen	Lymph Nodes	Body
4	37	110	108	88
8	18	52	69	78
12	12	35	18	91

[1] Ten to fifteen mice per point.

approximately unchanged. This suggests that CBV-3 infection does not act selectively on a specific class of lymphocytes. To test whether CBV-3-induced lymphoid atrophy was caused by virus replication in immunocytes, we checked for the presence of infectious centers in thymus, spleen, lymph node, and bone marrow cell suspensions. As shown in Table 3, virtually no infected cells were detectable in lymphoid organs at various times post-infection, with the exception of a small percentage of unidentified cells $(30/10^6)$ which were productively infected in the bone marrow. This amount of viral replication, however, does not seem sufficient to account for the large effects seen in lymphoid organs. Parallel experiments confirmed that even in vitro murine lymphoid cells do not allow detectable DBV-3 replication. In addition, we also tested the capability of CBV-3 to interfere directly with the antibody response to heterologous RBC in vitro. Spleen cell cultures infected in vitro consistently generated normal numbers of antibody-producing cells, no matter of the amount of infectious virus added. Taken together, these data strongly suggest that CBV-3-induced immunodeficiency and lymphoid atrophy are not mediated by the direct viral destruction of immunocytes.

Since elevated blood cortisol levels were found in the early phase of infection, an alternative possibility to explain, in part, virus-induced

Table 3. Virus-producing Cells in Various Organs
of CBV-infected Mice.

Source of Cells	$IC/10^6$ cells[1]
Pancreas	700,000
Peritoneal Cavity	2,250
Bone Marrow	30
Thymus	<1
Spleen	<1
Inguinal LN	<1

[1] IC: infectious centers. Test done three days after infection. Comparable results obtained on days 1, 2, and 4.

Table 4. Susceptibility to CBV-3-induced Atrophy of
         Lymphoid Organs

Mouse Strain	Mean Weight (% of Control)[1] Thymus	Spleen
BALB/c	17	43
C57BL/6	26	56
CBA	40	98
F1(BALB x CBA)	33	78
F1(C57 x CBA)	27	84

[1] 20 mice per group; sacrifice on day 10.

lymphoid atrophy was that the release of adrenal corticosteroids caused by
stress and/or by the acute destruction of thymus (6) might sufficiently
deplete the lymphoid organs of specific cell populations. However, infection

of adrenalectomized mice produced approximately the same level of lymphoid
atrophy as that seen in normal animals. To test whether non-specific metabolic alterations and/or malnutrition consequent to infection were responsible for the observed involution of lymphoid tissues, BALB/c mice were
infected with related Picornaviruses (i.e., CBV-1, CBV-5, and encephalomyocarditis virus). Infection with these agents failed to produce any marked
effects on lymphoid organs, although all of them reduced somewhat the thymus
weight. The observation that susceptibility to CBV-3-induced lymphoid
atrophy is genetically determined also suggests that this pathologic effect
does not represent a non-specific consequence of infection. As shown in
Table 4, different degrees of spleen atrophy were observed when various
mouse strains were infected with CBV-3. Histopathology showed, however,
that myocardial and pancreatic changes were of comparable severity in all
these mice. Thus, infection per se does not seem sufficient to trigger the
lymphoid atrophy, and lymphoid changes appear to derive from the specific
interaction of CBV-3 with some unidentified target tissue(s) that are
different in different mouse strains.

The observations that lymphoid atrophy cannot be prevented by treatment with various immunopotentiating agents (i.e., thymosin, isoprinosine,
or bestatin) and that these drugs actually aggravate the structural as well
as the functional damage, suggest that autoimmunity may be responsible in
part of the involution of lymphoid tissues. Though the mechanisms involved
are still unclear, the possible pathogenetic role of autoreactivity in CBV
infections has been already postulated with regard to chronic myocarditis
(7).

In conclusion, CBV-3 may produce a severe form of immunodeficiency in
susceptible mice that is associated with a permanent involution of the
entire lymphoid system. So far, this effect could not be attributed directly
to viral replication in lymphoid cells and seems mediated, in part, by indirect mechanisms, possibly immunopathologic in nature. These studies raise
the possibility that severe CBV infections may play a pathogenetic role in
some cases of acquired immunodeficiency.

ACKNOWLEDGMENTS

We thank Dr. Z. Gori for electron microscopy studies; Drs. B. Prabhakar and M. Campa for helpful comments and advice; and Mrs. L. Montagnani for technical assistance. This work was supported by a grant from the Italian National Research Council (Progetto Finalizzato Controllo delle Malattie da Infezione, contract No. 83.00626.52).

REFERENCES

1. M. H. Kaplan, S. W. Klein, J. McPhee, and R. G. Harper, Group B Coxsackievirus infections in infants younger than three months of age: a serious childhood illness, Rev. Infect. Dis. 5:1019 (1983).
2. J. H. S. Gear and V. Measroch, Coxsackievirus infections of the newborn, Progr. Med. Virol. 15:42 (1973).
3. A. Sebastiani, G. Fontana, and A. Balestrieri, Su due casi di polmonite pneumocistica del lattante associata ad infezione da virus Coxsackie B1, Arch. Ital. Sci. Med. Trop. Parass. 47:191 (1966).
4. M. Bendinelli, A. Ruschi, M. Campa, and A. Toniolo, Depression of humoral and cell-mediated immune responses by Coxsackieviruses in mice, Experientia 31:1227 (1975).
5. M. Bendinelli, D. Matteucci, A. Toniolo, A. M. Patane, and M. P. Pistillo, Impairment of immunocompetent mouse spleen cell functions by infection with Coxsackievirus B3, J. Infect. Dis. 146:797 (1982).
6. D. L. Healy, G. D. Hodgen, H. M. Schulte, G. P. Chrousos, D. L. Loriaux, N. R. Hall, and A. L. Goldstein, The thymus-adrenal connection: thymosin has corticotropin-releasing activity in primates, Science 222:1353 (1983).
7. R. J. Gudvangen, P. S. Duffey, R. E. Paque, and C. J. Gauntt, Levamisole exacerbates Coxsackievirus B3-induced murine myocarditis, Infect. Immun. 41:1157 (1983).

III. TUMOR VIRUS INFECTIONS AND IMMUNE RESPONSES

MAMMARY TUMOR VIRUS INFECTIONS AND IMMUNITY

Diana M. Lopez, Robert J. Pauley, and Ronald D. Paul

Department of Microbiology and Immunology
University of Miami School of Medicine
Miami, Florida

INTRODUCTION

Mammary tumorigenesis appears to be influenced by several factors including genetic background, hormones and the immune response. In animal models there is a correlation between infection with mouse mammary tumor virus (MMTV) and an increased incidence of spontaneous mammary tumors. Exogenous MMTV is transmitted from high mammary tumor incidence strains to certain low incidence strains through the milk (1) with the result of increased numbers of tumors in the latter. There is evidence suggesting that MMTV infection results in integration of this retrovirus into the mammary glandular tissues (2). In recent years the possibility has been explored, that expression of an endogenous counterpart of MMTV may be involved in the etiology of mammary tumors. The observation by Hageman et al. (3) of MMTV virions in mammary tumors arising in some low incidence mouse strains that had different characteristics from the classic exogenous milk transmitted virus, supports a role of endogenous MMTV in tumorigenesis.

In our laboratories we have investigated the modulating effects of the immune system in the initiation and development of mammary tumors. Our model system consists of two colonies of BALB/c mice: BALB/cCrgl, which harbor one partial copy and two complete proviral genomes of MMTV, and the syngeneic BALB/cfC3H, which in addition to the endogenous MMTV has been infected at birth with exogenous MMTV by foster nursing in C3H mice. BALB/-cCrgl breeders have an incidence of spontaneous mammary tumors of less than 3% at two years of age, whereas 95% of the BALB/cfC3H breeders develop mammary tumors by 24 months of age. A mammary tumor line, designated as D1-DMBA-3, has been transplanted, in our studies in the BALB/cCrgl colony. The D1-DMBA-3 tumor originated from a hyperplastic nodule appearing in BALB/c hormonally hyperstimulated and treated with 7,12-dimethylbenzanthracene (4), is immunogenic to the host of origin, and does not express MMTV related antigens. The BALB/cfC3H mice have been implanted in some studies with MMTV antigen-expressing spontaneous mammary tumors (SMT) naturally occurring in BALB/cfC3H breeders.

BLASTOGENIC RESPONSES TO TUMOR ASSOCIATED ANTIGENS (TAA) AND TO MMTV

BALB/cCrgl mice implanted with D1-DMBA-3, and BALB/cfC3H mice bearing spontaneous mammary tumors, have similar kinetics of blastogenic responses to purified membrane preparations of their respective tumors (TAA). Thus, spleen cells from mice of either colony have no response prior to transplantation, peaked reactivities two to three weeks after tumor implantation and loss of blastogenic reaction when tumors reach maximum size (5). A similar pattern of responses was observed in BALB/cfC3H splenocytes stimulated by purified preparations of MMTV in vitro. In contrast, splenocytes of normal BALB/cCrgl and BALB/cCrgl implanted with Dl-DMBA-3 mammary tumors, possess spleen lymphocytes that were capable of high levels of ^{3}H-thymidine incorporation upon exposure to purified preparations of MMTV irrespective of the stage of tumor development.

The results of studies designed to analyze the lymphoid cells responding to MMTV and TAA are presented in Table 1. It can be seen that nylon wool nonadherent cells from the two BALB/c colonies is the lymphocyte subclass that responds in blastogenesis to their TAA when they are bearing small spontaneous mammary tumors. Likewise, responses to MMTV antigens were observed in the nylon wool nonadherent spleen cells of the MMTV-positive BALB/-cfC3H mice bearing small SMT. As we previously described (6), all these responses sharply decline with increasing tumor burden. In contrast, the nylon wool nonadherent splenocytes of BALB/cCrgl appear to be non-responsive to MMTV antigens but SIg$^+$ nylon wool adherent spleen lymphocytes were capable of being stimulated by MMTV. The blastogenic response of these BALB/cCrgl B lymphocytes was present in normal BALB/cCrgl mice and was not altered by either tumor implantation or progression.

Several possibilities could account for the unalterable responsiveness of the BALB/cCrgl B lymphocytes to MMTV. Among these one could propose: a) horizontal transmission; b) stimulation by cell contaminants in the purified viral preparations; c) mitogen-like polyclonal activation of B

Table 1. Blastogenic Responses to TAA and to MMTV

Stimulus	Mice Population	BALB/cCrgl		BALB/cfC3H	
		Normal Mice	Tumor Bearers	Normal Mice	Tumor Bearers
TAA	Unseparated	505	5982	644	4048
	Nylon Non-Adherent	525	10226	597	9987
	Nylon Adherent	637	589	615	598
MMTV	Unseparated	11659	12033	1689	10141
	Nylon Non-Adherent	519	645	1328	14872
	Nylon Adherent	17854	16989	1456	1259

Results of ^{3}H-thymidine incorporation expressed as cpm above control. Standard deviations never exceeded 10%.

cells by MMTV; and d) sensitization to MMTV associated antigen(s) due to expression of an endogenous virus. Arguing against the first possibility is the fact that our BALB/cCrgl animals are geographically separated from any other animals and are handled by special personnel. In addition, the incidence of SMT in this colony never exceeded 3% at two years of age. More direct proof is afforded by the molecular biology studies presented in this chapter, where no additional copies of proviral MMTV can be detected in the various tissues of our BALB/cCrgl mice. One could rule out the second possibility, that the blastogenic stimulation observed in the spleen cells of BALB/cCrgl mice is due to host cell contaminants, by studies comparing MMTV from milk sources to the same MMTV grown in vitro in Crandall feline kidney cells. The same levels of reactions were observed when the spleen cells were stimulated with RIII-MMTV purified from milk or from infected cat cells (7). In connection with the third possibility that MMTV could be causing a non-specific polyclonal response in BALB/cCrgl mice, we have found indirect evidence that this is not the case. In the BALB/cfC3H colony, derived from BALB/cCrgl animals after foster nursing at birth on MMTV-positive C3H mice, no significant responsiveness to MMTV antigens could be detected in spleen cells, while the same preparations can be stimulated by the B cell mitogen, LPS (8). If MMTV is acting as a nonspecific mitogen in BALB/cCrgl mice, similar reactivities should have been observed in the two syngeneic colonies. In addition, in animals bearing large D1-DMBA-3 mammary tumors (5 to 10 g of weight), the responses to B- and T-cell mitogens are greatly depressed (9). We have found that the stimulation caused by MMTV antigen(s) remains stable in BALB/cCrgl mice even in the presence of a heavy tumor burden. Thus, the stimulation caused by MMTV in this mouse colony

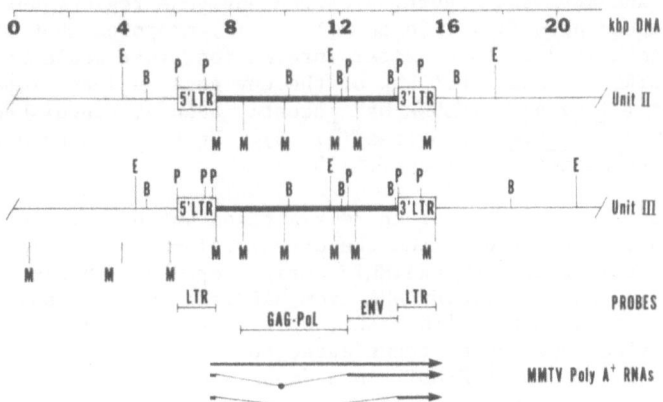

Fig. 1. Restriction of Map Units II and III of MMTV Proviral DNA in the BALB/c Strain. The EcoRI (E), BglII (B), PstI (P) and MspI (M) sites are mapped. MMTV DNA is indicated by the heavy line with the LTR region shown as open boxes, whereas flanking cellular DNA is indicated by the thin line. Noncontinuous lines to MspI sites indicated those sites that have not been specifically localized near Units II and III. The cloned MMTV DNA PstI fragments used as molecular hybridization probes (LTR, GAG-POL, ENV), which are aligned with the complementary regions of Units II and III, are shown below the restriction maps. The MMTV poly A⁺ RNAs, either the full length 9kb or the spliced 3.8kb and 1.7kb RNAs, are shown at the bottom as heavy lines, and are aligned to their complementary coding region.

appears to be quantitatively and qualitatively different from that obtained
with other mitogens such as PHA, Con A, and LPS. Regarding the last alternative, we have previously reported (10) that MMTV antigen(s) are present
in nylon wool adherent spleen cells from the BALB/cCrgl mouse strain. Double
label immunofluorescence studies unequivocally determined that the MMTV
antigen(s) appear to co-cap with surface immunoglobulins on the surface of
these B lymphocytes. Furthermore we also found that these MMTV antigens
were absent from the nylon wool nonadherent spleen population and from thymus
derived cells (10,11).

MMTV DNA ORGANIZATION AND RNA EXPRESSION IN MOUSE SPLEENS

Previous studies by Cohen and Varmus (12) have demonstrated that the
BALB/c strain, as well as all inbred mouse strains, contain multiple copies
of germinally-transmitted MMTV proviral DNA. BALB/c MMTV proviral DNA has
been characterized by restriction endonuclease mapping and molecular hybridization with either a MMTV complementary DNA (cDNA) (12-15) or cloned probes
of specific regions of the MMTV genome (16,17). The cloned subgenomic MMTV
DNA probes, the gag-pol, the env, and the LTR region probes used to determine
the restriction map of the two BALB/c genome size MMTV proviruses, designated
MMTV Unit II or mtv-8 and Unit III or mtv-9, are shown in Figure 1. The
two BALB/c genomic size MMTV proviruses are distinguished from each other
by the fact that the proviral DNAs are integrated within different regions
of cellular DNA, as evidenced by the unique size EcoRI fragments of Unit
II, 7.6 and 6.3 kbp, and Unit III, 7.2 and 9.1 kbp, and the specificity of
each fragment for hybridization with the gag-pol or env probes (17). In
addition, the BALB/c strain contains a subgenomic, or defective, MMTV provirus designated Unit I or mtv-6, that we have recently shown to contain
the LTR region and at least a portion of the env gene region, but lacks any
of the gag-pol sequences (17). Cohen et al. (13) proposed that MMTV Unit I
contains a maximum of 3.2 kbp of viral information, that would be consistent
with two MMTV LTRs and about 0.4 kbp of the env gene region. Importantly,
the BALB/c Unit I (mtv-6) MMTV DNA has recently been distinguished from the
genomic size Unit Ia (mtv-7) provirus (17,18). Unit Ia had been previously
described as a subgenomic provirus (14,15).

Based on the observations of an MMTV antigen on the surface of BALB/c
lymphocytes (10), we first examined the organization of MMTV DNA sequences
in tissues and cells that lack the MMTV antigen or that contain the MMTV
antigen. Briefly, total cellular DNA from BALB/c tissues or spleen cell
subpopulations, was digested with EcoRi, BglII or PSTI, size fractionated
by agarose gel electrophoresis, transferred to nitrocellulose filters, and
hybridized with either an α^{32}P-MMTV cDNA (data not shown) or the nick translated α^{32}P-MMTV gag-pol, env and LTR probes as previously described (17).
Identical size MMTV DNA-containing restriction fragments to those shown in
Figure 1, that hybridized with the specific MMTV DNA probes, and to Unit I
containing restriction fragments were observed in tissues and cells that
lack the MMTV antigen, BALB/c liver, mammary gland, carcinogen-induced mammary tumor, thymus and splenic nylon wool nonadherent cells, or that have
the MMTV antigen, BALB/c spleen and splenic nylon wool adherent cells (Table
2). Mammary tumors from BALB/c mice infected with the milk-transmitted
MMTV, BALB/cfC3H tumor, contained additional copies of MMTV proviral DNA
(Table 2). Therefore, there was no detectable amplification of the MMTV
DNA copy number, alteration in the cellular sites of integration, or alteration of the BALB/c MMTV proviral DNA organization in tissues or cells that
contain or lack the MMTV antigen.

We next sought to determine whether the expression of the MMTV antigen
on BALB/c spleen cells, which was absent from both normal or neoplastic
BALB/c mammary cells and from thymic cells, was due to the regulation of
MMTV RNA transcription. The amount of MMTV RNA, expressed as a percentage

Table 2. MMTV DNA in BALB/cCrgl Cellular DNA

Tissue	Fraction	MMTV DNA Units			
		I	II	III	Additional
Liver	Unseparated	+	+	+	None
Mammary Gland	Unseparated	+	+	+	None
Carcinogen-Induced Mammary Tumor	Unseparated	+	+	+	None
Thymus	Unseparated	+	+	+	None
Spleen	Unseparated	+	+	+	None
	Nylon wool nonadherent	+	+	+	None
	Nylon wool adherent	+	+	+	None
BALB/cfC3H Mammary Tumor	Unseparated	+	+	+	+

Table 3. MMTV RNA Expression in BALB/c Tissues

Tissue	MMTV*	Maximum Percent Hybridization[‡]
Thymus	0.0001%	14% @ 1×10^5 Equiv. Rot
Spleen	0.0015%	>90% @ 2.5×10^4 Equiv. Rot
Liver	$\leq$0.0001%	8% @ 1×10^5 Equiv. Rot
Retired Breeder Mammary Gland	0.0001%	26% @ 6×10^4 Equiv. Rot
Carcinogen-Induced Mammary Tumor	0.0001%	24% @ 1×10^4 Equiv. Rot
BALB/cfC3H	0.27%	100% @ 1×10^2 Equiv. Rot

*The level of MMTV RNA is expressed as a percentage of total cellular RNA, quantitified by RNA excess hybridization (19).

[‡]The maximum percent hybridization of the ^{3}H-MMTV cDNA observed during hybridization is specified, and the equivalent Rot at which the maximum percent hybridization was observed is specified. In most cases equivalent Rot values of greater than 5×10^4 could not be obtained under the hybridization conditions. About 3% mismatching between the MMTV cDNA and spleen RNA was observed; 70S MMTV RNA had a temperature of 86°, BALB/c spleen RNA had a temperature of 81.7°C.

of total cellular RNA was determined by comparing the kinetics of hybridization of total cellular RNA and a representative MMTV cDNA probe to hybridization between MMTV 70S RNA and probe (19). BALB/c liver, thymus, multiparous retired breeder mammary gland, and the D1-DMBA-3 carcinogen-induced
mammary tumor all contained MMTV RNA at (0.0001%) or below the limits of
detection, that demonstrated a very limited extent of hybridization to the
MMTV cDNA probe even at high equivalent Rot values (Table 3). In contrast,
virgin female BALB/c spleen contained a significant amount of MMTV RNA,
0.0015% of total cellular RNA (Table 3). The level of MMTV RNA in the BALB/c
spleen, however, was about 100-fold lower than the level of MMTV RNA observed in a BALB/cfC3H mammary tumor (Table 3) that contained additional
copies of the milk-transmitted MMTV DNA.

BALB/c spleen cells were separated into nylon wool nonadherent, T cell
enriched, or nylon wool adherent, B cell enriched, cell populations to determine if MMTV RNA expression is restricted to a specific subpopulation of
BALB/c spleen lymphocytes. Total cellular RNA was isolated and bound to a
nitrocellulose filter for hybridization with the $\alpha^{32}P$ MMTV DNA cloned probes
(Figure 2). The splenic T lymphocyte enriched subpopulations lacked detectable MMTV RNA (vertical lane 3). The splenic B lymphocyte subpoplations,
on the other hand, contained MMTV RNA, although at a level of less than
one-tenth the BALB/cfC3H mammary tumor (vertical lanes 4 and 5, respectively). Therefore, the level of MMTV RNA expression in BALB/c tissues and
splenic cell subpopulations correlates positively with the presence of MMTV
antigen(s) in the same tissues and splenic cell subpopulations. In

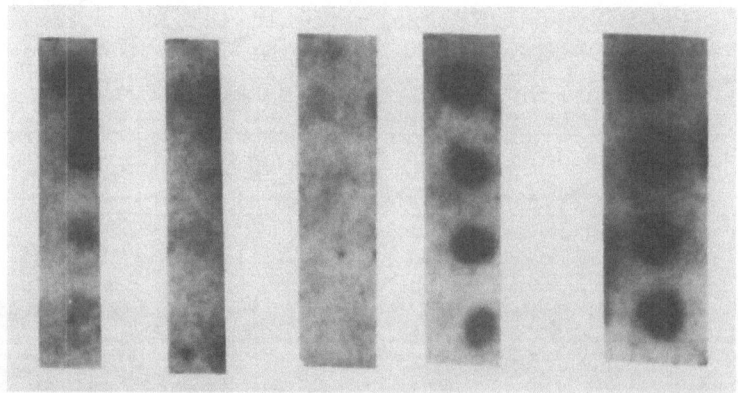

Fig. 2. MMTV RNA expression in BALB/c spleen cell subpopulations.
Total cellular RNA was prepared as previously described
(19), diluted to a concentration of 0.5 µg/ 1 in sterile
glass distilled water, except the BALB/cfC3H tumor RNA
which was diluted to 0.042 µg/ 1, then heat denatured.
The sample, 3 µl, and serial 1:1 dilutions were spotted
onto a nitrocellulose filter using RNA from a BALB/c
multiparous lactating mammary gland (column 1); a virgin
BALB/c liver (column 2); virgin BALB/c spleen cells
fractionated into nylon wool nonadherent, T cell enriched,
and nylon wool adherent, B cell enriched, subpopulations
(columns 3 and 4, respectively); and BALB/cfC3H mammary
tumor RNA (column 5). The filter was hybridized with a
mixture of the nick translated $\alpha^{32}P$-labelled, cloned
MMTV probes (gag-pol), env and LTR probes) as previously
described (17). The filter was autoradioraphed using
Kodak XAR film with a DuPont Cronex lightning plus intensifying screen.

combination, with the restriction mapping data (Table 2), these observations indicate that the germinally-transmitted MMTV provirus(es) are expressed in BALB/c splenic B lymphocytes.

MMTV poly A$^+$ RNA transcripts, which have been characterized by molecular sizing and in vitro translation (20-22) are of three types: the 9kb gag-pol and gag polypeptide precursor mRNA, the 3.8 kb env polypeptide precursor mRNA, which is spliced from the 9 kb mRNA, and the 1.7 kb LTR RNA, which is a spliced transcript containing predominately MMTV LTR sequences (Figure 1). It can be hypothesized that the most likely MMTV RNA transcript responsible for the accumulation of a MMTV antigen on the surface of BALB/c spleen cells is the 3.8 kb MMTV env mRNA. This hypothesis is indirectly supported by specific MMTV gp52 monoclonal antibody binding to BALB/c spleen cells. Direct support for this hypothesis has been provided by our recent observation of the 3.8 kb MMTV env mRNA in Abelson Murine Leukemia virus transformed BALB/c B cell lines (17). Studies are in progress to characterize the MMTV RNA transcripts in BALB/c spleen cells, which are in the poly A$^+$ RNA fraction (data not shown).

It is not possible, based on the data described above, to state which of the BALB/c germinally-transmitted MMTV proviral DNA are responsible for the expression of MMTV RNA sequences. To attempt to correlate between a specific germline MMTV provirus and MMTV RNA expression in the spleen several inbred mouse strains and recombinant inbred mice were examined for MMTV RNA expression and the MMTV DNA sequences were characterized by restriction mapping. Based on the restriction endonuclease mapping data shown in Figure 3

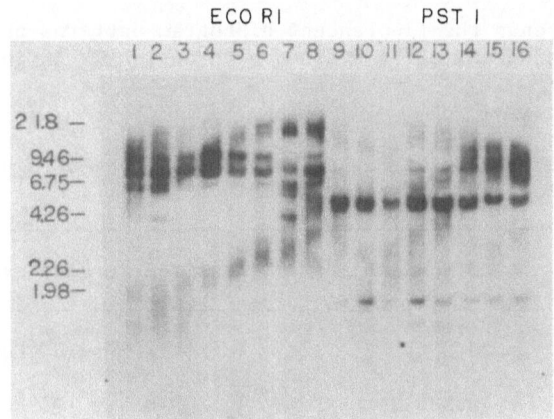

Fig. 3. Characterization of MMTV DNA in Different Mouse Strains and Recombinant Inbred Mice. DNA was prepared (17) from the liver of BXH-3 (lanes 1, 9), BXH-6 (lanes 2, 10), BXH-9 (lanes 3,11), C57BL/10J (lanes 4, 12), C57BL/6J (lanes 5, 13), CBA/CaJ (lanes 6, 14), C3H/HeJ (lanes 7, 15) and BALB/cCrgl (lanes 8, 16) mice. DNA, 10 µg, was digested with EcoRI (lanes 1-8) or PstI (lanes 9-16), eletrophoresed through 0.8% agarose and transferred to a nitrocellulose filter as described (17) except that 2.5 x 10^6 cpm/ml of a α^{32}P MMTV cDNA (19) at 650 cpm/pg was used as a hybridization probe. Following hybridization, the filter was washed (17) and MMTV DNA was visualized by autoradiography using Kodak XAR film with a DuPont Cronex lightning plus intensifying screen.

other studies in our laboratory using the cloned MMTV probes (17,18 and unpublished observations), and the work of other laboratories (12-16) we conclude that the C3H/HeJ strain contains MMTV proviral DNA Units I, Ia, II, V and IX (18), whereas C57BL/6J and CBA/CaJ contain Units II, III and X. In addition, several recombinant inbred mouse lines BXH-3, BXH-6, and BXH-9, which were derived from a cross of C57BL/6 and C3H/HeJ (23), were characterized for MMTV proviral DNA. BXH recombinant inbred mice all contained MMTV Units II and III, BXH-6 and BXH-9 contained in addition Unit V (Figure 3). MMTV RNA sequences were expressed at a low but detectable level in the spleen of all these mice (Table 4). Therefore, it is not possible to correlate MMTV RNA expression in the mouse spleen with a particular germ-line transmitted MMTV provirus, possibly because more than one MMTV provirus has the potential to be expressed in the mouse spleen.

DISSOCIATION OF MMTV-EXPRESSING AND MMTV-RESPONDING B-LYMPHOCYTE SUBSETS

PRESENT IN SPLEENS OF BALB/cCrgl MICE

As shown in the previous sections approximately one fourth of BALB/cCrgl B lymphocytes express antigen(s) of MMTV on their surface, although intact MMTV virions cannot be found in the tissues of these mice. Since both expression of the endogenous MMTV and blastogenic responsiveness appear to coincide in the nylon adherent population, the possibility of the existence of two B lymphocyte subsets, one expressing the putative sensitizing MMTV antigen(s) and the other responding to MMTV, was explored. Nylon adherent lymphocytes were stained with rabbit anti-MMTV and FITC-conjugated goat anti-rabbit IgG and positively selected by cell sorting in a FACS III instrument.

Figure 4 represents the fluorescent histogram patterns obtained with the unsorted nylon adherent cells stained with anti-MMTV antibody (B histo-

Table 4. MMTV RNA in the Spleen of Inbred Mouse Strains and Recombinant-Inbred Mouse Lines

Mouse Strain	MMTV RNA*	Maximum Percent Hybridization[+]
C3H/HeJ	0.0006%	83% @ 3×10^4 Equiv. Rot
C57BL/6J	0.0004%	70% @ 3×10^4 Equiv. Rot
C57BL/10J	0.0002%	56% @ 3×10^4 Equiv. Rot
BXH-3	0.0002%	34% @ 2×10^4 Equiv. Rot
BXH-6	0.0002%	15% @ 9×10^3 Equiv. Rot
BXH-9	0.0004%	56% @ 2×10^4 Equiv. Rot

*The level of MMTV RNA, expressed as a percentage of total cellular RNA, was quantitated by RNA excess hybridization.

[+]The maximum percent hybridization of the ^{3}H-MMTV cDNA observed during hybridization is specified, and the equivalent Rot at which the maximum percent hybridization was observed is specified. In most cases equivalent Rot values of greater than 5×10^4 could not be obtained under the hybridization conditions.

Table 5. Percent of MMTV Positive and MMTV Negative Cells in Unsorted and Sorted Populations

	Percent MMTV+	Percent MMTV−
Unsorted	29	71
Sorted for MMTV + Cells	87	13
Sorted for MMTV − Cells	5	95

gram). A negative control is presented in histogram A, which represents the nylon adherent cells stained with the prebleeds of the rabbits used to raise the polyvalent anti-MMTV antibody and the FITC conjugated second reagent. Histogram C indicates the population of MMTV negative cells, determined as the area where there is no overlap between the negative control and the unsorted nylon adherent population. Histogram D represents the MMTV positive population, which was collected from the point of intersect with line C to the channels expressing higher fluorescent intensity. The purity of the resulting nylon adherent subpopulations, submitted to the two-way cell sorting procedure, on the basis of their expression of MMTV antigen(s) on their surface is presented in Table 5. Cells sorted for the presence of MMTV antigens are 87% pure, while those cells sorted for absence of viral expression were 95% pure.

Blastogenesis studies using the B cell mitogen LPS and purified MMTV as stimuli, were performed with the populations derived from the cell sorting procedures (Figure 5). Unseparated BALB/cCrgl spleen cells as well as unsorted nylon wool adherent populations were included in these studies

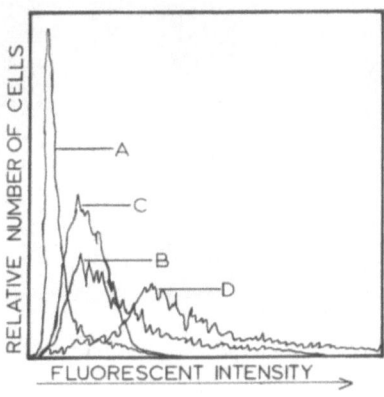

Fig. 4. Fluorescent histogram of the unsorted and FACS-III-sorted BALB/cCrgl nylon wool adherent spleen cells with sorting based on MMTV antigen expression. A. - Negative control; B. - unsorted nylon wool adherent cells; C. - MMTV-negative nylon wool adherent cells; D. - MMTV-positive nylon wool adherent cells.

Table 6. MMTV-gp52 Related Antigen in Human Spleens

| Cadaver Donors | Percentage of P7G6 Positive Cells | |
	Nylon Wool Non-Adherent	Nylon Wool Adherent
R.M. (f)	None	None
D.E. (f)	None	None
S.J. (f)	5.7	9.3
M.D. (m)	None	None
S.E. (m)	None	None

Percentage fluorescent cells with monoclonal mouse anti-MMTV-gp52 antibody and FITC conjugated anti-mouse SIg antibody as determined by FACS III analyses. Background fluorescence from the second antibody reagent was deducted by the FACS III instrument.

as reference points. The unseparated spleen lymphocytes have vigorous responses to both LPS and purified MMTV. Nylon wool non-adherent lymphocytes were not stimulated in the lymphocyte transformation assay when exposed to either LPS or MMTV, reconfirming previous results. In contrast, the

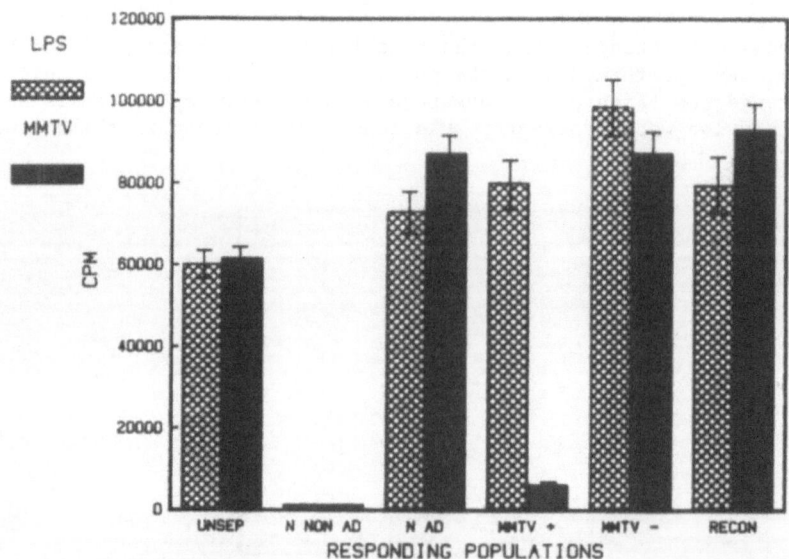

Fig. 5. Blastogenic responses in MMTV sorted Populations. Blastogenic responses of nylon wool adherent lymphocytes from normal BALB/cCrgl mice unsorted and after a two-way sort to separate MMTV positive from MMTV negative cells. Results are expressed as counts per minute per well of either MMTV or LPS stimulated cultures minus the background cpm of unstimulated cultures.

Table 7. MMTV-gp52 Related Antigen in Human Peripheral Blood
Lymphocytes.

Donor	Percentage of Positive Cells			
	LEU 4	SIg	P7G6	P2C2
D.L. (f)	71.4	22.2	7.5	10.4
L.H. (f)	76.5	24.1	7.1	6.2
B.S. (f)	62.0	27.0	8.1	11.1
S.K. (m)	53.5	19.2	6.2	7.0
R.P. (m)	52.5	29.7	6.3	14.7
M.D. (m)	64.4	26.4	10.0	17.3

Detection of an antigen cross reacting with two monoclonal
antibodies (P7G6 and P2C2) generated against MMTV gp52 in
peripheral blood leukocytes of normal human subjects. Included
as reference are the levels of T and B lymphocytes, indicated
by the presence of the Leu4 antigen or SIg in their surfaces.

nylon wool adherent cells had enhanced levels of responses to these two
reagents in comparison to the unseparated spleen cells. When the cells
expressing MMTV antigens were tested in this cell mediated immune assay, a
high stimulation was observed with the B-cell mitogen LPS but no responses
could be observed with MMTV. Strikingly, the MMTV-negative nylon wool
adherent cells appear to be fully responsive to both the LPS and the viral
antigens. Cultures reconstituted to represent the levels of MMTV-positive
and MMTV-negative nylon wool adherent cells before the sorting procedure,
i.e. 29% MMTV-positive cells and 71% MMTV-negative cells, had blastogenic
responses that are essentially the same as observed in the nylon wool adherent non-sorted populations. These data indicate that in normal BALB/cCrgl
mice antigen expression of the endogenous MMTV retrovirus is restricted to
a nylon wool adherent cell subset which is different from those B lymphocytes
responding in blastogenesis to the viral antigens.

EXPRESSION OF MMTV-RELATED ANTIGENS IN HUMAN LYMPHOID CELLS

An association between mouse mammary tumor virus and human carcinoma
of the breast has been suggested by the immunological studies of several
laboratories including ours (24-28). Furthermore, there have been reports
of virus-like particles in human milk and in fresh human breast carcinomas
(29). Using immunohistochemical techniques, Mesa-Tejada et al. (30) detected
a MMTV-cross-reacting antigen in human breast carcinomas and Dion et al.
(31) isolated a glycoprotein cross-reactive with the MMTV gp52 molecule
from pooled human milk. More recently, Callahan et al. (32) and May et al.
(33) detected sequences related to the MMTV genome in human DNA.

In order to explore the possibility that such genetic information related to MMTV may be expressed in human cells we utilized two monoclonal
antibodies against the major glycoprotein of MMTV (gp 52) developed by Massey
et al. (34) in immunofluorescence studies with human lymphoid cells. A

series of experiments were performed utilizing nylon wool adherent and nylon wool non-adherent human spleen cells from cadaver donors, obtained from accident victims through the Tissue Typing Bank of the University of Miami. As seen in Table 6, of five patients tested with monoclonal antibody P7G6, only one female patient demonstrated a positive reaction (5.7% in the nylon wool non-adherent vs. 9.3% in the nylon wool adherent population). It should be noted that these preparations of human nylon wool adherent and non-adherent cells had substantial contamination of T and B lymphocytes, respectively, as indicated by fluorescent markers, i.e. anti-Leu4 and anti-human SIg antibodies.

Peripheral blood monoclonal cells were isolated from the blood of six healthy donors, three females and three males as previously described (27). Table 7 contains the results of those studies performed as described in Table 6 and analyzed by flow cytometry. All subjects tested regardless of sex possessed lymphocytes that had antigenic determinants in their surface cross reactive with two different monoclonal antibodies against different epitopes of MMTV gp52, the major external glycoprotein of mouse mammary tumor virus.

At present we cannot exclude the possibility that these results may be a case of "molecular mimicry." It is conceivable that the epitope recognized by the monoclonal antibodies against gp52 is not actually related to MMTV. Alternatively, one could postulate that, because DNA sequences related to MMTV are present in human cells, these related sequences are being expressed in a subset of peripheral blood leukocytes. Obviously molecular biologic studies investigating this alternative would have to be performed before one could arrive at a firm conclusion; nevertheless, the parallel between retroviral expression in animal models and in humans raises the question of a potential role of those antigens in normal lymphoid cell growth and differentiation.

ACKNOWLEDGMENTS

This work was supported by Public Health Service grants CA-25583, CA-28999 and CA-27890 from the National Cancer Institute. The excellent technical assistance of Mantley Dorsey, Jr. and Lynn Herbert is gratefully acknowledged. We thank Wynn Howard for typing this manuscript.

REFERENCES

1. H. B. Andervont, The influence of foster nursing upon the incidence of of spontaneous mammary cancer in resistant and susceptible mice, J. Natl. Cancer Inst. 1:147 (1940).
2. J. C. Cohen, P. R. Shank, V. L. Morris, R. Cardiff, and H. E. Varmus, Integration of the DNA of mouse mammary tumor virus in virus-infected normal and neoplastic tissue of the mouse, Cell 16:333 (1979).
3. P. Hageman, J. Calafat, and J. H. Daams, The mouse mammary tumor viruses, in: "RNA Viruses and Host Genome in Oncogenesis," P. Emmelot and P. Bentvelzen, eds., North-Holland Publishing Company, Amsterdam and London (1972).
4. D. Medina and K. B. DeOme, Response of hyperplastic alveolar nodule outgrowth line D1 to mammary tumor virus, nodule-inducing virus and prolonged humoral stimulation acting singly and in combination, J. Natl. Cancer Inst. 42:303 (1969).
5. D. M. Lopez, M. M. Sigel, and V. Charyulu, Kinetics of responses to tumor antigens and mouse mammary tumor virus in BALB/cCrgl and BALB/cfC3H mice, J. Natl. Cancer Inst. 66:191 (1981).
6. M. M. Sigel, D. M. Lopez, and G. Ortiz-Muniz, In vitro immune responses

to viral and tumor antigens in murine breast cancer, Cancer Res. 36:748 (1976).

7. D. M. Lopez, V. Charyulu, and M. M. Sigel, Subset of spleen lymphocytes from BALB/cCrgl mice stimulated by mouse mammary tumor virus, Cancer Res. 41:813 (1981).

8. D. M. Lopez and R. D. Paul, Analysis of the lymphoid cells responding to viral and tumor associated antigens in spleens of syngeneic mouse mammary tumor systems with low and high oncogenic potentials, J. Natl. Cancer Inst. 69:1403 (1982).

9. M. M. Sigel, D. M. Lopez, and G. Ortiz-Muniz, Migration inhibition and blastogenic reactions with viral and tumor antigens in transplantable mammary tumor systems, Annals N.Y. Acad. Sci. 276:358 (1976).

10. V. Charyulu, M. S. Sigel, D. L. Durden, and D. M. Lopez, Mouse mammary tumor virus (MMTV) antigen(s) are present in B lymphocytes of BALB/c mice, Int. J. Cancer 24:813 (1979).

11. D. M. Lopez, M. M. Sigel, V. Charyulu, G. Ortiz-Muniz, J. Schlom, and B. Lozzio, Cell-mediated immunity to MMTV antigen(s): its relevance to host defenses against mammary tumors, in: "Advances in Breast Cancer Research," M. J. Brennan, C. M. McGrath, M.A. Rich, eds., Academic Press, New York (1979).

12. J. C. Cohen and H. E. Varmus, Endogenous mammary tumor virus DNA varies among wild mice and segregates during inbreeding, Nature 278:418 (1979).

13. J. C. Cohen, J. E. Majors, and H. E. Varmus, Organization of mouse mammary tumor virus-specific DNA endogenous to BALB/c mice, J. Virol. 32:483 (1979).

14. V. L. Traina, B. A. Taylor, and J. C. Cohen, Genetic mapping of endogenous mouse mammary tumor viruses: locus characterization, segregation and chromosomal distribution, J. Virol. 40:735 (1981).

15. V. Traina-Dorge and J. C. Cohen, Molecular genetics of mouse mammary tumor virus, Current Topics in Microbiology and Immunology 106:35 (1983).

16. B. Groner, E. Buetti, H. Diggelmann, and N. E. Hynes, Characterization of endogenous and exogenous mouse mammary tumor virus proviral DNA with site-specific molecular clones, J. Virol. 36:734 (1980).

17. R. J. Pauley, W. P. Parks, and B. J. Popko, Expression and demethylation of germinally-transmitted BALB/c mouse mammary tumor virus DNA in Abelson MuLV B-lymphoid cell lines, Virus Research (1984, in press).

18. B. J. Popko and R. J. Pauley, Organization and expression of mouse mammary tumor virus sequences in normal and neoplastic C3Hf/HeSed Tissues, J. Virol. 50:328 (1984).

19. R. J. Pauley, D. Medina, and S. H. Socher, Murine mammary tumor virus expression during mammary tumorigenesis in BALB/c mice, J. Virol. 29:483 (1979).

20. J. P. Dudley and H. E. Varmus, Purification and translation of murine mammary tumor virus mRNAs, J. Virol. 39:207 (1981).

21. D. L. Robertson and H. E. Varmus, Structural analysis of the intracellular RNAs of murine mammary tumor virus, J. Virol. 30:576 (1979).

22. D. A. Wheeler, J. S. Butel, D. Medina, R. D. Cardiff, and G. L. Hager, Transcription of mouse mammary tumor virus: identification of a candidate mRNA for the long terminal repeat gene product, J. Virol. 46:42 (1983).

23. B. A. Taylor, Recombinant inbred strains: use in gene mapping, in: "Origins of Inbred Mice," H. Morse, ed., Academic Press, New York (1978).

24. M. M. Black, D. H. Moore, B. Shore, R. E. Zachrau, and H. P. Leis, Jr., Effect of murine milk samples and human breast tissues on human leukocyte migration indices, Cancer Res. 34:1054 (1974).

25. C. L. Wiseman, J. M. Bowen, J. M. Davis, E. M. Hersh, B. W. Brown, and G. R. Blumenschein, Human lymphocyte blastogenesis responses to mouse

mammary tumor virus, J. Natl. Cancer Inst. 64:425 (1980).

26. N. K. Day, S. S. Witkin, N. H. Sarkar, D. Kinne, D. J. Jussawalla, A. Levin, C. C. Hsia, N. Geller, and R. A. Good, Antibodies reactive with murine mammary tumor virus in sera of patients with breast cancer: geographic and family studies, Proc. Natl. Acad. Sci. U.S.A. 78:2483 (1981).

27. D. M. Lopez, W. P. Parks, M. a. Silverman, and J. A. Distasio, Lymphoproliferative responses to mouse mammary tumor virus in lymphocyte subsets of breast cancer patients, J. Natl. Cancer Inst. 67:353 (1981).

28. J. L. McCoy, A. Tagliabue, R. E. Ames, Y. A. Teramoto, G. B. Cannon, C. Alford, R. B. Herberman, and J. Schlom, Indirect leukocyte migration inhibition in breast cancer and benign breast disease patients by mouse mammary tumor virus grown in feline kidney cells, J. Natl. Cancer Inst. 72:569 (1984).

29. D. H. Moore, J. Charney, B. Kramarsky, E. Y. Lasfargues, N. H. Sarkar, M. J. Brennan, J. H. Burrows, S. M. Sirsat, J. C. Paymaster, and A. B. Waidya, Search for a human breast cancer virus, Nature 229:611 (1971).

30. R. Mesa-Tejada, I. Keydar, M. Ramanarayan, T. Ohno, C. Fenoglio, and S. Spiegelman, Detection in human breast carcinomas of an antigen immunologically related to a group-specific antigen of mouse mammary tumor virus, Proc. Natl. Acad. Sci. 75:1529 (1978).

31. A. S. Dion, D. C. Farwell, A. A. Pomenti, and A. J. Girardi, A human protein related to the major envelope protein of murine mammary tumor virus: identification and characterization, Proc. Natl. Acad. Sci. 77:1301 (1980).

32. R. Callahan, W. Drohan, S. Tronick, and J. Schlom, Detection and cloning of human DNA sequences related to the mouse mammary tumor virus genome, Proc. Natl. Acad. Sci. 79:5503 (1982).

33. F. E. May, B. R. Westley, H. Rockefort, E. Buetti, and H. Diggelman, Mouse mammary tumor virus related sequences are present in human DNA, Nucleic Acids Res. 11:4127 (1983).

34. R. J. Massey, L. O. Arthur, R. C. Nowinski, and G. Schochetman, Monoclonal antibodies identify individual determinants on mouse mammary tumor virus glycoprotein gp52 with group, class or type specificity, J. Virol. 34:635 (1980).

MOUSE MAMMARY TUMOR VIRUS AND HUMAN BREAST CANCER: RELATIONSHIP OF PRESENCE OF gp52 IN BREAST TISSUE TO CIRCULATING ANTIBODY TO MuMTV

Katsuhiko Machida[1], Maxine Watson[1], Hideki Teshima[2], Kokichi Kikuchi[3], Lien Shou[4], Ambrose Wasunna[5], Frank Gatchell[6], Karl Boatman[7], Robert A. Good[8], and Noorbibi K. Day

[1]Oklahoma Medical Research Foundation, Oklahoma City, OK
[2]Kyushu University, Fukuoka, Japan; [3]Sapporo Medical College Sapporo, Japan; [4]National Defense Medical Center, Taipei, Taiwan; [5]Kenyatta Hospital, Nairobi, Kenya; [6]Presbyterian Hospital, Oklahoma City, OK; [7]Baptist Medical Center, Oklahoma City, OK, [8]University of South Florida College of Medicine, Department of Pediatrics/St. Petersburg, St. Petersburg, FL

INTRODUCTION

Prior investigations involving cellular immune responses, morphological studies and molecular hybridization analyses have suggested a link between mouse mammary tumor virus (MuMTV) and human breast cancer (1,2). With new methods developed in our laboratory for complement-dependent antibody specific release of reverse transcriptase from lysed virus (3) or binding of IgG to the purified MuMTV particles by an enzyme linked immunoassay, we have shown that 25-30% of sera of breast cancer patients in America have antibodies to MuMTV. Frequency of occurrence of positive antibody titers among breast cancer patients is differently distributed around the world (4). We have also shown that human breast cyst fluids contain low concentrations of IgG and IgA (5). The IgA:IgG ratios in individual breast cyst fluids ranged from 1:0.6 to 1:4. These levels are considerably higher than their ratio in serum (1:7). IgA from 33% of the breast cyst fluids examined and IgG from 10% of the fluids reacted with MuMTV. Antigen reactive with antiserum of MuMTV core protein p28 was located in a 165,000 g pellet of breast cyst fluids (6). Particles resembling the cores of retroviruses were observed in fractions having a buoyant density of 1.24 g/ml (6). These fractions also possessed DNA polymerase activity and reacted with MuMTV p28 antiserum, but not with murine leukemia virus p30 antiserum (6). We also found that among the families studied in which breast cancer occurred with high frequency antibody to MuMTV was present among family members (4). In the present study we have extended our previous observations of familial breast cancer to 20 families. In addition, we have studied the relationship of circulating antibody levels to MuMTV in human breast cancer to the presence of gp52 antigen in breast tissue obtained from the same patient.

MATERIAL AND METHODS

Patient Population

Breast cancer patients and their family members used for our study

were as follows: a) 62 breast cancer patients who were from families where breast cancer occurred with high frequency according to the family history; b) 107 breast cancer patients without a family history of breast cancer; c) 84 family members without breast cancer (45 females and 39 males) of 20 breast cancer patients obtained from a); and d) 218 healthy female and 42 male controls without a family history of breast cancer. The majority of American participants were residents of Oklahoma. In addition, paired samples, i.e., breast tissue and blood obtained from women with breast cancer (16 American, 11 Taiwanese, 4 Japanese and 3 East African) were included in the study.

Serum Samples

Blood samples (10-15 ml) without anticoagulants were drawn under sterile conditions and the separation of sera was performed by previously described methods (7), divided into 300 µl aliquots and stored at-70°C until used.

Virus and Viral Components

MuMTV (0.35 mg of protein/ml, Lot 1400) derived from Mm5mt/Cl cells and purified by sucrose density gradient centrifugation was obtained from Frederick Cancer Research Center, Bethesda, Maryland. The isolation of gp52 and p27 from virus was performed according to published procedures (8,9,10).

Titrations of Antibody to MuMTV by Enzyme Linked Immunosorbent Assay (ELISA)

Sera were assayed using ELISA for antibody reaction with MuMTV according to methods described previously (3,11).

Radioimmunoassay (RIA) for Detection of gp52 Antigen in Serum

gp52 was first isolated from MuMTV by column chromatography according to the method of Marcus et al. (8). The final product gave a single band on PAGE. Monospecific antibody to purified gp52 was raised in rabbits. The RIA was carried out using ^{125}I gp52 as follows: 100 µl of test sera was added to 200 µl of rabbit anti-gp52 antibody (final dilution 1:5,000) and incubated for four hours at room temperature. Next 100 µl of ^{125}I (18,000 cpm) was added to each sample and the mixtures were incubated for four hours at room temperature. 90 µg of rabbit IgG (Cappel) was next added to each tube followed by the addition of 500 µl of appropriately diluted goat antirabbit IgG and the mixtures were incubated at 4°C overnight. The precipitated protein was pelleted by centrifugation for ten minutes at 2000 rpm in a Beckman JB-6 centrifuge, and the resulting pellet was washed twice with 0.1M phosphate buffered saline (pH 7.0). The radioactive iodine in the precipitate was counted directly in a gamma spectrometer. Serial dilutions of unlabeled gp52 (0.01-100 ng) were used to determine the standard content of gp52 in the solution. The content of gp52 in the serum sample was estimated from comparison with this standard curve of unlabeled gp52. To check the effects of antibody to MuMTV in human sera on this radioimmunoassay system, immunoglobulins in human sera were absorbed with rabbit IgG against human IgM, IgG and IgA (Cappel). 200 µl of human serum was added to the 200 µl of rabbit IgG against human immunoglobulins and incubated at 37°C for two hours at 4°C overnight. The resulting precipitate was removed by centrifugation. The supernatant was tested by radioimmunoassay and the result compared with one of the unabsorbed samples.

Immunohistochemical Staining

The immunohistochemical staining of human breast cancer tissue was performed using methods described by Keydar et al. (12) and Heyderman and

Neille (13) with minor modifications. The dewaxed sections were treated with the following chemicals to suppress endogenous peroxidase activity: 1M periodic acid in distilled water was applied for five minutes, and 0.02% fresh sodium borohydrate in water was applied for two minutes. After each treatment, the sections were washed with water for five minutes. The sections were incubated with normal sheep serum (1:10 in 1% bovine serum albumin) at room temperature for 20 minutes. After a gentle rinse in 0.01M PBS-T for 15 minutes, the sections were incubated with the primary antibodies (rabbit antibody to MuMTV or rabbit antibody to gp52 at 50 μg/ml in 0.01M PBS) for 45 minutes at room temperature. After three washes for five minutes each with 0.01M PBS, sheep antibody to rabbit IgG (1:20 diluted with PBS) was applied for 45 minutes at room temperature. After washing as before, the sections were submerged for ten minutes at room temperature in a saturated solution of 3,3'-diaminobenzidine (Sigma, 50 mg of free base in 100 ml of PBS) to which hydrogen peroxide (0.003%) had been added just prior to use. The sections were then washed, sometimes lightly counterstained in diluted methylene blue, dehydrated in graded alcohols and xylene, and mounted with Permount.

Analysis of Results

The results of antibody analyses against MuMTV are expressed (a) as the mean of individual values of antibody to MuMTV in each group and (b) as the percentage of individuals in each group with increased levels of antibody to MuMTV at 1:30 dilution of sera. In previous studies, 98% of 50 healthy women in New York showed values below 0.400 by ELISA. We used identical methods of analysis in the present study as described previously and the sera that showed over 0.400 by ELISA were considered to have an increased level of antibody to MuMTV. The two-sample test was used to detect differences between mean MuMTV antibody levels of each group.

RESULTS AND DISCUSSION

Study of Circulating MuMTV Antibody Levels in Sera by Breast Cancer Patients in Oklahoma

Twenty-three percent of patients with breast cancer (176 studied) had circulating antibody to MuMTV compared to 8% of the healthy population (260 individuals) p = 0.001.

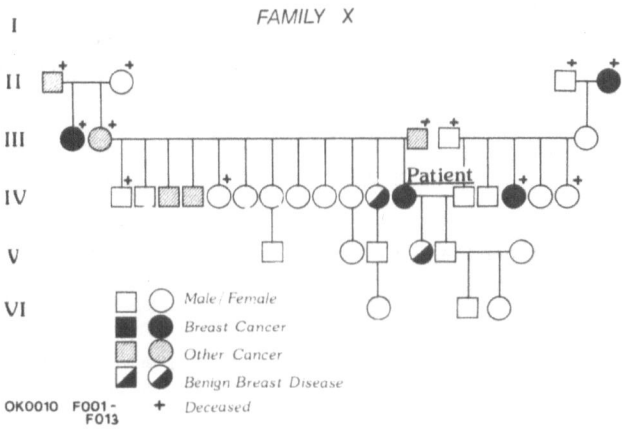

Figure 1. Pedigree of a Patient with Breast Cancer

Study of MuMTV Antibody Levels in Sera of Healthy Family Members of Patients with Familial Breast Cancer

Family of 20 families with familial breast cancer were studied. A typical pedigree is shown in Figure 1. A significantly higher percentage of female members (43%) when compared with male members (23%) had elevated levels of antibody to MuMTV. Nine of 13 daughters (69%), four of ten sons (40%), ten of 16 sisters (63%) and one of five brothers (20%) showed elevated levels of MuMTV antibody in their sera. These results indicate that the presence of antibody to MuMTV may be related to hormonal influences (14,15), antigenic stimulation, and/or sex chromosome linked immune response genes or other factors. The specificity of the antibody in these studies was determined as described previously (3).

Levels of Circulating Antigen to gp52 in Human Breast Cancer Sera

Using a competitive radioimmunoassay and purified gp52 we established a method for the detection of circulating antigen to gp52 in human breast cancer. The sensitivity of the test was 3 ng. the interference of the antibody to MuMTV was below ten percent when absorbed sera were used and their values compared with unabsorbed sera. Our results using the above methods showed that no differences were observed in any of the different categories of sera tested including controls. Ritzi et al. (16) have shown that plasma of C3H/HeJ mice bearing mammary tumors had high levels of gp52 (over 100 ng/ml) when compared with plasma of non-tumor bearing mice (<10 ng/ml). They also showed that ^{125}I gp52 injected intravenously into mice was quickly removed from the circulation. It is possible in our experiments that either the methods we have used are not sensitive enough, or the antigens related to MuMTV are trapped by phagocytes, lymphocytes or other cells and hence undetectable in the circulation.

Presence of gp52 Antigen in Breast Cancer Tissue

Using a polyclonal antibody and/or monoclonal antibody to gp52 and whole virus, a total of 34 paired samples of tissue and sera obtained from the same individual (16 American, 11 Taiwanese, four Japanese and three East African) with breast cancer were studied. Table 1 shows the results obtained. Four of 18 patients that had gp52 related antigens in the sections of breast tissue also had low levels of circulating antibody. To date, we have not detected the presence of gp52 antigen in tissue in association with elevated levels of antibody to MuMTV in sera. Although the number of patients in this study is still small, the results have been consistent. Based on the above observation, it is attractive to postulate that the circulating antibody is either absorbed to antigen present in the tissue and hence the antigen is not detectable by an immunohistochemical technique or the circulating antibody is complexed to circulating antigen, thus making it difficult with the techniques used to detect antibody in the circulation. These questions are currently under investigation.

CONCLUSIONS

1. Studies in Oklahoma and prior studies from New York show that approximately one quarter of breast cancer patients have increased levels of antibody to MuMTV.

2. Some breast cancer patients from Oklahoma, as well as those from New York frequently have pg52 antigen demonstrable in the breast cancer tissue.

Table 1. Relationship Between the Presence of gp52 Antigen in Breast
Tissue and Circulating Antibodies Against MuMTV

Antigen*/Antibody**	American	Japanese	Taiwan	African
Ag-positive/Ab low level (in breast tissue)	4/18(22%)***	0/4	0/11	0/3
Ag-positive/Ab high level	0/18	0/4	0/11	0/3
Ag-negative/Ab low level	12/18(67%)	2/4(50%)	4/11(36%)	0/3
Ag-negative/Ab high level	2/18(11%)	2/4(50%)	7/11(64%)	3/3(100%)

* Detection of antigen (gp52) in tissue = performed by immunoperoxidase
staining.
** Levels of anti-MuMTV = measured by enzyme linked immunosorbent assay.
Low level is below 0.400 and high level is over 0.400 by ELISA.
***Top number = number of patients in category. Bottom number = number of
patients in study.
Parenthesis = % of persons per category

3. Healthy members of breast cancer families often had increased antibody titer to MuMTV and healthy females in these families had increased
titers more frequently than males.

4. gp52 antigen was not readily demonstrated in any breast cancer
sera tested.

5. In studies of women with breast cancer, the presence of demonstrable
gp52 antigen in the tissues was associated with low titers of anti-MuMTV
antibody in the sera.

ACKNOWLEDGMENTS

This work was supported in part by Public Health Service Grant CA-34016
awarded by the National Cancer Institute, the New-Land Foundation, and The
Eleanor Naylor Dana Trust.

REFERENCES

1. A. B. Vaidya, M. M. Black, A. S. Dion, and D. H. Moore, Homology
    between human breast tumor RNA and mouse mammary tumor virus genome,
    Nature (London) 249:565 (1974).
2. S. Spiegelman, I. Keydar, R. Mesa-Tejada, T. Ohno, M. Ramamarayaman, R.
    Nayak, J. Bausch, and C. Fenoglio, Possible diagnostic implications
    of a mammary tumor virus related protein in human breast cancer,
    Cancer 46:879 (1981).
3. S. S. Witkin, R. A. Egeli, N. H. Sarkar, R. A. Good, and N. K. Day,
    Virolysis of mouse mammary tumor virus by sera from breast cancer
    patients, Proc. Natl. Acad. Sci. U.S.A. 76:2984 (1979).
4. N. K. Day, S. S. Witkin, N. H. Sarkar, D. Kinne, D. J. Jussawalla, A.

Levin, C. C. Hsia, N. Geller, and R. A. Good, Antibodies reactive with murine mammary tumor virus in sera of patients with breast cancer: geographic and family studies, <u>Proc</u>. <u>Natl</u>. <u>Acad</u>. <u>Sci</u>. <u>U.S.A.</u> 78:2483 (1981).

5. S. S. Witkin, N. H. Sarkar, D. W. Kinne, R. A. Good, and N. K. Day, Antibodies reactive with the mouse mammary tumor virus in sera of breast cancer patients, <u>Intl</u>. <u>J</u>. <u>Cancer</u> 25:721 (1980).

6. S. S. Witkin, N. H. Sarkar, D. W. Kinne, C. N. Bread, R. A. Good, and N. K. Day, Antigens and antibodies cross-reactive to the murine mammary tumor virus in human breast cyst fluid, <u>J</u>. <u>Clin</u>. <u>Invest</u>. 67:216 (1981).

7. N. K. Day, J. B. Winfield, J. B. Winchester, T. Gee, H. Teshima, and H. G. Kunkel, Evidence for immune complexes involving antilymphocyte antibodies associated with hypocomplementaemia in chronic lymphocytic leukemia (CLL), <u>Clin</u>. <u>Exp</u>. <u>Immunol</u>. 26:189 (1976).

8. S. L. Marcus, R. Kopelman, and N. H. Sarkar, Simultaneous purification of murine mammary tumor virus structure proteins: analysis of antigenic reactivities of native gp34 by radioimmunocompetition assay, <u>J</u>. <u>Virol</u>. 31:341 (1979).

9. N. H. Sarkar, A. A. Pomenti, and A. S. Dion, Replication of mouse mammary tumor virus in tissue culture I. Establishment of a mouse mammary tumor cell line, virus characterization and quantitation of virus production, <u>Virology</u> 77:12 (1977).

10. E. Ritzi, A. Baldi, and S. Spiegelman, The purification of a gs antigen of the murine mammary tumor virus and its quantitation by radioimmuno-assay, <u>Virology</u> 75:188 (1976).

11. S. S. Witkin, N. H. Sarkar, R. A. Good, and N. K. Day, An enzyme-linked immunoassay for the detection of antibodies to the mouse mammary tumor virus: application to human breast cancer, <u>J</u>. <u>Immunol</u>. <u>Methods</u> 32:85 (1980).

12. I. Keydar, R. Mesa-Tejada, M. Ramamarayaman, T. Ohno, C. Fenoglio, R. Hu, and S. Spiegelman, Detection of viral proteins in mouse mammary tumor by immunoperoxidase staining of paraffin sections, <u>Proc</u>. <u>Natl</u>. <u>Acad</u>. <u>Sci</u>. <u>U.S.A.</u> 76:1524 (1978).

13. E. Heyderman and A. M. Nenille, A shorter immunoperoxidase technique for the demonstration of carcinoembryonic antigen and other cell products, <u>J</u>. <u>Clin</u>. <u>Path</u>. 30:138 (1977).

14. M. P. Osborne, P. P. Rosen, M. L. Lesser, M. R. Schwartz, C. J. Menendez-Botet, J. H. Fishman, D. W. Kinne, and E. J. Beattie, The relationship between family history, exposure to exogenous hormones, and estrogen receptor protein in breast cancer, <u>Cancer</u> 51:2134 (1983).

15. L. D. Cowan, L. Gordis, J. A. Tonascia, and G. S. Jones, Breast cancer incidence in women with a history of progesterone deficiency, <u>Amer</u>. <u>J</u>. <u>Epidemiol</u>. 114:209 (1981).

16. E. Ritzi, D. S. Martin, R. L. Storfi, and S. Spiegelman, Plasma levels of a viral protein as a diagnostic signal for the presence of tumor: the murine mammary tumor model, <u>Proc</u>. <u>Natl</u>. <u>Acad</u>. <u>Sci</u>. <u>U.S.A.</u> 73:4190 (1976).

RETROVIRUS-INDUCED IMMUNODEFICIENCY IN MICE

Mauro Bendinelli, Donatella Matteucci, and Antonio Toniolo

Institute of Epidemiology, Hygiene and Virology and
Institute of Microbiology, University of Pisa, Pisa, Italy

INTRODUCTION

In the 25 years that have elapsed since the Friend murine leukemia complex (FLC) was first reported to be immunodepressive in mice (1), many different retroviruses, both acutely and slowly tumorigenic, have been etiologically linked with the occurrence of immunodeficiency in a variety of naturally and experimentally infected hosts, including man (Table 1). The mechanisms whereby the immunodepressive changes are brought about by such viruses remain, however, largely unknown.

Just as individual retroviruses may transform different cell types, it is likely that they impair the immune system by different routes. There are no doubts, however, that knowing in one model system the precise cellular and subcellar mechanisms which lead to immunodeficiency would represent a considerable step forward in the understanding of retrovirus-induced immunodeficiency in general and in the development of appropriate therapeutic strategies. At least two thirds of the literature generated so far in the field deal with the murine system and with FLC in particular (2,3). Though even in this highly investigated model the general picture still looks blurred, a critical appraisal of the many interesting points that have been established seems worthwhile. A complete coverage of the abundant findings in this expanding area is, however, beyond the scope of this article.

THE MODEL

The reasons why FLC (there are two main forms of FLC, anemia- or polycythemia-inducing, but their immunodepressive effects are seemingly alike) has been the preferred model for the study of retrovirus-induced immunodeficiency are manyfold (4). To us, a major reason of interest has been the opportunity of comparing the immunodepressive action of the slowly tumorigenic helper virus with that of the acutely tumorigenic entire complex. It is well known that FLC is composed by a defective component (SFFV) and a replication-competent helper virus (F-MuLV), whose leukemogenic effects have been the subject of extensive investigation (5). Very briefly, in susceptible mice such as BALB/c strain FLC causes an early erythroblastosis of the spleen which is followed by the development of erythroleukemia in five to seven weeks, whereas F-MuLV induces an early mild hyperplasia of the spleen and lymphatic leukemias in seven to ten months.

Table 1. A List of Retroviruses That Have Been Etiologically
Linked to Immunodeficiency

Host	Chronic Viruses	Acute Viruses
Chicken	Avian leukosis virus (various subgroups)	Avian erythroblastosis virus Avian myeloblastosis virus Avian sarcoma virus Reticuloendotheliosis virus
Mouse	Murine leukemia virus (AKR, Friend, Graffi, Gross, Moloney, DMBA, 334C), murine mammary tumor virus	Friend leukemia complex Rauscher leukemia complex Murine sarcoma virus
Rat	Murine leukemia virus (Moloney)	
Cat	Feline leukemia virus	
Baboon	Baboon endogenous virus	
Macaque	Mason-Pfizer monkey virus, other type D retroviruses	
Man	Human T lymphotropic virus-3/ Lymphadenopathy-associated virus	

Table 2 summarizes the effects of FLC and F-MuLV on the immunological
reactivity of leukemia susceptible mice. As established by a number of
investigations, in either infection the extent of immunological impairment
observed is influenced by many variables including the host's genotype, the
dose of the infecting virus, the nature and the dose of the antigen used to
monitor the immunoresponsiveness. Another factor of major importance is
the part of the immune system which is involved in the response and consequently the route of antigen administration, the spleen representing the
organ which is by far more affected by either infection. The reasons for
this compartmentalization have not been extensively studied and a limitation of most data discussed in the following sections is that they have
been obtained working almost exclusively with spleen cells. Furthermore,
in both infections ongoing immune responses as well as established immunity
are relatively spared, and a number of data point to the conclusion that
the immunologic events most intensively impaired are those related to the
inductive stages of humoral and cell-mediated responses.

Animals infected with either viral preparation also exhibit a highly
enhanced susceptibility to superinfecting bacteria and viruses (Table 3).
In addition, the lesions produced by infectious agents in such animals may
be considerably different from those produced by the same agents in intact
animals; for example, an absence of inflammatory cell infiltration has been
noticed (unpublished observations).

However, as shown by Table 2, the immunodepression induced by F-MuLV
shares with that induced by FLC only those manifestations that are already

Table 2. Effects of FLC and F-MuLV on Major Parameters of Immunological Responsiveness in BALB/c Mice (2,4,6).

Parameter	FLC	F-MuLV
Background antibody production	reduced (D)[a]	unchanged
Primary antibody responsiveness	reduced (E)[b]	reduced
Secondary antibody responsiveness	reduced (E)	reduced
Immunological maturation	reduced (D)	reduced
Delayed hypersensitivity	reduced (D)	NT[c]
Contact sensitivity	reduced (D)	unchanged
Graft rejection	reduced (D)	NT
T cytotoxic responsiveness	reduced (D)	NT
Resistance to superinfection	reduced	reduced
Resistance to tumor grafts	reduced	NT

[a] D = delayed effect
[b] E = early effect
[c] NT = not tested

present in the early phases of FLC infection. A second major difference (not apparent from Table 2) is that FLC-induced immunodepression progresses until the animals succumb (though it may wane in infections sustained by regressing strains of FLC), whereas F-MuLV-induced immunodepression is very profound in the early stages of infection, but subsequently gradually subsides and the responsiveness stabilizes at about half the normal values for the life span of the infected mice. This, coupled with the fact that the titer of the helper virus exceeds that of the defective component by ten to 100-fold, has lead us to attribute an important role to F-MuLV in the overall early immunodepressive effects of the entire complex, and to consider the rapid leukemic changes that develop following FLC infection a major cause for the observed differences. Evidence from other systems also indicates that helper viruses can play a pivotal role in the immunosuppressive role of oncoviral complexes (7).

Additional findings relevant to the following discussion are that: 1) cell-mediated responses appear not to be significantly affected by F-MuLV and to be depressed by FLC appreciably later than humoral responses; 2) antibody responses to T-independent antigens are relatively little affected as compared to T-dependent antibody responses: 3) inoculation of a B cell mitogen such as LPS together with the antigen brings T-dependent antibody response to normal or near-normal levels. Though the latter effect is less evident in mice infected with FLC than in F-MuLV-infected animals, the result is important because it also says that the immunodepression induced by such viruses is at least partly reversible.

CELLULAR BASIS

Much work has been devoted to the study of the cellular deficits responsible for the reduced immunoresponsiveness of FLC and F-MuLV-infected mice.

Table 3. Effect of FLC and F-MuLV on the Susceptibility of Mice to Some Superinfecting Agents

| Superinfection[a] | | Mortality in Mice Pretreated with | | | | | |
| Agent | Dose (CFU or PFU) | No Virus | | FLC | | F-MuLV | |
		%	MDD[b]	%	MDD	%	MDD
S. typhimurium	1.6×10^2	0	-	71	10	100	7
	1.6×10	0	-	37	6	100	7
Ps. aeruginosa	1.3×10^5	0	-	43	2	71	2
Coxsackie B3	3.0×10^7	87	14	100	10	100	10
EMC virus	3.0×10^3	0	-	30	13	50	8

[a]Leukemia susceptible mice of CD-1 or BALB/c strains were infected with 10^3 FFU (S^+L^-) of F-MuLV or FLC ten days before intraperitoneal challenge with indicated superinfecting agents (10-20 mice per group).
[b]MDD = mean day of death

Tables 4-6 summarize the data bearing on the functionality of single immuno-competent cell classes as emerged from such studies. Due to the high level of integration existing within the immune response system, a general problem with these kinds of data is that one cannot be certain that a given change observed is intrinsic to the cell type affected or rather reflects altera-tions of other cell types. This limitation, together with the existence of conflicting reports (all but rare in cellular immunology), makes available information on the cellular basis of the immunodeficiency difficult to interpret.

Thus, it has yet proven impossible to establish which of the changes observed pertain in a critical way to the genesis of the immunodeficiency and which merely represent side effects. The problem is compounded as it is likely that multiple cellular pathways converge in the generation of the immunodeficiency and assume different weight depending on variables such as

Table 4. Effect of FLC and F-MuLV Infections on Some T Cell Functions (6,8,9).

Function	FLC	F-MuLV
Antigen-driven blastogenesis	reduced	unchanged
Antigen-driven MIF production	reduced	unchanged
Expression of cytotoxic activity	reduced	NT
Acquisition of cytotoxic potential	reduced	NT
Mitogen-driven blastogenesis	reduced	unchanged
Help to T-dependent antibody responses	NT	unchanged
Expression of Thy-1 antigen	reduced	reduced

NT = not tested

Table 5. Effect of FLC and F-MuLV Infections on Some B Cell Functions
(9,10,11)

Function		FLC	F-MuLV
In vitro antibody responses	T-dep.	strongly reduced	
	T-indep.	reduced	
Ongoing antibody synthesis		reduced	unchanged
Antibody secretion		unchanged	NT
Antigen binding		unchanged	NT
LPS blastogenesis		reduced	unchanged
Surface Ig expression		reduced	
Surface Ig capping		reduced	

NT = not tested.

the time interval from the initiation of infection. The following generalizations seem, however, possible:

1. Both inducer and effector functions of T lymphocytes do not appear
to be grossly altered by F-MuLV. By contrast, substantial damages of in
vitro correlates of cell-mediated responses have been documented in FLC-infected mice (Table 4). However, similar to the depression of cell-mediated
responses of intact mice, the latter changes develop later than the depression of the antibody response and may, in part at least, be secondary to
the development of neoplasia. The reduced expression of Thy-1 antigen (as
measured by the binding of fluoresceinated antibody) which has been observed
in animals infected with either viral preparation (9), does not seem to
correlate with significant functional derangements. T cells exert some of
their activities through the secretion of diffusible factors. Nevertheless,
in preliminary studies we have detected no changes in the production of,
and in the response to IL-2 following FLC and F-MuLV infections.

2. B cell functions show substantial alterations (Table 5). However,
findings that the reduced antibody responsiveness to T-dependent antigens
of F-MuLV-infected mice is overcome, both in vivo and in vitro, by simple
manipulations such as the administration of a polyclonal B cell mitogen
(12) or of exogenous macrophages (13) suggest that B cells are not irrever-
sibly damaged. Thus, their functional deficit might reflect an intrinsic
disturbance of B cells (such as, for example, an elevation of the threshold
for activation which, in turn, might be correlated with the reduced expression of antigen receptors (9), but might also be due to defects of other
elements needed for their triggering or regulation.

In keeping with the latter possibility, several functions of B lymphocytes which are independent of the cooperation of other cell types, such
as the binding of erythrocyte antigens (10) and the secretion of antibody
(2), were found to be appreciably disturbed only in leukemic FLC-infected
mice. On the other hand, findings that ongoing antibody responses and LPS
blastogenesis are depressed in leukemic animals (2,4) indicate that considerable siderable damage of potential antibody-forming cells in the spleen
or of their precursors in the bone marrow may be produced by the neoplastic
process.

3. As clearly shown by cross-recombination experiments (13), macrophages present a prompt and consistent loss of their ability to cooperate

Table 6. Effect of FLC and F-MuLV Infections on Some Macrophage
Functions (13).

nonimmune phagocytosis	unchanged	unchanged
Fc-dependent phagocytosis	conflicting data	unchanged
expression of Fc receptors	unchanged	unchanged
spread on surfaces	reduced	unchanged
motility on surfaces	reduced	NT
killing of ingested bacteria	reduced	NT
cooperation in antibody response	reduced	reduced
negative regulation of antibody response	unchanged	unchanged

NT = not tested.

normally with lymphocytes in the generation of antibody responses. Reportedly, in FLC-infected mice these cells exhibit a number of additional dys-
functions (Table 6), but many such data are open to criticism on the ground
that the viral preparations used were not shown to be free of LDH virus, a
contaminant known to impair the reticuloendothelial system selectively.

The impairment of the accessory functions of macrophages has been well
documented both in FLC and F-MuLV-infected mice. However, while the addition
of few a exogenous macrophages effectively restored the antibody responsiveness of F-MuLV-infected spleen cells in vitro and in vivo, the same treatment was much less effective in the case of FLC-infected mice. This again
suggests that additional mechanisms may be operative and, possibly, dominant
in the course of FLC infection. Whether such additional mechanisms are
exclusively linked to the rapid leukemogenic activity of FLC remains to be
determined.

Indirect evidence indicates that in F-MuLV-infected mice it is the
preparation of antigen for presentation to lymphocytes that is impaired
(13). Although it has recently been suggested that macrophages of FLC-infected mice produce reduced amounts of "antibody response helper factors,"
(14) we have found no defects in the ability of FLC and F-MuLV-infected
spleen cells to produce IL-1 constitutively or in response to LPS stimulation in vitro (data not shown). The expression of Ia-antigen by such cells
in infected mice has yet to be investigated.

4. Suppressor cells have been identified as important determinants in
the genesis of immunodeficiency in general. However, existing data tend to
exclude the activation of professional suppressor cells as a major factor
contributing to the immunodepression induced by FLC and F-MuLV. Although
spleen cells of both FLC and F-MuLv-infected mice were shown to suppress
the antibody response of normal lymphoid cultures, the cells responsible
for such effect were identified as virus-producing B cells or as leukemia
cells whose action appeared to be mediated by virus-related products (see
below). In fact, there are data suggesting that FLC infection may damage T
suppressor cells or their precursors (15). Recently, macrophage-like cells
have been implicated in the suppression of normal NK activity which occurs
when FLC-infected spleen cells are admixed in vitro with uninfected lymphoid
cells (16), but further studies are needed to evaluate the significance of
this finding.

5. It is important to stress here that the cells of the immune response
system are not the only effectors involved in bodily defenses which may be
perturbed by infection. Not only NK activity but also the production of

interferon was found to be strongly decreased in FLC-infected mice [17].
Even though these aspects have been little investigated, it appears likely
that other nonspecific effectors of natural resistance may be negatively
influenced by infection. It is clear that any impairment at this level may
be of importance in determining the reduced resistance to superinfection
and tumors exhibited by the infected animals.

MECHANISMS OF IMMUNOCOMPETENT CELL ALTERATION

When considering the possible means whereby a given viral infection
can lead to altered functioning of immunocompetent cells one is faced with
a basic question: are the observed changes caused by a direct interaction
of the infecting virus with the affected cells, or are they generated via
less direct pathways [18]? In the case of FLC and F-MuLV infections, however, the preponderance of available data suggest rather clearly that direct
mechanisms are of paramount importance. Such evidence can be summarized as
follows:

1. Both F-MuLV and SFFV replicate effectively in the immunocompetent
cell classes that appear functionally most compromised by the infection,
that is in B lymphocytes and macrophages [19,20]. Indeed, replication in
the latter cells may begin very early postinfection [20]. In addition, the
permissiveness of B lymphocytes increases following blastogenic activation,
and this may imply that those cells which are actively engaged in immune
responses may be preferentially infected [21]. The imbalance of soluble
thymic factors production that occurs during FLC infection has also been
correlated with a wave of viral replication in the thymus [22];

Table 7. Effect of a Cell-free Preparation of FLC on the Antibody Responsiveness of Normal Lymphoid Cultures[a].

Dose of FLC Added[b]	% Suppression[c]
undiluted	80
10^{-1}	68
10^{-2}	57
10^{-3}	50
10^{-4}	17
undiluted, 1 h at 60°C	45
undiluted, + 10^4 ergs UV	59
undiluted, + anti-FLC mouse serum[d]	13
undiluted, + control mouse serum	67

[a]Spleen cells of BALB/c mice (10^7/culture) were supplemented with
the indicated material, stimulated with 2×10^6 sheep red cells
at time 0, and tested for direct antibody-forming cells (PFC) 5
days later. Four to six cultures per group.
[b]Plasma from three-week infected mice partially purified by
differential centrifugation.
[c]As compared to untreated cultures (control response: 5896± 713
PFC/culture).
[d]Before addition to the cultures, the virus was preincubated with
the indicated serum for 1 h at 37°C. Sera alone had no effects
on the response.

Table 8. Some Indirect Mechanisms Whereby FLC and F-MuLV
Might Derange Immune Functions.

Production of immunoregulatory soluble factors (interferon,
prostaglandins, cytokines, lymphotoxins, etc.)
Antigenic competition
Action of anti-MuLV antibody on immunocompetent cells (27)
Immunocomplexes
Altered lymphocyte circulation
Stress and other disease-associated physiopathological changes

---

2. The already mentioned suppression of antibody response by infected
spleen cells in vitro was found to be mediated by virus-producing cells and
was entirely prevented by the presence of virus-specific antibody (23);

3. The addition of cell-free preparations of virus consistently depressed the responsiveness of normal uninfected cells (Table 7) in a dose-dependent manner (interestingly, a partial purification of the virus was a pre-
requisite for suppression to occur, possibly suggesting the existence of
substances exerting opposite effects in the viral preparations);

4. Structural components of MuLV and other retroviruses have repeatedly been shown to modulate immunocompetent cell behavior very effectively.
For example, virions and semipurified components of FLC and of the related
Rauscher leukemia complex have been shown to enhance spontaneous lymphocyte
blastogenesis and to suppress lymphoproliferative responses to mitogens
(24,25), while disaggregated virions and the protein p15E from several MuLV
have been seen to inhibit macrophage accumulation at sites of inflammation
(26). In line with such findings, in the study summarized in Table 7 heat
and ultraviolet treatments of FLC that abolished the infectivity abated its
suppressive activity only partially.

It should be stressed, however, that direct and indirect mechanisms
are not mutually exclusive. The fact that immunocompetent cell derangement
results from direct interaction with the virus and/or viral product does
not preclude the possibility that indirect mechanisms participate in the
generation of the overall immunodeficiency. For example, there are a
variety of other events linked with infection and disease (Table 8) that
might be conducive to the aberrant activation of immunoregulatory cells and
circuits. Although as already mentioned, no activated professional suppressor cells have been consistently detected in infected animals, the suppression of lymphoproliferative responses exerted by FLC in vitro has been attributed to a complex chain of events ultimately resulting in the activation
of suppressor cells (25). A further suggestion that indirect mechanisms
may indeed play some role in the genesis of FLC-induced immunodeficiency
comes from the failure of virus-rich cell-free preparations and sonicates
of infected cells (Table 9) to reproduce the suppression of NK activity
exerted by infected spleen cells in vitro.

Finally, as already noted, it is conceivable that at least some immunodepressive manifestations observed in the leukemic stages of FLC infection
are secondary to the tumorous process. This might impede the normal development of immune responses not only due to dilution of immunocompetent cells
in the lymphoid organs by the rapidly proliferating neoplastic cells, but
also by a variety of other mechanisms. The production of soluble immunodepressive factors is a likely possibility (29). For example, we have found
that in culture, selected clones and subclones of FLC-transformed cells

Table 9. Suppression of Natural Cytolysis of Uninfected
Splenocytes by FLC-infected Spleen Cells[a]

Infected Cell/ Effector Ratio[b]	% Suppression[c]	
	Viable Cells	Sonicated Cells[d]
3 : 1	64	18
2 : 1	33	12
1 : 1	28	- 4
0.5 : 1	8	-20

[a] 18 h assay against 10^4 YAC-1 cells; E : T = 50.
control specific cytotoxicity: 28 ± 2.
[b] Effectors: splenocytes from five-week old FLC-infected
BALB/c mice. Infected cells: spleen cells from BALB/c
mice infected with FLC 16 days earlier. Filler cells:
uninfected splenocytes precultured for 24 h to abate
their cytotoxic activity; when required, filler cells
were sonicated before addition to effector cells.
[c] Inhibition of lysis as compared to equivalent mixtures of
effector and filler cells.
[d] Three cycles of sonication on ice.

release soluble factors which suppress the development of antibody responses
in vitro and that such effect is entirely unrelated to the production of
infectious virus and of viral envelope glycoprotein gp71 (Table 10).

CONCLUSIONS

In this article we have briefly reviewed our current understanding of
the pathogenesis of the immunodeficiency induced in mice by the viruses of
the FLC. Although the model still contains many unknowns, there are two
major conclusions that, in our opinion, can be safely drawn. One is that,
among the multiple alterations of immunocompetent cells described in the
animals infected with this viral complex, the impairment of antigen presenting cells holds a prominent position. It is tempting to speculate that
such a lesion is a unifying determinant in the genesis of many manifestations
of this immunodepression.

The second is that the direct interaction of the infecting virus with
immunocompetent cells is an important factor in the derangement of the immune
system. Although there are indications that the mere physical contact with
the virions or virion components is sufficient to perturb both lymphocytes
and macrophages, it seems likely that the virus must replicate within them
in order for these cells to become grossly or permanently malfunctioning.
In any case, at least before the onset of neoplasia, indirect mechanisms
(Table 8) appear to play a very secondary role.

It is difficult to say how much these conclusions apply to other forms
of retrovirus-induced immunodeficiency. The moderate impairment of T cells
observed in FLC-infected mice seems to distinguish this from other retrovirus-induced immunodeficiencies whose cellular basis have been investigated.
In several instances the major deficits have been seen to dwell at the level
of T cells (2,3,30), and HTLV-3/LAV, the retrovirus presently thought to be
responsible for AIDS, is cytopathic for the OKT4[+] helper-inducer subset
(31,32).

Table 10. Suppression of Antibody Response in vitro by Culture
Fluids of Individual Subclones of the FLC-transformed
Producer Line 3BM-78 (28).

Supernatant	% Suppression[a]	gp71 (ng P/ml)[b]	F-MuLV (FFU/ml)[c]	SFFV (Foci/ml)[d]
clone 01	18	2,850	195	30
02	60	493	210	30
03	58	2,647	10	15
04	24	1,020	100	15
05	11	6,453	55	0
06	47	1,767	105	TNC[e]
07	17	3,147	10	TNC
08	0	3,266	85	TNC
09	3	3,800	75	0
10	17	11,860	20	63

[a]The supernatants, normalized to contain 10^6 cell/ml, were added to
normal DBA/2 spleen cells stimulated with TNP-horse red blood cells.
The cultures were assayed for anti-TNP antibody-producing cells (PFC)
five days later. Average of three separate experiments; mean control
value: $2,413 \pm 118$ PFC/10^6 cells.
[b]Competition RIP with specific goat anti-FLV gp71.
[c]S^+L^- assay.
[d]Spleen foci produced in DBA/2 mice.
[e]TNC = too numerous to count.

It should be recalled, however, that a large number of retroviruses
infecting widely different animal species have been shown to replicate
effectively in the cells of the monocyte-macrophage lineage (33). Thus,
impairment of the nonspecific, yet necessary, accessory functions performed
by such cells might be a common denominator in the genesis of retro-virus-
induced immunodeficiencies. Macrophages are now known to play a key role
in many retroviral infections (33,34) and, interestingly, in AIDS the pattern of infectious complications suggests severe monocyte defects (35).
However, as taught by the FLC model, the impairment of the fine accessory
functions of macrophages might occur also in the absence of detectable defects in other, more primitive, activities of these cells.

ACKNOWLEDGMENTS

This work was supported by grants from CNR, special project "Oncology,"
and the Ministry of Education.

REFERENCES

1. J. L. Old and D. A. Clarke, Reticuloendothelial function in mice
infected with the Friend leukemia virus, Fed. Proc. 18:589 (1959).
2. S. Specter and H. Friedman, Viruses and immune response, Pharmac. Ther.
A. 2:595 (1978).
3. J. Cerny and M. Essex, Mechanisms of immunosuppression by oncogenic RNA
viruses, in: "Naturally Occurring Biological Immunosuppressive
Factors and their Relationship to Disease," R. H. Neubauer, ed., CRC
Press, Cleveland (1979).

4. M. Bendinelli, Rapporti tra sistema immunitario e virus di Friend, in:
    "Virus Oncogeni ad RNA," C. De Giuli-Morghen, ed., Piccin, Padova
    (1981).
5. N. Teich, J. Wike, T. Mak, A. Bernstein, and W. Hardy, Pathogenesis of
    retrovirus-induced disease, in: "RNA Tumor Viruses," R. Weiss, N.
    Teich, H. Varmus, and J. Coffin, eds., Cold Spring Harbor
    Laboratory, Cold Spring, NY (1982).
6. E. V. Genovesi, D. Livnat, and J. J. Collins, Immunotherapy of murine
    leukemia. VII. Prevention of Friend leukemia virus-induced
    immunosuppression by passive serum therapy, Int. J. Cancer 30:609
    (1982).
7. B. J. Rup, J. D. Hoelzer, and H. R. Bose, Helper virus associated with
    avian acute leukemia viruses inhibits the cellular immune response,
    Virology 116:61 (1982).
8. B. N. Dracott, N. Wedderburn, and M. J. Doenhoff, The immunodepressive
    effect of Friend virus. III. Effects on spleen T cells, Immunology
    33:573 (1977).
9. M. Bendinelli and H. Friedman, Immunodepression by Rowson-Parr virus in
    mice: lymphocyte markers and the capping response of spleen and
    lymph node cells after infection, Infect. Immun. 14:613 (1976).
10. J. Halasa, H. Friedman, and W. S. Ceglowski, Rosette-forming cells in
    spleens of immunosuppressed leukemic mice, J. Reticuloendothe. Soc.
    11:468 (1981).
11. B. N. Dracott, N. Wedderburn, and M. J. Doenhoff, The immunodepressive
    effect of Friend virus. IV. Effects on spleen B lymphocytes,
    Immunology 34:679 (1978).
12. M. Bendinelli, M. Campa, A. Toniolo, and C. Garzelli, An analysis of
    the role of lymphatic leukemia virus in the immunodepression exerted
    by Friend complex in leukemia-resistant C57BL/6 mice, J. Gen. Virol.
    39:243 (1978).
13. M. Bendinelli, D. Matteucci, A. Toniolo, and H. Friedman, Macrophage
    involvement in leukemia virus-induced tumorigenesis, Adv. Exp. Biol.
    Med. 121B:493 (1980).
14. R. C. Butler, J. M. Frier, M. S. Chapekar, M. O. Graham, and H.
    Friedman, Role of antibody response helper factors in
    immunosuppressive effects of Friend leukemia virus, Infect. Immun.
    39:1260 (1983).
15. E. Garaci, G. Migliorati, T. Jezzi, A. Bartocci, L. Gioia, C. Rinaldi,
    and E. Bonmassar, Impairment of in vitro generation of cytotoxic or
    T suppressor lymphocytes by Friend leukemia virus infection in mice,
    Int. J. Cancer 28:367 (1981).
16. D. J. Moody, S. Specter, M. Bendinelli, and H. Friedman, Suppression of
    natural killer cell activity by Friend murine leukemia virus, J.
    Natl. Cancer Inst. 72:1349 (1984).
17. J. De Maeyer-Guignard, Mouse leukemia: depression of serum interferon
    production, Science 177:797 (1972).
18. M. Bendinelli, Immunomodulation in viral infections: virus or
    infection-induced? in: "Immunomodulation: New Frontiers and
    Advances," H. H. Fudenberg, H. D. Whitten, and F. Ambrogi, eds.,
    Plenum Press, New York (1984).
19. D. D. Isaak, J. A. Price, C. L. Reinisch, and J. Cerny, Target cell
    heterogeneity in murine leukemia virus infection. I. Differences in
    susceptibility to infection with Friend leukemia virus between B
    lymphocytes from spleen, bone marrow and lymph nodes, J. Immunol.
    124:1822 (1979).
20. A. Toniolo, D. Matteucci, M. P. Pistillo, Z. Gori, and M. Bendinelli,
    Early replication of Friend leukemia viruses in spleen macrophages,
    J. Gen. Virol. 49:203 (1980).
21. J. Cerny and D. D. Isaak, Interactions of murine leukemia virus (MuLV)
    with isolated lymphocytes. IV. The role of mitogen-induced cellular
    DNA synthesis in virus infection and replication, Int. J. Cancer
    23:260 (1979).

22. G. Tonietti, G. B. Rossi, V. Del Gobbo, N. Accinni, A. Ranucci, F. Titti, M. G. Premrov, and E. Garaci, Effects of in vivo Friend leukemia virus infection on levels of serum thymic factors and on selected T-cell functions in mice, Cancer Res. 43:4355 (1983).

23. M. Bendinelli, D. Matteucci, A. Toniolo, and H. Friedman, Suppression of in vitro antibody response by spleen cells of mice infected with Friend-associated lymphatic leukemia virus, Infect. Immun. 24:1 (1979).

24. M. Bendinelli and H. Friedman, B and T lymphocyte activation by murine leukemia virus infection, Adv. Exp. Med. Biol. 121B:91 (1980).

25. V. Kumar and M. Bennett, Genetic resistance to Friend virus-induced erythroleukemia and immunosuppression, Curr. Top. Microbiol. Immunol. 92:65 (1981).

26. G. J. Cianciolo, T. J. Matthews, D. P. Bolognesi, and R. Snyderman, Macrophage accumulation in mice is inhibited by low molecular weight products from murine leukemia viruses, J. Immunol. 124:2900 (1980).

27. H. P. Senn and R. Papoian, Mitogenic effect of anti-Friend leukemia virus antiserum on T cells, Eur. J. Immunol. 13:824 (1983).

28. R. Revoltella, L. Bertolini, and C. Friend, In vitro transformation of bone marrow cells by the polycythemic strain of Friend leukemia virus, Proc. Natl. Acad. Sci. U.S.A. 76:1464 (1979).

29. I. Kamo and H. Friedman, Immunosuppression and the role of suppressive factors in cancer, Adv. Cancer Res. 25:271 (1977).

30. M. D. Daniel, N. W. King, L. N. Letvin, R. D. Hunt, P. K. Sehgal, and R. C. Desrosiers, A new type D retrovirus isolated from Macaques with an immunodeficiency syndrome, Science 223:602 (1984).

31. R. C. Gallo, S. Z. Salahuddin, M. Popovic, G. M. Shearer, M. Kaplan, B. F. Haynes, T. J. Palker, R. Redfield, J. Oleske, B. Safai, G. White, P. Foster, and P. D. Markham, Frequent detection and isolation of cytopathic retroviruses (HTLV-III) from patients with AIDS and at risk for AIDS, Science 224:500 (1984).

32. D. Klatzmann, F. Barre-Sinoussi, M. T. Nugeyre, C. Dauguet, E. Vilmer, C. Griscelli, F. Brun-Vezinet, C. Rouzioux, J. C. Gluckman, J. C. Chermann, and L. Montagnier, Selective tropism of lymphadenopathy associated virus (LAV) for helper-inducer T lymphocytes, Science 225:59 (1984).

33. M. Bendinelli, The reticuloendothelial system in infection with RNA tumor viruses, in: "The Reticuloendothelial System: A Comprehensive Treatise, Volume 10, Infection," M. Escobar and J. P. Utz, eds., Plenum Press, New York (in press).

34. J. A. Price and R. E. Smith, Inhibition of concanavalin A response during osteopetrosis virus infection, Cancer Res. 42:3617 (1982).

35. J. G. Sincovics, F. Gyorkey, J. L. Melnick, and P. Gyorkey, Acquired immune deficiency syndrome (AIDS): speculations about its etiology and comparative immunology, Rev. Inf. Dis. (in press).

IMMUNOSUPPRESSION BY HUMAN AND FELINE RETROVIRUSES

M. Essex and L. Kitchen

Department of Cancer Biology
Harvard University School of Public Health
Boston, Massachusetts

Among retroviruses which infect several species including humans, to date two groups have been firmly linked with immunodeficiency in addition to leukemia: feline leukemia viruses and human T-cell leukemia viruses. A mutant strain of HLTV is suspected to play a key etiological role in the development of the acquired immune deficiency syndrome (AIDS).

A family of T-lymphotropic retroviruses, designated the feline leukemia viruses (FeLV) infect cats under natural conditions and cause leukemia in this species. However, more cats infected with FeLV die as a result of immune suppression and opportunistic infections than develop leukemia or lymphoma (1,2). Cats infected with FeLV may develop thymic atrophy (3), impaired cell-mediated immune responses (4), lymphopenia (1), and depressed humoral immune responses despite the presence of hypergammaglobulinemia (5). Lethal opportunistic infections with selected viral, bacterial, protozoan, and fungal agents usually occur in the form of peritonitis, pneumonia, septicemia and/or encephalitis (1,2). Malignancies other than T-cell leukemia/lymphoma also occur (1,2,6). The varied clinical outcomes associated with FeLV infection relate in part to differences in the strain of infecting virus; however, a different host response to a virus of similar virulence must also be considered.

The family of human T-cell lymphotropic retroviruses (HTLV) refers to a group of related retroviruses that preferentially infects T-helper cells. HTLV has been etiologically linked with mature T-cell malignancies of adults endemic to certain areas of southern Japan, the Caribbean, and Africa (7-9). There are two lines of evidence for HTLV-induced immunosuppression. First, existing data suggest clinically important (but not necessarily lethal) immunosuppression resulting from infection with HTLV in otherwise unremarkable Japanese adults. In studies recently conducted in southwestern Japan on the island of Kyushu, non-opportunistic infections occurred at higher rates in anti-HTLV antibody positive individuals than in the age-matched healthy adults from the same city (10). The procedure used, indirect membrane immunofluorescence with HTLV-infected Hut-102 and MT-2 cells, has been described in detail (11,12,13). Representative positives were confirmed for reaction specificity with both gag gene and env gene proteins by immuno-precipitation using lysates of cells metabolically labeled with ^{35}S-cysteine (11-14). While the prevalence rate of antibodies to HTLV and related antigens was 16% in the general healthy adult population, it was 42% in patients

Table 1. Examples of Opportunistic Disease Processes that Occur
in AIDS Patients

Viral Diseases: disseminated cytomegalovirus infections
                           progressive Herpes simplex infections

Bacterial Diseases: Mycobacterium avium tuberculosis
                           nocardiosis

Protozoan Diseases: toxoplasmosis
                           Pneumocystis carinii pneumonia
                           cryptosporidiosis

Fungal Diseases: Cryptococcal meningitis
                           Aspergillus pneumonia
                           Candida infections of oral cavity and esophagus

Neoplastic Diseases: Kaposi's sarcoma (associated with viral agents
                             such as cytomegalovirus or hepatitis B virus?)
                           Lymphoma (associated with viral agents such as
                             Epstein-Barr virus or HTLV?)
                           Rectal carcinomas (associated with viral agents
                             such as papilloma?)

---

with acute infectious diseases, and almost 100% in patients with T-cell
leukemia. The increased rate of infectious diseases in HTLV-infected individuals was apparently not due to hospital-related blood transfusions.
Whether the HTLV carrier state in Japan is associated with alterations in
lymphocyte populations has yet to be determined.

HTLV VARIANT: A CANDIDATE AGENT FOR AIDS

The second major line of evidence to support HTLV-induced immunosuppression is its suspected role in the development of AIDS. Since 1981,
this unprecedented epidemic form of lethal and transmissible immunodeficiency
has dramatically emerged in the United States, Europe, Haiti and central
Africa. Patients with AIDS suffer from prominent defects of the T-lymphocyte
arm of the immune system, although they also have evidence of B-cell dysfunction. Pneumocystis carinii pneumonia, other opportunistic infections, and
Kaposi's sarcoma are the most conspicuous illnesses subsequent to this profound state of immune compromise (Table 1). Two years after the onset of
clinical disease, which follows a prolonged incubation period of one to
perhaps five years, the case-fatality rate may exceed 90% (15).

Although a comprehensive picture of the pathogenesis of this complicated
syndrome remains elusive, data gathered over the past three years have yielded considerable insight concerning the putative agent, and information thus
far is consistent with HTLV-induced disease. First, because AIDS has been
noted in different groups at the same time [promiscuous homosexual men within
in major metropolitan areas of the U.S. (16), I.V. drug abusers, hemophiliacs, Haitians (17), children of high risk mothers (18), and recipients of
blood transfusions(19)], a single recently introduced or recently mutated
virus or other infectious agent is the most likely cause of this disease.

Second, the striking diversity of opportunistic infections (viral,
fungal, protozoal, mycobacterial, etc.) in afflicted patients suggests that
the underlying immunodeficiency is due to a single agent.

Third, although the means of spread of disease in Haiti and central Africa is not entirely clear at this time, epidemiological studies in the United States indicate that the transmission of AIDS is similar to that of hepatitis B virus. Because cases are observed in I.V. drug abusers and hemophiliacs, transmission by blood and/or blood products and/or contaminated needles is suspected. Because the disease occurs most often in promiscuous homosexual men, and clusters of cases are observed involving sexual contact, it appears that the agent is transmitted via sexual contact, and transmitted better by males than by females when exposure to blood products or contaminated needles is not involved. However, it appears that AIDS is less easily transmissible than is HBV; single needlestick accidents have not yet definitely resulted in AIDS in the recipient.

Several viruses which are known to infect humans have similar modes of transmission, including HTLV. HTLV is thought to be spread by blood transfusion (20,21) and from carrier mothers to their infants (22), and reportedly males infect females more efficiently than females do males (22). It is clear that HTLV is only poorly transmissible since only 5-30% of people in endemic areas such as southwestern Japan become infected during their lifetimes, and in adjacent areas of the country only one percent or less of the populations becomes infected (23,24,25).

Fourth, cell-mediated immunity is severely depressed in AIDS, resulting in absolute lymphopenia and reduced subpopulations of helper T-lymphocytes (OKT4 cells) (26-29), and HTLV is highly tropic for OKT4 cells (30). While other lymphoid cell populations can become infected, the frequency at which this occurs is much lower, even though infection appears to require cell-to-cell contact.

Fifth, HTLV appears to be endemic to southern Africa and Haiti, regions that have been considered possible sites for the origin of the AIDS agent (31). Since an increased incidence of AIDS has not been reported in the rest of the Caribbean basin and in southwestern Japan, both regions that have relatively high rates of infection with HTLV, if an HTLV variant leads to AIDS it would probably be a relatively recent mutant strain and much more lethal than the wild type in Japan. T-cell leukemias occur in only a small fraction of the individuals that become infected with HTLV in Japan, and most remain asymptomatic carriers throughout life. A similar asymptomatic carrier state is found in most people that become infected with the Epstein-Barr herpes-virus, except that the latter infection is much more prevalent throughout the world and limited to B rather than T cells (32).

Sixth, and probably most compelling, the overall clinical picture in AIDS--opportunistic infections, depressed cell mediated immunity, and decreased humoral immune responses despite hypergammaglobulinemia--is strikingly analogous to the disease FeLV induces in cats.

EVIDENCE FOR HTLV INFECTION IN AIDS PATIENTS AND RELATED RISK GROUPS

Three different approaches have been used to identify exposure to HTLV in AIDS patients: nucleic acid hybridization experiments to detect proviral DNA in patients' lymphocytes, virus isolation, and seroepidemiological methods. Using HTLV-specific probes and Southern blotting hybridization, integrated provirus was found in lymphocyte DNA from two of 33 patients examined in one study (33). However, upon repeat examination at a later date, the two positive AIDS cases were negative indicating that the numbers of positive cells had decreased to subdetectable levels or were eliminated from the host as the disease progressed. While this is compatible with the knowledge that HTLV infections are usually limited to a fraction of the OKT4 cells, and this cell population is known to be decreased or eliminated in advanced AIDS, it also suggests that the usefulness of this experimental approach is limited, at least for use with blood lymphocytes from seriously ill AIDS cases. An independent study using Southern blotting hybridization confirmed that HTLV-related sequences are undetectable in lymphocytes from at least 90% of the AIDS patients examined (34).

The approach of virus isolation using cultures established from AIDS patients has been more successful. Direct cultivation of T cells from AIDS cases using T-cell growth factor (TCGF) and/or co-cultivation with susceptible cord blood lymphocyte revealed T-cell associated HTLV and/or HTLV antigens in three AIDS patients in initial studies (35). Since that time, many more cultures from AIDS patients have been examined and found to contain HTLV (R. Gallo, personal communication). Some culture positive cases lack demonstrable antibodies to HTLV antigens, indicating that at least some patients are antibody negative because of such possibilities as an insufficient humoral response rather than an absence of exposure to the virus.

Using the seroepidemiological approach, more than 150 serum samples from clinically confirmed AIDS cases have been tested for antibody to HTLV using the immunofluorescence technique (Table 2). When the patients' sera were examined only once, particularly at a late stage of disease, only 30-40% were positive for antibodies to HTLV-MA. However, the antibody positive patients represented all major cities in the United States as well as several cities in Europe, and included patients from all major risk groups [homosexual men, I.V. drug abusers, hemophiliacs, Haitians, infant cases of high risk parents (17,18)], and individuals who apparently acquired the disease by blood transfusion (9). Perhaps of even greater importance, of those individuals where multiple serum samples were available from intervals of several weeks, the proportion of positives detected in at least one sample from a given patient was greatly increased. Two examples are given in Table 3. The authenticity of these results were verified by their reproducibility; while some samples from selected patients were positive and some negative, the result obtained on a given sample from a specific date was regularly reproducible, and the presence of antibodies to HTLV proteins in the positive samples could be confirmed using other procedures. These results, together with the viral isolation data discussed previously, indicate that serological studies based on the examination of a single sample

Table 2. Prevalence of Antibodies to HTLV-MA in Patients with
          AIDS, Patients with Lymphadenopathy, and Various
          Control Groups

Clinical Status	Number Tested	Number Positive	Percent Positive
AIDS cases	159	60	38
AIDS cases with multiple sequential samples	17	13	77
LAS cases	92	24	26
Kidney transplant patients	93	2	2.2
Systemic lupus erythematosus	17	0	0
Random blood donors and lab workers	345	1	0.3
Healthy homosexuals	126	1	0.8
Asymptomatic hemophiliacs	172	21	12

Table 3. Detection of Antibodies to HTLV-MA in Two AIDS
Patients Samples at Multiple Intervals

Patient Number	Weeks After Initial Sample								
	0	2	4	6	8	10	12	14	16
1	–	–	ND	ND	+	+	–	ND	–
2	–	+	–	–	–	–	+	ND	ND

from each patient results in a significant under-representation of the true positivity rate.

Multiple explanations can be considered for such variations in the presence of detectable antibodies. First, AIDS patients demonstrate inadequate humoral immune responses to specific antigens even in the presence of hypergammaglobulinemia which is apparently caused by the non-specific mitogenic stimulation of B cells (36). Second, AIDS patients have high levels of circulating immune complexes, and it seems likely that fluctuations would occur in the levels of immune complexes, yielding variable amounts of antibody available for detection. Third, it has been observed that the major antibodies to HTLV-related proteins in AIDS patients are IgM rather than IgG, whereas most HTLV infected primarily have anti-HTLV IgG antibodies (37). This is compatible with observations that sera from AIDS patients are less likely to be positive when examined late in the disease, and that the antibodies are more sensitive to freezing and thawing than might be expected. The specificity of the antibodies for the env gene glycoproteins was confirmed by showing that representative samples react with the protein portion of the deglycosylated molecules (13). Also, while AIDS patients often have high titers of antibodies to viruses such as the Epstein-Barr virus (EBV) and cytomegalovirus (CMV), as do matched healthy homosexual controls (38), AIDS patients with low titers of antibodies to these viruses are just as likely to have detectable anti-HTLV-MA as are AIDS patients with high titers of antibodies to EBV and CMV (39).

Analysis of serum samples from 92 cases of lymphadenopathy in homosexual males revealed that 24 or 26% were positive (11,12). However, one percent or less of various control groups were positive for anti-HTLV-MA (See Table 2). This included not only healthy homosexual males, but also patients with systemic lupus erythematosus and with chronic active hepatitis. Also of 93 patients with kidney transplants and drug-induced immunosuppression, only two were positive for antibodies to HTLV-MA. The relative absence of antibodies in lupus patients and transplant patients lends further credence to the specificity of the test, since these individuals generally demonstrate high titers of antibodies to agents such as CMV and EBV, which frequently infect patients with drug-induced immunosuppression, in addition to those suffering from AIDS.

Asymptomatic hemophiliacs were also examined for the presence of anti-HTLV-MA, since they represent a risk group for AIDS development, and also receive concentrated blood components from thousands of donors (14). About 12% of asymptomatic hemophiliacs examined have antibodies to HTLV-MA, and the specificity of the antibodies to HTLV proteins has been confirmed by immunoprecipitation and by blocking tests to show that the antibodies from healthy hemophiliacs react with the same proteins detected with antibodies from Japanese T-cell leukemia patients (14). More than 170 hemophiliacs have been examined from four U.S. cities.

Since hemophiliacs receive blood components from such large numbers of donors, the possibility that they might receive units from healthy HTLV-carrier individuals of Caribbean origin may be an important consideration. Furthermore, since a significant proportion of the hemophiliacs from New York had evidence of antibodies to HTLV-MA prior to 1980, it seems likely that most were only exposed to a conventional strain of HTLV rather than a putative "AIDS mutant" (40). However, asymptomatic hemophiliacs with anti-HTLV-MA appear to have reduced levels of T4 cells when compared to antibody negative hemophiliacs (40). This would be analogous to the observation, mentioned previously, that Japanese patients with a higher rate of infectious disease residing in endemic areas also appear to have higher rates of infection with HTLV.

Serum samples from transfusion-associated AIDS cases and from individuals who donated to the cases approximately two years before disease development have also been examined for anti-HTLV-MA antibodies (41). Three of eight cases of transfusion associated AIDS had evidence of antibodies to HTLV-MA, and antibodies were found in at least one donor per set from nine to twelve "donor sets" examined. Donors who gave blood to such transfusion-associated cases were found to be anti-HTLV-MA positive significantly more often than were random blood donors, and the anti-HTLV-MA positive donors were usually but not always (i.e., in six of nine sets) "suspicious" in terms of carriage of the putative AIDS agent, based on such characteristics as male homosexuality, I.V. drug abuse, and/or the presence of abnormal T-helper/T-suppressor lymphocyte ratios. In still another category of patients, namely infants with AIDS, we also found that more than 50% were positive for anti-HTLV-MA (41).

POSSIBLE MECHANISMS OF DISEASE

Several possible explanations could be considered to address the issue of how an HTLV variant might cause AIDS at the cellular and/or host level. First, HTLV-infected T4 cells might be attacked by a specific immune and/or autoimmune mechanism. Possible targets for such immune mechanisms might be the gp61 or gp45 component of HTLV-MA and/or class I HLA antigens of the A and B haplotypes. While most or all cultured HTLV carrier lines express HTLV-MA at the cell surface, these proteins are not found at detectable levels in freshly biopsied tumor cells from adult T-cell leukemia patients (41). The expression of such antigens in large numbers of peripheral T4 cells in vivo presumably could result in the destruction of that population since antibodies from patients and HTLV healthy carriers alike are cytotoxic for the HTLV-MA positive cultured cells (42). A similar mechanism might be envisioned for the potential elimination of HTLV-infected T4 cells that present an "alien" set of HLA antigens in vivo (43). Second, since one of the virion structural proteins p19, appears to mimic certain cell proteins involved in thymic differentiation, a similar autoimmune type of mechanism directed to this putative target might be imagined (44). Third, HTLV, like most retroviruses, has potential for a cytopathic effect, such as the formation of syncitia in vitro in appropriate cell types (45). Thus, the possibility that some strain(s) of HTLV could cause T4 cell destruction in vivo cannot be ruled out. Fourth, since HTLV clearly causes altered expression of such cell surface proteins as the TCGF receptor, it seems logical that altered lymphokine feedback responses might occur that would interfere with stabilization of T4 cell levels.

Finally, since some clones of HTLV-infected cells have been shown to be specifically sensitive to cytotoxic lymphocyte lysis in an HLA-linked manner, the presence of such cells and/or virus strains could lead to destruction of important components of the immune system.

CONCLUSION

While a virulent strain of HTLV may be necessary for the development of AIDS, asymptomatic carriers of the "AIDS agent" can be infectious. As evident in the transfusion-related AIDS studies, at the time of donation the donors to the AIDS cases were not noticeably symptomatic. Also, it would seem likely that there were other recipients of the implicated donors and these individuals have not yet been reported to develop clinical disease (46). As with other infectious diseases, and as is probably the case with FeLV, the immunological and/or genetic state of the host at the time of transmission and during the long incubation period probably influences the outcome of the infection.

REFERENCES

1. M. Essex, W. Hardy, Jr., S. Cotter, R. Jakowski, and A. Sliski, Naturally occurring persistent feline oncornavirus infections in the absence of disease, Infect. Immun. 11:470 (1975).
2. D. P. Francis, M. Essex, R. Jakowski, S. Cotter, T. Lerer, and W. Hardy, Jr., Increased risk for lymphoma and glomerulonephritis in a closed population of cats exposed to feline leukemia virus, Amer. J. Epidemiol. 11:337 (1980).
3. E. A. Hoover, L. Perryman, and G. Kociba, Early lesions in cats inoculated with feline leukemia virus, Cancer Res. 33:145 (1973).
4. L. E. Perryman, E. Hoover, D. Yohn, Immunological reactivity of the cat: immunosuppression in experimental feline leukemia, J. Natl. Cancer Inst. 49:1357 (1972).
5. Z. Trainin, D. Wernicke, H. Ungar-Waron, and M. Essex, Suppression of the humoral antibody response in natural retrovirus infections, Science 220:858 (1983).
6. K. Weijer, J. Colofat, J. Daams, P. Hageman, and W. Misdorp, Feline malignant mammary tumors. II. Immunologic and electron microscopic investigations into a possible viral etiology, J. Natl. Cancer Inst. 52:673 (1974).
7. B. Poiesz, F. Ruscetti, M. Reitz, B. Kalyanaraman, and R. Gallo, Isolation of a new type C retrovirus (HTLV) in primary uncultured cells of a patient with Sezary T-cell leukemia, Nature 294:268 (1981).
8. M. Reitz, Jr., B. Poiesz, F. Ruscetti, and R. Gallo, Characterization and distribution of nucleic acid sequences of a novel type C retrovirus isolated from neoplastic human T lymphocytes, Proc. Natl. Acad. Sci. 77:7415 (1980).
9. B. Poiesz, F. Ruscetti, A. Gazdar, P. Bunn, J. Minna, and R. Gallo, Detection and isolation of type-C retrovirus particles from fresh and cultured lymphocytes of a patient with cutaneous T-cell lymphoma, Proc. Natl. Acad. Sci. 77:7415 (1980).
10. M. Essex, M. McLane, N. Tachibana, D. Francis, and T. H. Lee, Seroepidemiology of HTLV in relation to immunosuppression and the acquired immunodeficiency syndrome, in: "Human T-Cell Leukemia/Lymphoma Viruses," R. C. Gallo, M. Essex, and L. Gross, eds., Cold Spring Harbor Press, Cold Spring Harbor, New York (1984).
11. M. Essex, M. McLane, T. Lee, L. Falk, C. Howe, J. Mullins, C. Cabradilla, and D. Francis, Antibodies to cell membrane antigens associated with human T-cell leukemia virus in patients with AIDS, Science 220:859 (1983).
12. T. H. Lee, T. Homma, K. Schultz, M. McLane, N. Tachibana, C. Howe, and M. Essex, Antigens expressed by human T-cell leukemia virus trans-

formed cells, in: "Human T-Cell Leukemia/Lymphoma Viruses," R. C. Gallo, M. Essex, and L. Gross, eds., Cold Spring Harbor Press, Cold Spring Harbor, New York (1984).

13. T. Lee, J. Coligan, T. Homma, M. F. McLane, N. Tachibana, and M. Essex, Human T-cell leukemia virus associated membrane antigens (HTLV-MA): identity of the major antigens recognized following virus infections, Proc. Natl. Acad. Sci. 81:3856 (1984).

14. M. Essex, M. F. McLane, T. H. Lee, N. Tachibana, J. Mullins, J. Kreiss, C. Kasper, M.-C. Poon, A. Landay, S. Stein, D. Francis, C. Cabradilla, D. Lawrence, and B. Evatt, Antibodies to human T-cell leukemia virus membrane antigens (HTLV-MA) in hemophiliacs, Science 221:1061 (1982).

15. J. E. Groopman, Kaposi's sarcoma and other neoplasms, in: "The Acquired Immunodeficiency Syndrome," M. S. Gottlieb, moderator, Ann. Intern. Med. 99:208 (1983).

16. Anonymous, A cluster of Kaposi's sarcoma and Pneumocystis carinii among homosexual male residents of Los Angeles and Orange Counties, California, Morb. Mortal. Weekly Rep. 31:305 (1982).

17. D. Francis, J. Curran, and M. Essex, Epidemic acquired immune deficiency syndrome: epidemiologic evidence for a transmitted agent, J. Natl. Cancer Inst. 71:1 (1983).

18. J. Oleske, A. Minnefor, R. Cooper, K. Thomas, A. dela Cruz, H. Ahdieh, I. Guerrero, V. Joshi, and F. Desposito, Immune deficiency syndrome in children, J. Amer. Med. Assoc. 249:2345 (1983).

19. J. Curran, D. Lawrence, H. Jaffe, J. Kaplan, L. Zyla, M. Chamberland, R. Weinstein, K.-J. Lui, L. Schonberger, T. Spira, W. Alexander, G. Swinger, A. Ammann, S. Solomon, D. Auerback, D. Mildvan, R. Stoneburner, J. Jason, H. Haverkos, and B. Evatt, Acquired immunodeficiency syndrome (AIDS) associated with transfusions, New Eng. J. Med. 310:60 (1984).

20. I. Miyoshi, M. Fujishita, H. Taguchi, Y. Ohtsuki, T. Akagi, Y. Morinoto, and A. Nagasaki, Caution against blood transfusion from donors seropositive to adult T-cell leukemia-associated antigens, Lancet 1:1074 (1982).

21. W. Saxinger and R. Gallo, Possible risk to recipients of blood from donors carrying serum markers of human T-cell leukemia virus, Lancet 1:1074 (1982).

22. Y. Hinuma, Association of retrovirus (ATLV) with adult T-cell leukemia: review of serologic studies, Gann 28:211 (1982).

23. Y. Hinuma, H. Komoda, T. Chosa, T. Kondon, M. Kohakura, T. Takenaka, M. Kikuchi, M. Ichimaru, K. Hunoki, I. Sato, R. Mutsuo, Y. Takiuchi, H. Uchinio, and M. Hanaoka, Antibodies to adult T-cell leukemia-virus-associated antigen (ATLA) in sera from patients with ATL and controls in Japan: a nation-wide seroepidemiologic study, Int. J. Cancer 29:631 (1982).

24. M. Robert-Guroff, Y. Nakao, K. Notake, Y. Ito, A. Sliski, and R. Gallo, Natural antibodies to human retrovirus HTLV in a cluster of Japanese patients with adult T-cell leukemia, Science 215:975 (1982).

25. M. F. McLane, N. Tachibana, G. deThe, C. Howe, T. H. Lee, J. Azocar, V. Kalyanaraman, R. Gallo, and M. Essex, Distribution of antibodies to human T-cell leukemia virus-associated cell membrane antigen (HTLV-MA), in: "Leukemia Reviews International," M. A. Rich, ed., Marcel Dekker (1983).

26. R. Stahl, A. Friedman-Kien, R. Dubin, M. Marmor, S. Zolla-Pazner, Immunologic abnormalities in homosexual men: relationship to Kaposi's sarcoma, Am. J. Med. 73:171 (1982).

27. F. Siegal, C. Lopez, G. Hammer, et al., Severe immunodeficiency in the male homosexuals, manifested by chronic perianal ulcerative herpes simplex lesions, N. Eng. J. Med. 305:1439 (1981).

28. M. Gottlieb, R. Schroff, H. Schanker, et al., Pneumocystis carinii pneumonia and mucosal candidiasis in previously healthy homosexual

men: evidence of a new acquired cellular immunodeficiency, N. Eng. J. Med. 305:1425 (1981).

29. H. Masur, M. Michelis, J. Green, et al., An outbreak of community-acquired Pneumocystis carinii pneumonia: initial manifestation of cellular immune dysfunction, N. Eng. J. Med. 305:1431 (1981).

30. M. Popovic, P. Sarin, M. Robert-Guroff, V. Kalyanaraman, D. Mann, J. Minowada, and R. Gallo, Isolation and transmission of human retrovirus (human T-cell leukemia virus), Science 219:856 (1983).

31. R. Gallo, personal communication.

32. M. Periera, J. Blake, and A. Macrae, EB virus antibody at different stages, Brit. Med. J. 4:526 (1969).

33. E. Gelman, M. Popovic, D. Blayney, H. Masur, G. Sidhu, R. Stahl, and R. Gallo, Proviral DNA of a retrovirus, human T-cell leukemia virus, in two patients with AIDS, Science 220:862 (1983).

34. J. Mullins and M. Essex, unpublished observations.

35. R. Gallo, P. Sarin, E. Gelman, M. Robert-Guroff, E. Richardson, V. Kalyanaraman, D. Mann, G. Sidhu, R. Stahl, S. Zolla-Pazner, J. Leibowitch, and M. Popovic, Isolation of human T-cell leukemia virus in acquired immune deficiency syndrome, Science 220:865 (1983).

36. H. Lane, H. Masur, L. Edgar, G. Whalen, and A. Fauci, Abnormalities of B lymphocyte activation and immunoregulation in patients with the acquired immune deficiency syndrome, N. Eng. J. Med. 309:453 (1983).

37. J. Godsmit, personal communication.

38. M. Roger, D. Morens, J. Stewart, R. Kaminski, T. Spira, P. Feorino, S. Larsen, D. Francis, M. Wilson, L. Kaufman, and The Task Force of Acquired Immune Deficiency Syndrome, National case-control study of Kaposi's sarcoma and Pneumocystis carinii pneumonia in homosexual men: Part 2, laboratory results, Ann. Intern. Med. 99:151 (1983).

39. D. Francis and M. Essex, Unpublished observations.

40. B. Evatt, D. Stein, D. Lawrence, M. F. McLane, J. McDougal, T. H. Lee, T. Spira, C. Cabradilla, J. Mullins, D. Francis, and M. Essex, Antibodies to human T-cell leukemia virus associated membrane antigens (HTLV-MA) in hemophiliacs: evidence for infection prior to 1980, Lancet 2:698 (1983).

41. M. Essex, Unpublished observations.

42. C. Howe, M. F. McLane, T. H. Lee, N. Tachibana, and M. Essex, Cytotoxic antibodies in patients with adult T-cell leukemia-lymphoma, in: "Leukemia Reviews International," M. A. Rich, ed., Marcel Dekker (1983).

43. D. Mann, M. Popovic, P. Sarin, C. Murray, M. Reitz, D. Srong, B. Haynes, R. Gallo, and W. Blattner, Cell lines producing human T-cell leukemia virus show altered HLA expression, Nature 305:58 (1983).

44. B. Haynes, M. Robert-Guroff, R. Metzgar, G. Franchini, V. Kalyanaraman, T. Paulker, and R. Gallo, Monoclonal antibody against human T-cell leukemia virus p19 defines a human thymic epithelial antigen acquired during ontogeny, J. Exp. Med. 157:907 (1983).

45. H. Hoshino, M. Shimoyama, M. Miwa, and T. Sugimura, Detection of lymphocytes producing a human retrovirus associated with adult T-cell leukemia by syncitia induction assay, Proc. Natl. Acad. Sci. 80:7337 (1983).

46. J. Bove, Transfusion-related AIDS (editorial), New Eng. J. Med. 310:115 (1984).

VIRUS INTERACTIONS WITH THE HOST:

PAST, PRESENT AND FUTURE DEVELOPMENTS

John J. Trentin

Division of Experimental Biology
Baylor College of Medicine
Houston, Texas

ADENOVIRUS ONCOGENESIS: CURRENT STATUS

The first demonstration of the oncogenicity of a human virus was the induction of malignant transplantable tumors by injection of human adenovirus Type 12 into newborn hamsters (1), or mice (2). Tumors arose early at any of several sites of injection, and sometimes remotely, usually in the liver, resulting in death from tumor growth in from 29 to 108 days (3). The tumors were histologically undifferentiated malignant neoplasms (4). They contained virus-induced transplantation antigens (5) and newborn hamsters could be passively protected against tumor induction by immunization of the mothers before pregnancy (6).

It soon became apparent that:

1) Several but not all of the more than thirty serotypes of human adenovirus were either strongly or weakly oncogenic in newborn hamsters (7,8,9,10,11).

2) Although adeno 12 virus could not be recovered from the tumors, a significant portion of the messenger ribonucleic acid of the tumors, or of in vitro transformed cells, is virus specific (12).

3) In addition to transplantation antigen, the tumor cells contained a virus-induced and virus-specific intranuclear neoantigen (T-antigen) that could be demonstrated by complement fixation (13,14), immunofluorescence (15,16), and immunodiffusion (17) with serum of adeno-12 tumor bearing hamsters.

Some of the adenoviruses, such as Type 2, that are capable of transforming cells in vitro are, paradoxically, "non-oncogenic" in vivo. Because of the T-antigen was not responsible for the virus-induced transplantation immunity (T cell mediated), it was presumed to be of only diagnostic significance. However, since the more recent discovery of the important role of natural killer (NK) cells in lysis of tumor cells and defense against cancer (18), some interesting new work indicates that the adenovirus Type 2 T-antigen may be responsible for adeno-2 being "non-oncogenic" in vivo by rendering the adeno-2 tumor cells susceptible to lysis by NK cells (19,20,21).

When it became apparent that the adeno 12-induced T-antigen of hamster tumors and of mouse tumors were cross-reactive and apparently identical, we used adeno 12-induced hamster T-antigen, and adeno 12 tumor-bearing hamster serum to test respectively for adeno 12 T-antibody and T-antigen in sera of 269 patients, most of whom had some type of neoplastic disease, and of 103 normal controls (22) and in 91 human tumors and 21 control tissues (23). No specific evidence for adenovirus oncogenesis was found.

More recently, by much more advanced nucleic acid hybridization methods, Maurice Green and associates have, over a number of years, conducted an extensive search of human cancer DNA's for groups A through E human adenovirus transforming gene sequences. Depending on the adenovirus groups, they have examined from one-half to three-fourths of the types of cancers found in the United States, as high sensitivity for the adeno groups A, B, and C, but lesser sensitivity for groups D and E. To date they have found no evidence for human adeno 12 transforming genes sequences (24).

From one point of view these results are perhaps not surprising. To date a number of oncogenic adenovirus serotypes have been found in several non-human species tested including bovine (25), avian (26), and simian. Six out of 18 of the simian adenovirus types tested were oncogenic (27). In each case oncogenicity has been demonstrated only "out of species," usually in hamsters, but also in mice, rats, and mastomys. In vitro transformation appears to work best in rat embryo cells. "Out of species" the adenoviruses usually have an incomplete replication cycle, allowing survival of infected and transformed cells, rather than a complete and lytic replication cycle as "in species." However, by the same token, man is often in contact with other species which have oncogenic adenoviruses of their own, for which man is "out of species." Chicken embryo lethal orphan (CELO) virus is highly oncogenic in hamsters, and is found in market eggs. Much research should be directed toward the potential oncogenicity for man of non-human adenoviruses with which man is in contact, such as those of the avian, bovine, simian, canine, feline, murine and other species.

Over the years, an interesting series of investigations have been reported suggesting that even the human adenoviruses may possibly be responsible for certain of the less common human tumor types, namely tumors of neurogenic origin. Ogawa et al., as early as 1966, reported a neuroectodermal origin of hamster tumors induced by human adenovirus 12 in the peripheral nervous system (28), with the induction of medulloblastomas in the central nervous system of hamsters and mice (29). Albert et al. demonstrated that the neural retina of young adult hamsters could be transformed in vitro by adeno 12 (30). Based on these findings, Mukai and associates were able to induce retinoblastomas by intraocular injection of adeno 12, first in rats (31), and then in baboons (32). Based on this, Byrd et al. (33), succeeded in transforming human embryo retinoblasts in vitro by transfection with cloned adenovirus 12 DNA. The retinoblast cell line so produced contained many copies of the adeno 12 transforming region, expressed virus specific proteins, and when inoculated into athymic mice formed tumors resembling retinoblastomas.

Mak et al., using electrophoretic and blotting methods similar to those of Green and Wold (24), isolated and analyzed the RNA and DNA of six human retinoblastoma established cell lines or transplanted tumors in nude mice by blotting with ^{32}P-labelled adeno 12 DNA, and failed to find viral sequenced (34). In contrast, Ibelgaufts et al. (35), using "a highly sensitive in-situ hybridization technique," analyzed 32 human tumors, mainly neurogenic, with ^{3}H-labelled DNA from adenovirus types 2 and 12 of the human, and oncogenic bovine adenovirus type 3 and avian CELO adenovirus, under conditions that detect complementary RNA. Adenovirus-related RNA was reported in 62% of all tumors tested. These dissimilar results of the Green group and the Ibelgaufts group await future clarification, and may depend on questions of sensitivity versus specificity of the different nucleic acid hybridization methods used by each group.

ATHEROSCLEROSIS: IS THIS NO. 1 KILLER SIMPLY A BENIGN SMOOTH

MUSCLE CELL TUMOR?

The basic histopathology of atherosclerosis begins as nodular, then confluent, overgrowth of smooth muscle cells in the intima of the muscular arteries. This proliferation of smooth muscle cells has been described as a key event in the genesis of the lesions of atherosclerosis (36). Initially the intima is relatively acellular. The smooth muscle cells that invade and thicken it to the point of occlusion of the lumen, are believed to originate from the muscular medial layer by passage through the elastic lamina. Earl Benditt, pathologist, astutely observed that the proliferating intimal smooth muscle cells were atypical not only in location, but in size, in a preponderance of associated collagen rather than elastin, and in the absence of intercellular junctions. He wondered if they were transformed, and sought to test this by means of the glucose-6-phosphate dehydrogenase (G6PD) isoenzymes, previously used for this determination in the case of tumors (37).

G6PD is determined by a gene on the X chromosome. In women heterozygous for this enzyme, the maternal and the paternal X chromosome each control production of a slightly different isoenzyme distinguishable by electrophoretic mobility. In each cell only one X chromosome, at random, remains active, the other becomes the inactive Barr body (the Lyon phenomenon). Depending on whether the maternal or paternal X chromosome of a given cell remains active, that cell will produce only one or the other isoenzyme. Since in normal tissues of heterozygous women half of the cells produce the A form and half the B form of the isoenzyme, normal tissues have equal amounts of both forms. However, since tumors, both malignant and benign, invariably arise as monoclonal progeny of a single transformed cell, they have been found to have only one or the other of these two marker isoenzymes. In G6PD-heterozygous women with multiple benign smooth muscle tumors of the uterus, approximately half of the tumors have only the A form, and the other half the B form of the isoenzyme (38). The data clearly indicated multicentric origin of these monoclonal leiomyomas, each of unicellular origin.

In 1973 Benditt and Benditt reported that when multiple individual atheromata of women heterozygous for G6PD were dissected out and tested, each usually contained only one or the other isoenzyme, whereas the intervening tissue usually contained both (39). In 1975, Pearson et al. confirmed these findings (40). In the combined data of both publications, approximately half of the atheromata were of the A type, half of the B type. Based on these findings, Benditt and Benditt postulated that transforming agents such as viruses and chemical mutagens may be atherogenic. What he apparently did not know, was that as early as 1950 Paterson and Cottral reported that in spontaneous epizootics of infectious avian lymphomatosis (Marek's disease) there is an associated increased incidence of coronary arteriosclerosis, and that tracheal washings from infected chickens, given to clean chickens, increased the incidence and severity of coronary arteriosclerosis (41). Stimulated by Benditt and Benditt's observation and prediction, by 1977 Albert et al. reported that two chemical carcinogens, dimethylbenzathracine and benzopyrene were atherogenic in chickens (42). Since Paterson's early transmission of coronary arteriosclerosis by infectious material from chickens with Marek's disease, the infectious agent of Marek's disease has been isolated and identified as a herpesvirus, known as Marek's disease virus (MDV). In 1978 the Fabricants and their associates reported that MDV, in addition to inducing lymphoma, is highly atherogenic in chickens, even on a low cholesterol diet (43). They reported moreover, that the arteriosclerosis induced by Marek's disease virus closely resembles that of man (44). The addition of high cholesteroldiet aggravated the arteriosclerosis, converting the MDV-induced proliferative lesions to fatty-proliferative lesions. But given alone, MDV caused a much higher incidence of arteriosclerosis on a low fat diet, than did a high cholesterol diet in the absence of MDV.

153

It is well established that high fat, high cholesterol diets are athero-genic in man and in animals, and that genetic factors control susceptibility to diet-induced hypercholesterolemia and atherogenesis (45). But MDV is highly atherogenic in chickens even on a low cholesterol diet. What then is the correlation between cholesterol atherogenesis and viral induced athero-genesis? There are several possibilities. Cigarette smoking is known to be a high risk factor for atherosclerotic heart disease as well as broncho-genic carcinoma. Cigarette smoke contains known premutagens including benz-pyrene and methylcholanthrene, which have been shown to be transported in the blood by the same low density and very low density lipoproteins that contain cholesterol (46). Alternatively, or additionally, hypercholester-olemic diets have been shown to induce a broad immunosuppression with impair-ment of host immune response to viral, bacterial and tumor cell challenge (47). Finally, chicken arterial smooth muscle cell cultures, when infected with MDV, develop a lipid metabolic imbalance that both qualitatively and quantitatively resembles that seen in human arteriosclerotic arteries (48).

All of this stimulated the search for human herpesvirus in human athero-sclerotic tissue. There are five known herpesviruses of man: herpes simplex (HSV) types 1 and 2, herpes Varicella-zoster, Cytomegalovirus (CMV), and Epstein-Barr virus (EBV). In 1983 Melnick et al. (49) reported that 25% of smooth muscle cell cultures derived from either atherosclerotic carotid endarterectomy specimens, or from grossly uninvolved punch biopsy specimens obtained during coronary artery bypass surgery, reacted by immunofluorescence with antisera to CMV but not to HSV-1, or 2. Replicating CMV was not de-tected by electron microscopy, and infectious CMV could not be recovered by co-culture with permissive human fibroblasts, suggesting latency (49). On the other hand, Benditt et al. (50) reported evidence, by in situ hybridiza-tion, for the presence of herpes simplex viral mRNA in 13 specimens of human arterial tissue from atheromatous patients. In some of the specimens, all of the cells in discrete foci of intimal cell proliferation were positive, whereas the medial cells were negative. None of the specimens were found to contain mRNA of CMV, EBV or MDV. They next cultured smooth muscle cells from human fetal aorta and inoculated them with HSV, CMV and EBV. HSV-1 and 2 caused rapid and classic cytopathic effects and in situ hybridization gave strongly positive results with HSV-1 and 2. For CMV and EBV they re-ported negative results. It is apparent that much work remains to be done in this challenging new aspect of atherosclerosis research.

PASSENGER RETROVIRUS IN THE EBV-PRODUCING B95-8 CELL LINE

Our own work in this area has included the use of the B95-8 cell line, the most widely used source of high transforming EBV. Dr. J. Tumilowicz of our laboratory discovered, in electron micrographs of this cell line, not only the expected herpes virus particles, but also retrovirus particles which resembled a type D retrovirus. To determine if it was in this cell line when we first received it, we obtained another shipment from the same laboratory, the laboratory of origin of this EBV-transformed marmoset lympho-cyte cell line. Immediately on receipt cells were fixed and again found to have Type D particles, as well as type A intracytoplasmic immature particles. Reverse transcriptase studies revealed RNA-directed DNA polymerase (RDDP) with a preference for Mg^{2+} rather than Mn^{2+}, typical of Type D retrovirus. B95-8 cells obtained from two other sources in the U.S.A. also showed evi-dence for retrovirus by either electron microscopy, or presence of RDDP (51). One of these showed retrovirus only by the presence of RDDP, whereas type D particles were not found. We later learned that Popovic et al. (52) had earlier found type E retrovirus in B95-8 cells from European sources but not from the U.S.A. Since they found the retrovirus to be highly related to squirrel monkey retrovirus, and we found it in B95-8 from the laboratory of origin, it is possible that this is a simian retrovirus that was in the marmoset lymphocytes originally transformed by EBV.

Cardiovascular disease and cancer are the number one and number two causes of death, respectively in the United States. Atherosclerosis is responsible for the large majority of cardiovascular deaths. Although high-fat, high-cholesterol diets are known to be conducive to atherosclerosis, and to a few kinds of cancer such as breast and colon cancer, the basic etiology of these two major causes of death has been thought to be quite separate and independent. The finding that human atheromata are monoclonal (39,40), a characteristic of virtually all tumors, benign as well as malignant, raises the realistic possibility that they may have etiologic factors in common. This has been reinforced by the demonstration that two known carcinogenic hydrocarbons (42) and MDV (43,44) a herpesvirus that causes lymphomatosis and coronary artery sclerosis in avian epizootics, each are atherogenic. The reports of CMV antigen and HSV mRNA in arteries of atherosclerotic humans (49,50) suggest herpesviruses as possible atherogenic agents in man.

If any of the herpes or other viruses can be proven to be a cause of human atherosclerosis, the possibility of prevention by immunization is indeed real and exciting. But, one might ask, why has not immunoprevention of human cancer progressed farther and faster, even though there are several candidate human tumor viruses, such as EBV, CMV, HSV-2, adenoviruses, and papovaviruses? Each of these has been associated with only a small part of the totality of human cancers. Moreover, the risks associated with attenuated live virus vaccines, and the cells they grow in (as witness the recent discovery of a retrovirus in the EBV-producing B95-8 cell line) have been impediments. But real progress is being made in the development of subunit glycoprotein vaccines for infectious diseases (53). And more human tumors are being shown to be associated with viruses, and therefore infectious, although fortunately not highly contagious. One of the latest of these is human T cell leukemia and its associated retrovirus, HTLV. In this instance, as discussed in other chapters of this book, HTLV Type III, possibly a recent mutant, is believed to be the primary cause of acquired immune deficiency syndrome (AIDS). Because of the rapid escalation in the number of new cases of AIDS, the high mortality rate, and the evidence for spread of this disease to the general public by blood and blood products, there is understandably great incentive for development of both a screening test for the virus, and a vaccine. Since HTLV is a cancer virus, it may well become the first of the human "cancer vaccines," although, ironically it will be developed primarily for AIDS, in which the tumor manifestations usually appear to be associated with previously latent CMV or EBV, being activated by HTLV-induced immunosuppression! But it is the herpes virus that appear to be associated with most of the spontaneously occurring tumors in nature, in both man and animals, as witness: Lucké virus and frog kidney carcinoma; Marek's disease virus and highly contagious lymphomatosis of poultry; EBV and African lymphoma, nasopharyngeal carcinoma (in China) and infectious mononucleosis, a self-limiting "neoplastic" disease (U.S.A.); CMV and Kaposi's sarcoma; HSV-2 and cervical cancer. Perhaps we are expecting too much too soon, as has been the case for tumor immunotherapy (54). But tumor immunoprevention may be closer at hand.

The poultry research people are farthest ahead in the area of cancer preventive vaccines. For largely economic reasons, they have identified the causative agent of Marek's disease (avian lymphomatosis) as a herpes virus (MDV), and have developed both an attenuated MDV vaccine, and a live virus vaccine using the related herpes virus of turkeys (HVT). HVT is now routinely used to immunize newly hatched chicks. Thereby, infectious avian lymphomatosis, a neoplastic disease that had previously devastated the poultry industry with recurring epizootics, has been virtually eliminated (55). Still more recently, it has been reported (56) that vaccination of chicks with HVT also protects them against the atherosclerosis induced by MDV! The poultry researchers have given us a proven and every day working model for control of herpes virus induced lymphoma, and a promising one for control of herpes virus induced atherosclerosis. If any of the human herpesviruses can be conclusively shown to be causative for human atherosclerosis, the basis for the majority of cardiovascular morbidity and mortality, including myocardial infarction and stroke, then herpes virus vaccines may someday control that part of both the number one and number two killer diseases in the United States and other developed nations!

REFERENCES

1. J. J. Trentin, Y. Yabe, and G. Taylor, The quest for human cancer viruses. A new approach to an old problem reveals cancer induction in hamsters by human adenovirus, Sci. 137:835 (1962).
2. Y. Yabe, L. Samper, E. Bryan, G. Taylor, and J. J. Trentin, Oncogenic effect of human adenovirus, type 12, in mice, Sci 143:46 (1964).
3. Y. Yabe, L. Samper, G. Taylor, and J. J. Trentin, Cancer induction in hamsters by human type 12 adenovirus. Effect of route of injection, Proc. Soc. Exp. Biol. Med. 113:221 (1963).
4. H. J. Spjut, G. L. Van Hoosier, Jr., and J. J. Trentin, Neoplasms in hamsters induced by adenovirus type 12, Arch. Pathol. 83:199 (1967).
5. J. J. Trentin and E. Bryan, Virus-induced transplantation immunity to human adenovirus type 12 tumors of the hamster and mouse, Proc. Soc. Exp. Biol. Med. 121:1216 (1966).
6. J. J. Trentin, Immunization against tumors induced by human adenovirus, in: "Viruses Inducing Cancer," Walter J. Burdette, ed., University of Utah Press (1966).
7. J. J. Trentin, G. L. Van Hoosier, Jr., and L. Samper, The oncogenicity of human adenoviruses in hamsters, Proc. Soc. Exp. Biol. Med. 127:683 (1968).
8. R. J. Heubner, W. P. Row, and W. T. Lane, Oncogenic effects in hamsters of human adenovirus Type 12 and 18, Proc. Natl. Acad. Sci. U.S. 48:2051 (1962).
9. A. J. Girardi, M. R. Hilleman, and R. E. Zwickey, Tests in hamsters for oncogenic quality of ordinary viruses including adenovirus Type 7, Proc. Soc. Exp. Biol. Med. 115:1141 (1964).
10. M. S. Pereira, H. G. Pereira, and S. K. R. Clarke, Human adenovirus Type 31. A new serotype with oncogenic properties, Lancet 1:21 (1965).
11. R. J. Huebner, J. J. Casey, R. M. Chanock, and K. Scholl, Tumors induced in hamsters by a strain of adenovirus Type 3: sharing of tumor antigens and "neoantigens" with those produced by adenovirus Type 7 tumors, Proc. Natl. Acad. Sci. U.S. 54:381 (1965).
12. K. Fujinaga and M. Green, The mechanism of viral carcinogenesis by DNA mammalian viruses: Viral-specific RNA in polyribosomes of adenovirus tumor and transformed cells, Proc. Natl. Acad. Sci. U.S. 55:1567 (1966).
13. M. D. Hoggan, W. P. Rowe, P. H. Black, and R. J. Huebner, Production of "tumor-specific" antigens by oncogenic viruses during acute cytolytic infections, Proc. Natl. Acad. Sci. U.S. 53:12 (1965).
14. G. L. Van Hoosier, Jr., S. Stinebaugh, and J. J. Trentin, CF reactions with human adenovirus type 12 (A-12) hamster and mouse tumors and observations on human sera and tumors, Fed. Proc. 23:130 (1964).
15. J. H. Pope and W. P. Rowe, Immunofluorescent studies of adenovirus 12 tumors and of cells transformed or infected by adenoviruses, J. Exptl. Med. 120:577 (1964).
16. J. D. Levinthal, C. Ahmad-Zadeh, G. L. Van Hoosier, Jr., and J. J. Trentin, Immunofluorescence of human adenovirus type 12 in various

cell types, Proc. Soc. Exp. Biol. Med. 121:405 (1966).

17. L. D. Berman and W. P. Rowe, A study of the antigens involved in adenovirus 12 tumorigenesis by immunodiffusion techniques, J. Exptl. Med. 121:955 (1965).

18. R. B. Herberman and J. R. Ortaldo, Natural killer cells: their role in defense against disease, Science 214:24 (1981).

19. J. L. Cook, J. Hauser, C. T. Patch, A. M. Lewis, Jr., and A. S. Levine, Adenovirus 2 early gene expression promotes susceptibility to effector cell lysis of hybrids formed between hamster cells transformed by adenovirus 2 and simian virus 40, Proc. Natl. Acad. Sci. U.S. 80:5995 (1983).

20. J. L. Cook and A. M. Lewis, Jr., Differential NK cell and macrophage killing of hamster cells infected with non-oncogenic or oncogenic adenovirus, Science 124:612 (1984).

21. J. M. Sheil, P. H. Gallimore, S. G. Zimmer, and M. L. Sopori, Susceptibility of adenovirus 2-transformed rat cell lines to natural killer (NK) cells: direct correlation between NK resistance and in vivo tumorigenesis, J. Immunol. 132:1578 (1984).

22. G. L. Van Hoosier, Jr. and J. J. Trentin, Reactivity of human sera with adenovirus type-12 hamster tumor antigens in the complement-fixation test, J. Natl. Cancer Inst. 40:249 (1968).

23. K. J. McCormick, G. L. Van Hoosier, Jr., and J. J. Trentin, Attempts to find human adenovirus type-12 tumor antigens in human tumors, J. Natl. Cancer Inst. 40:255 (1968).

24. M. Green and W. S. M. Wold, Search for adenovirus genetic information in normal and malignant human tissues, in: "Viruses Associated with Human Cancer," L. A. Phillips, ed., Marcel Dekker, Inc., New York (1983).

25. J. H. Darbyshire, Oncogenicity of bovine adenovirus Type 3 in hamsters, Nature 211:102 (1966).

26. P. S. Sarma, R. J. Huebner, and W. T. Lane, Induction of tumors in hamsters with an avian adenovirus (CELO), Science 149:1108 (1965).

27. R. N. Hull, I. S. Johnson, C. G. Culbertson, C. B. Reimer, and H. F. Wright, Oncogenicity of the simian adenoviruses, Science 150:1044 (1965).

28. K. Ogawa, A. Tsutsumi, K. Iwata, Y. Fujii, M. Okmori, K. Taguchi, and Y. Yabe, Histogenesis of malignant neoplasms induced by adenovirus type 12, Gann 57:43 (1966).

29. K. Ogawa, K. Hamaya, Y. Fujii, K. Matsuura, and T. Endo, Tumor induction by adenovirus Type 12 and its target cells in the central nervous system, Gann 60:3837.

30. D. M. Albert, A. S. Rabson, and A. J. Dalton, In vitro neoplastic transformation of uveal and retinal tissue by oncogenic DNA viruses, Invest. Ophthalmol. 7:357 (1968).

31. S. Kobayashi and M. Mukai, Retinoblastoma-like tumors induced by human adenovirus Type 12 in rats, Cancer Res. 34:1646 (1974).

32. N. Mukai, S. S. Kalter, L. B. Cummins, V. A. Matthews, T. Nishida, and T. Nakajima, Retinal tumor induced in the baboon by human adenovirus 12, Science 210:1023 (1980).

33. T. Byrd, K. W. Brown, and P. H. Gallimore, Malignant transformation of human embryo retinoblasts by cloned adenovirus 12 DNA, Nature 298:69 (1982).

34. S. Mak, I. Mak, B. L. Gallie, R. Godbout, and R. A. Phillips, Adenovirus-12 genes undetectable in human retinoblastoma, Int. J. Cancer 30:697 (1982).

35. H. Ibelgaufts, K. W. Jones, N. Maitland, and J. F. Shaw, Adenovirus-related RNA sequences in human neurogenic tumors, Acta. Neuropathol. (Berlin) 56:113 (1982).

36. R. Ross and J. A. Glomset, Atherosclerosis and the arterial smooth muscle cell. Proliferation of smooth muscle is a key event in the genesis of the lesions of atherosclerosis, Science 180:1332 (1973).

37. P. J. Fialkow, The origin and development of human tumors studied with cell markers, New Eng. J. Med. 291:26 (1974).

38. D. Lindner and S. M. Gartler, Glucose-6-phosphate dehydrogenase mosaicism: utilization as a cell marker in the study of leiomyomas, Science 150:67 (1965).

39. E. P. Benditt and J. M. Benditt, Evidence for a monoclonal origin of human atherosclerotic plaques, Proc. Natl. Acad. Sci. U.S. 70:1753 (1973).

40. T. A. Pearson, A. Wang, K. Solez, and R. H. Heptinstall, Clonal characteristics of fibrous plaques and fatty streaks from human aortas, Amer. J. Pathol. 81:379 (1975).

41. J. C. Paterson and G. E. Cottral, Experimental coronary sclerosis. III Lymphomatosis as a cause of coronary sclerosis in chicken, Arch. Pathol. 49:699 (1950).

42. R. E. Albert, M. Vanderlaan, F. J. Burns, and M. Nishizumi, Effect of carcinogens on chicken atherosclerosis, Cancer Res. 37:2232 (1977).

43. C. G. Fabricant, J. Fabricant, M. M. Litrenta, and C. R. Minick, Virus-induced atherosclerosis, J. Exp. Med. 148:335 (1978).

44. C. R. Minick, C. G. Fabricant, J. Fabricant, and M. M. Litrenta, Atherosclerosis induced by infection with a herpesvirus, J. Amer. Pathol. 96:673 (1979).

45. J. D. Morrisett, H. S. Kim, J. R. Patsch, S. K. Datta, and J. J. Trentin, Genetic susceptibility and resistance to diet-induced atherosclerosis and hyperlipoproteinemia, Artheriosclerosis 2:312 (1982).

46. E. P. Benditt, The origin of atherosclerosis, Scientific American 236:#2,74 (1977).

47. W. L. Kos, R. M. Loria, M. J. Snodgrass, D. Cohen, T. G. Thorpe, and A. M. Kaplan, Inhibition of host resistance by nutritional hypercholesteremia, Infection and Immunity 26:658 (1979).

48. C. G. Fabricant, D. P. Hajjar, and C. R. Minick, Herpesvirus infection enhances cholesterol and cholesteryl ester accumulation in cultured arterial smooth muscle cells. Amer. J. Pathol. 105:176 (1981).

49. J. L. Melnick, G. R. Dressman, C. H. McCollum, B. L. Petrie, J. Burek, and M. E. DeBakey, Cytomegalovirus antigen within human arterial smooth muscle cells, Lancet, Sept. 17 (1983).

50. E. P. Benditt, T. Barrett, and J. T. McDougall, Viruses in the etiology of atherosclerosis, Proc. Nat. Acad. Sci. 80:6386 (1983).

51. J. J. Tumilowicz, G. E. Gallick, J. L. East, J. J. Trentin, and R. B. Arlinghaus, Presence of retrovirus in the B95-8 Epstein-Barr virus-producing cell line from different sources, In Vitro 20:486 (1984).

52. M. Popovic, V. S. Kalyanaraman, M. S. Reitz, M. G. Sarngadharan, Identification of the RPMI 8226 retrovirus and its dissemination as a significant contaminant of some widely used human and marmoset cell lines, Int. J. Cancer 30:93 (1982).

53. M. R. Hilleman, Vaccines for the decade of the 1980's and beyond, S. Afr. Med. Jour. 61:691 (1982).

54. J. J. Trentin, Tumor immunotherapy in experimental animals: current status and prospectus, Annals N.Y. Acad. Sci. 227:716 (1976).

55. Multiple authors and articles, in: "Avian Diseases; Special Issue; Control of Marek's Disease," Vol. 16, No. 1, pp. 1-200 (1972).

56. C. G. Fabricant, J. Fabricant, C. R. Minick, and M. M. Litrenta, Herpesvirus-induced atherosclerosis in chickens, Fed. Proc. 42:2476 (1983).

VIRUSES, CANCER AND IMMUNITY

Ronald B. Herberman

Biological Response Modifiers Program
National Cancer Institute
Frederick, Maryland

The main theme of this book is on the interactions of viruses with the immune system. As a tumor immunologist, I would like to address this chapter to the many analogies between interactions of the immune system with viruses on the one hand and cancer on the other. As a framework for specific discussion of such interactions, two main questions might be identified: (i) What effects do cancer and viruses have on the immune system? and (ii) What effects does the immune system have on cancer and on virus infections? There is abundant information about the reciprocal nature of these interactions. The presence of tumors or viruses in the host can have profound effects on the immune system and, conversely, the immune system can play a key role in defense against cancer and virus infections.

First, let us consider the effects of cancer and viruses on the immune system. Such effects might be either stimulatory or inhibitory. In regard to stimulatory effects, one might categorize these into three types:

1. Induction of specific immune responses. Most viruses can be shown to be immunogenic and induce T cell-mediated immunity and humoral immunity in the host. Similarly, many tumors can be demonstrated to have tumor-associated antigens, which can elicit specific T cell-mediated immunity and/or antibodies. In experimental tumor systems, such immunogenicity has been particularly associated with tumors induced by oncogenic viruses. However, tumors induced by chemical carcinogens are also frequently quite immunogenic. Of particular current concern, in view of the possible analogy to human tumors, is whether spontaneous tumors have tumor-associated antigens and might under certain circumstances be immunogenic (for detailed discussion of this issue, see references 1-4). In regard to the T cell-mediated immunity, the cytolytic T cells induced by various tumors as well as those induced by viruses generally exhibit MHC restriction, i.e., they react only with target cells sharing some or all of the antigenic determinants of the major histocompatibility complex (5). However, in at least some virus-induced murine tumor systems, this MHC restriction does not appear to be complete (e.g., 6).

2. In addition to stimulation of specific immune response, both tumor cells and viruses have been shown to be able to strongly augment the natural immune system. For example, probably because of their interferon-inducing capability, inoculation of animals with any of a wide variety of viruses leads to rapid and potent augmentation of natural killer (NK) cell activity

(7). Similarly, soon after inoculation of various tumor cells, NK reactivity
can be shown to be substantially increased (8).

3. More generally, both viruses and cancer may have potent immunoregulatory effects by means of their ability to stimulate the production of a
variety of cytokines. It has recently been found that such stimulation of
cytokine production does not depend on specific T cell-mediated immunity.
Large granular lymphocytes (LGL), the small subpopulation of cells which
account for NK activity, as well as macrophages or monocytes, can be stimulated by various viruses or tumor cell lines to release substantial amounts
of alpha and/or gamma interferon (9,10). In addition, LGL can be stimulated
to produce a variety of other cytokines, including interleukin 2 (IL-2),
interleukin 1 (IL-1), B-cell growth factor (BCGF), NK cytotoxic factor and
other factors with direct antitumor effects, and colony-stimulating factor
(11-14).

In addition to the above described stimulatory effects, both viruses
and tumor cells can have a profound depressive or inhibitory effect on
various components of the immune system. First, potent inhibition of immune
reactivity may be due to direct effects on lymphoid cells. As demonstrated
extensively by Drs. Herman Friedman and Walter Ceglowski, and discussed in
detail elsewhere in this volume, infection of lymphoid cells by viruses can
interfere with their functional activity. Similarly, tumors involving
various cell types in the immune system can be profoundly immunosuppressive,
since the transformed cells may be functionally inactive and may crowd out
the other functional elements of the immune system. In addition to such
direct effects, the immunodepression associated with viruses or cancer may
be due to the induction of suppressor cells or factors. It should be noted
that two major types of suppressor cells have been identified in association
with either virus infections or tumor growth. In addition to suppressor T
cells, which may specifically interfere with immune reactivity against the
inducing agent or may cause a more general immunosuppression (15,16), viruses
or tumor cells may induce suppressor macrophages, which may potently inhibit
cell-mediated immune responses and/or humoral immune responses (17,18). It
is of interest that the initial observations of tumor-associated suppressor
macrophages came from studies with an oncogenic virus in mice, the Moloney
sarcoma virus (19). Some of the nonspecific immunosuppression induced by
cancer or viruses may be mediated by soluble factors. Prostaglandins of
the E series have been shown to be released in considerable amounts from
activated macrophages and these may strongly inhibit specific immune
responses and also NK and macrophage functions (e.g., 20).

I would now like to turn to the issue of the effects of the immune
system on cancer and virus infections. It has been proposed that a properly
functioning immune system is responsible for effective resistance against
the development and progressive growth of tumors and also for effective
resistance against viruses and other microbial infections. This concept
is generally referred to as the immune surveillance hypothesis (21-23). In
his formulation of the hypothesis, Burnet specified the T cell as the effector cell responsible for immunologic surveillance (23). In some situations,
deficiencies in T cells or in their functions have been associated with a
much higher risk of developing serious disease. The many serious problems,
including Kaposi's sarcoma and various opportunistic infections, with the
acquired immune deficiency syndrome (AIDS), as discussed in detail elsewhere
in this book, are a striking example of the apparent importance of T cell-
mediated immunity. However, deficiencies in T cell-mediated immunity have
not been found to be associated with a generalized increase in susceptibility to virus infections or development of tumors, and this has led to
considerable skepticism about the validity of the immune surveillance hypothesis. As I have discussed in detail elsewhere (24), it seems important to
update the immune surveillance hypothesis to allow for the possible central

involvement of other aspects of the immune system. Such an updated hypothesis might be stated as follows: Transformed cells, viruses, and other microbial agents express surface antigens or other structures that can be recognized by one or more components of the immune system. One or more of these components of the natural and/or induced immunologic effector mechanisms can then eliminate the transformed or infected cells or at least impede the progressive course of disease. The principal revision in this hypothesis is the inclusion of the possible involvement of the natural immune system in defense against cancer and other diseases. Over the last several years, there has been increasing awareness of the potential important role of the natural immune system in resistance against disease. The natural immune system has some important attributes which make it likely to be involved as an initial line of defense against disease. Natural effector cells have spontaneous cytotoxic reactivity and can thereby react immediately against foreign materials. In addition, the components of the natural immune system, in contrast to specific immune reactivity, can be augmented very rapidly by various stimuli, e.g., interferon and other cytokines.

This updated version of the immune surveillance hypothesis leads to several testable predictions:

1. Tumor cells and microbial agents, or cells infected by such agents, have surface structures recognized by one or more effectors.

2. Tumor cells or affected target cells will be susceptible to lysis or growth inhibition by one or more of the effector mechanisms.

3. One or more of the relevant effector cells should be able to enter the site of tumor growth or infection.

4. Augmentation of the relevant effector mechanism(s) will decrease the incidence of progressive tumors or infections.

5. Depression of relevant effector mechanisms by various immunosuppressive treatments will increase the incidence of tumors or infections.

6. Restoration of the depressed effector activity will decrease the incidence of such disease.

Many investigators have suggested that macrophages play a central role in immune surveillance (e.g., 25, 26). There are substantial data to support several of the above predictions regarding a possible role of macrophages. A wide variety of tumor cells and microbial agents have been shown to be susceptible to lysis or growth inhibition by macrophages and large numbers of macrophages often accumulate in neoplastic or infectious lesions (27, 28). Further, treatment with immunomodulators which augment macrophage-mediated cytotoxic activity have resulted in decreased tumor growth and, conversely, various immunosuppressive regimens which result in inhibition of macrophage reactivity have interfered with host resistance against tumors (e.g., 29). However, it should be noted that there are some major limitations to such evidence. First, there is remarkably little evidence that macrophages have cytotoxic activity against primary, freshly harvested tumor cells, as opposed to established tumor cell lines. Secondly, silica and carrageenan, and virtually all of the other depressive treatments that have been used, may not be entirely selective in their effects. In fact, they may cause increases in some functions, particularly suppressor activity, by macrophages or other cells (30).

There is substantial evidence for an important role of NK cells in in vivo resistance against established cell lines of tumors, particularly those that show susceptibility to in vitro cytolysis by NK cells (summarized in

31). In addition, there are several types of evidence that conform to the predictions of the immune surveillance hypothesis:

1. NK cells have been shown to be able to accumulate at sites of inflammation (32) and in small primary as well as transplanted tumors (33).

2. NK cells have a natural and also rapidly activatable ability to lyse a variety of primary autochtonous tumors (e.g., 34, 35).

3. There is considerable evidence for the ability of NK cells to eliminate metastatic tumor cells and thereby resist tumor spread.

4. An increased tumor incidence (primarily lymphomas) has been found in individuals with depressed NK activity [beige mice (36), patients with Chediak-Higashi syndrome (37), and immunosuppressed transplant recipients (38)]. Some carcinogens (urethane, γ or X-irradiation, and dimethylbenzan-thracene) have been shown to cause early, profound depression of NK activity (39-41).

The most convincing data relate to the important role of NK cells in host resistance against metastases. The observation that NK cells appear to be mainly responsible for the rapid elimination of intravenously inocu-lated tumor cells provided the initial indication that this effector mech-anism might provide a very effective control of hematogenous spread of tumors (42). Experimental support for this possibility first came from the finding that cells from the lung metastases of a transplantable tumor in mice were more resistant to NK activity than locally growing tumor cells (43). An important role of NK cells in resistance against metastatic growth of trans-plantable tumors has been further supported by observations that suppression or augmentation of NK activity of mice was associated with parallel altera-tions in resistance to artificial metastases produced by intravenous inocula-tion of tumor cells (44-46). The patterns of results obtained in these studies suggested that NK cells may primarily influence metastatic spread of tumors by acting during the phase of hematogenous dissemination, presum-ably by their ability to eliminate rapidly the tumor cells from the circula-tion of capillary beds. As further confirmation of the association between depressed NK activity and increased metastases, Barlozzari et al. (47) have shown that selective restoration of NK activity in rats by adoptive transfer of highly purified large granular lymphocytes was accompanied by increased resistance to pulmonary metastases. Similarly, Warner and Dennert (48) showed that adoptive transfer of a clone of cultured lymphoid cells with NK-like activity protected against development of pulmonary or liver metastases.

Direct evidence for a possible role of NK cells in immune surveillance is quite limited and relates mainly to two models of carcinogenesis. With regard to the first model, there are several indications for a role of NK cells in protection against urethane-induced lung tumors in mice. This carcinogen produces lung tumors in only some strains of mice and was shown to cause transient and marked depression of NK activity in a susceptible strain (39) but not in resistant strains (49). However, it is clear that genetically determined susceptibility to depression of NK activity by ure-thane is only one of the factors determining the strain distribution. C57BL/6 mice were found to be highly resistant to urethane-induced lung tumors (50). The resistance to lung carcinogenesis even in the NK-deficient strain is probably attributable to the known genetic resistance of the lung tissues of C57BL/6 mice to transformation by urethane (51). In further studies in A/J mice, which are highly susceptible to induction of lung tumors by urethane, a further reduction in NK activity by treatment with cyclophos-phamide led to a significantly higher tumor incidence (50).

The second carcinogenesis system that has received considerable attention is the induction of thymic lymphomas by multiple low doses of irradiation of C57BL/6 mice. Development of tumors in this system appears to be dependent on a complex series of factors, and it has been difficult to demonstrate a clear contribution of NK cells to the overall process of leukomogenesis (52). However, NK cells did appear to be involved in protection against the transplantation of preleukemic bone marrow cells from donors which received fractionated doses of irradiation. Recipients of the preleukemic bone marrow that were irradiated with 400 R were susceptible to leukemia and in parallel were found to have depressed NK activity. Whereas unirradiated C57BL/6 recipients were resistant, unirradiated C57BL/6 beige recipients were found to be susceptible to induction of leukemia by the transferred bone marrow cells. As further evidence for the possible role of NK cells in this transplantation system, spleen cells of nude mice, which have high NK activity, protected against the transfer of leukemia, whereas spleen cells from mice with low NK activity did not protect. Further positive evidence for a role of NK cells in resistance against leukomogenesis has come from the studies of Warner and Dennert (48). They found that adoptive transfer of cloned cells with NK-like activity, during a four-week period after the last dose of fractionated irradiation, conferred substantial protection against the development of leukemia. Despite such suggestive positive evidence for a role of NK cells, a series of other experiments (52) has indicated that non-NK-related factors seemed to have a more important influence on the incidence of leukemia than did the levels of NK activity.

In addition to the increasing evidence for an important role of NK cells in natural resistance against tumor growth, recently considerable evidence has accumulated for an important role of NK cells in natural resistance against various microorganisms. Most compelling has been a series of studies performed along the same lines as those described above for resistance to metastases, in which alterations in NK activity were shown to result in substantial changes in natural resistance against virus infections. Significant correlations between levels of NK activity and natural resistance have been demonstrated for infections by cytomegalovirus (53), herpes simplex virus (54), and hepatitis virus (55) in mice.

It is important to note that more than one effector mechanism may be involved in protection against tumors or microbial infections. In addition to possible separate contributions by two or more effector mechanisms, in many instances the activity of a particular effector mechanism may be dependent on the action or other form of collaboration from another component of the immune system. The best-known example of such a collaboration is antibody-dependent cell-mediated cytotoxicity (ADCC), in which natural or induced antibodies cooperate with effector cells. In addition to the well-known cytokine production by macrophage and T cells, NK cells have been shown to secrete a variety of cytokines (interferons, IL-1, IL-2, CSF, BCGF) (56-59) and this function might contribute to the role of NK cells in resistance to tumors or infections.

Another aspect to consider with regard to the possible involvement of multiple effector cells is the possibility of sequential contributions by natural effector cells and immune T cells. Because of their spontaneous levels of reactivity and/or their ability to be rapidly activated, NK cells and macrophages might be viewed as a first line defense against small numbers of transformed cells or infected cells. If these natural effector cells are not completely effective in eliminating tumor cells or infectious agents, immune T-cell reactivity might be induced and be responsible for the subsequent elimination of control of disease.

CONCLUSIONS

In the context of the updated, broad formulation of the hypothesis, immune surveillance does not appear to exist, at least for certain types of tumors and microbial infections. This conclusion is based primarily on the considerable evidence that various forms of immunodepression have been associated with an increased incidence of tumors and infections. A major challenge to immunologists is to determine the possible effector mechanism(s) involved in immune surveillance. This task will undoubtedly continue to be quite difficult despite further studies along the lines outlined above. One problem is that most augmenting and suppressive treatments are not entirely selective for one effector mechanism. Furthermore, the lack of effect of a selective treatment on disease incidence might be attributable to the compensatory protection from an alternative effector mechanism. Conversely, a positive effect of a selective suppressive treatment on disease incidence might only reflect the cooperative involvement of that effector mechanism, with a different mechanism actually being the effector of resistance.

With regard to the potential of immunomodulation for prophylaxis or therapy of cancer or infectious diseases, the questions of the overall efficacy of immune surveillance, or of the most relevant effector mechanisms in such resistance, are of secondary importance. Although natural host defenses may be inadequate to protect against some diseases, because of insufficiently low levels of reactivity, augmentation of one or more effector mechanisms may inhibit and even abrogate malignant development or infections. More studies focused on this important, practical issue are required.

REFERENCES

1. H. B. Hewitt, Animal tumor models and their relevance to human tumor immunology J. Biol. Resp. Modif. 1:107 (1982).
2. R. B. Herberman, Counterpoint: Animal tumor models and their relevance to human tumor immunology, J. Biol. Resp. Modif. 2:39 (1983).
3. H. B. Hewitt, Second Point: Animal tumor models and their relevance to human tumor immunology, J. Biol. Resp. Modif. 2:210 (1983).
4. R. B. Herberman, Second counterpoint: Animal tumor models and their relevance to human tumor immunology, J. Biol. Resp. Modif. 2(3):217 (1983).
5. C. P. Doherty, R. V. Blanden and R. M. Zinkernagel, Specificity of virus-immune effector T cell for H-2K or H-2D compatible interactions: implications for H-antigen diversity, Transpl. Rev. 29:89 (1976).
6. H. T. Holden and R. B. Herberman, Cytotoxicity against tumor-associated antigens not H-2 restricted, Nature, 268:250 (1977).
7. R. B. Herberman, M. E. Nunn, H. T. Holden, S. Staal and J. Y. Djeu, Augmentation of natural cytotoxic reactivity of mouse lymphoid cells against syngeneic and allogenic target cells, Int. J. Cancer, 19:555 (1977).
8. J. Y. Djeu, K.-Y. Huang and R. B. Herberman, Augmentation of mouse natural killer activity and induction of interferon by tumor cells in vivo, J. Exp. Med. 151:781 (1980).
9. J. Y. Djeu, N. Stocks, K. Zoon, G. J. Stanton, T. Timonen and R. B. Herberman, Positive self regulation of cytotoxicity in human natural killer cells by production of interferon upon exposure to influenza and herpes viruses, J. Exp. Med. 156:1222 (1982).
10. J. Y. Djeu, T. Timonen and R. B. Herberman, Production of interferon by human natural killer cells in response to mitogens, viruses and bacteria, in: "NK Cells and Other Natural Effector Cells," R. B. Herberman, ed., Academic Press, New York, (1982).

11. T. Kasahara, J. Y. Djeu, S. F. Dougherty and J. J. Oppenheim, Capacity of human large granular lymphocytes (LGL) to produce multiple lymphokines: interleukin 2, interferon and colony stimulating factor, J. Immunol. 131:2379 (1983).

12 W. Domzig and B. M. Stadler, The relation between human natural killer cells and interleukin 2, in: "NK Cells and Other Natural Effector Cells, R. B. Herberman, ed., Academic Press, New York (1982).

13. G. Scala, P. Allavena, J. Y. Djeu, T. Kasahara, J. R. Ortaldo, R. B. Herberman and J. J. Oppenheim, Human large granular lymphocytes are potent producers of interleukin-1, Nature, 309:56 (1984).

14. R. B. Herberman, P. Allavena, G. Scala, J. Djeu, T. Kasahara, W. Domiz, A. Procopio, I. Blanca, J. Ortaldo and J. J. Oppenheim, Cytokine production by human large granular lymphocytes (LGL), in: "Natural Killer Activity and Its Regulation," T. Hoshino, H. S. Koren and A. Uchida, eds., Excerpta Medica Ltd. Tokyo (1984).

15. S. Fujimoto, M. I. Greene and A. H. Sehon, Regulation of the immune response to tumor antigens. I. Immunosuppressor cells in tumor-bearing hosts, J. Immunol. 116:791 (1976).

16. M. L. Kripke and M. S. Fisher, Immunologic parameters of ultraviolet carcinogensis, J. Natl. Cancer Inst. 57:211 (1976).

17. H. Kirchner, M. Glaser, H. T. Holden, B. R. Fernbach and R. B. Herberman, Suppressor cells in tumor-bearing mice and rats, Biomedicine 24:371 (1976).

18. S. Broder, L. Muul and T. A. Waldmann, Suppressor cells in neoplastic disease, J. Natl. Cancer Inst. 61:5 (1978).

19. H. Kirchner, T. M. Chused, R. B. Herberman, H. T. Herberman and D. H. Larvin, Evidence of suppressor cell activity in spleens of mice bearing primary tumors induced by Moloney sarcoma virus, J. Exp. Med. 139:1473 (1974).

20. M. J. Brunda, R. B. Herberman and H. T. Holden, Inhibition of murine natural killer cell activity by prostaglandins, J. Immunol. 124:2682 (1980).

21. P. Ehrlich, Uber den jetzigen Stand der Karcinomaforschung, in: "The Collected Papers of Paul Ehrlich," Vol. II, F. Himmelweit, ed., Permagon Press, London (1957).

22. F. M. Burnet, Cancer--a biological approach, Brit. Med. J. 1:779 841 (1957).

23. F. M. Burnet, The concept of immunological surveillance, Prog. Exp. Tumor Res. 13:1 (1970).

24. R. B. Herberman, Immune surveillance hypothesis:updated formulation and possible effector mechanisms, in: "Progress in Immunology V," Y. Yamamura and T. Tade, eds., Academic Press, Tokyo (1983).

25. D. O. Adams and R. Snyderman, Do macrophages destroy nascent tumors? J. Natl. Cancer Inst. 62:1341 (1979).

26. J. B. Hibbs, Jr., H. A. Chapman, Jr. and J. B. Weinberg, The macrophage as an antineoplastic surveillance cell: biological perspectives, J. Reticuleondothel. 24:549 (1978).

27 R. Evans, Macrophages in syngeneic animal tumors, Transplantation 14:468 (1972).

28. C. L. Gauci and P. Alexander, The macrophage content of some human tumors, Cancer Lett. 1:20 (1975).

29. K. C. Norbury and M. L. Kripke, Ultraviolet-induced carcinogenesis in mice treated with silica, trypan blue or pyran copolymer, J. Reticuloendothel. Soc. 26:826 (1979).

30. G. Cudkowicz and P. S. Hochman, Do natural killer cells engage in regulated reactions against self to ensure homeostasis? Immunol. Rev. 44:13 (1979).

31. R. B. Herberman and W. T. Holden, Natural cell-mediated immunity, Adv. Cancer Res. 27:305 (1978).

32. J. M. Ward, F. Argilan and C. W. Reynolds, Immunoperoxidase

localization of large granular lymphocytes in normal tissues and lesions of athymic nude rats, J. Immunol. 131:132 (1983).

33. J. M. Gerson, Systemic and in situ natural killer activity in tumor-bearing mice and patients with cancer, in: "Natural Cell-Mediated Immunity Against Tumors," R. B. Herberman, ed.,New York (1980).

34. S. A. Serrate and R. B. Herberman, Natural cell-mediated cytotoxicity against spontaneous mouse mammary tumors, in: "NK Cells and Other Natural Effector Cells," R. B. Herberman, ed., Academic Press New York (1982).

35. S. A. Serrate, B. M. Vose, T. Timonen, J. R. Ortaldo and R. B. Herberman, Association of human natural killer cell activity against human primary tumors with large granular lymphocytes, in: "NK Cell and Other Natural Effector Cells," R. B. Herberman, ed., Academic Press, New York (1982).

36. J. F. Loutit, K. M. S. Townsend and J. F. Knowles, Tumor surveillence in beige mice, Nature 285:66 (1980).

37. P. B. Dent, L. A. Fish, J. F. White and R. A. Good, Chediak Higashi syndrome. Observations on the nature of the associated malignancy, Lab. Invest. 15:1634 (1966).

38. M. Lipinski, T. Tursz, H. Kreis, Y. Finale and J. L. Amiel, Dissociation of natural killer cell activity and antibody-dependent cell-mediated cytotoxicity in kidney allograft recipients receiving high-dose immunosuppressive therapy, Transplantation 29:214 (1980).

39. E. Gorelik and R. B. Herberman, Inhibition of the activity of mouse NK cells by urethane, J. Natl. Cancer Inst. 66:543 (1981).

40. D. R. Parkinson, R. P. Brightman and S. D. Waksal, Altered natural killer cell biology in C57BL/6 mice after leukomogenic split-dose irradiation, J. Immunol. 126:1460 (1981).

41. R. Ehrlich, M. Efrati and I. P. Witz, Cytotoxicity and cytostasis mediated by splenocytes of mice subjected to chemical carcinogens and of mice bearing tumors, in: "Natural Cell-Mediated Immunity Against Tumors," R. B. Herberman, ed., Academic Press, New York (1980).

42. C. Riccardi, P. Puccetti, A. Santoni and R. B. Herberman, Rapid in vivo assay of mouse NK cell activity, J. Natl. Cancer Inst. 63:1041 (1979).

43. E. Gorelik, M. Fogel, M. Feldman and S. Segals, Differences in resistance of metastatic tumor cells and cells from local tumor growth to cytotoxicity of natural killer cells, J. Natl. Cancer Inst. 63:1397 (1979).

44. N. Hanna and I. Fidler, Relationship between metastic potential and resistance to natural killer cell-mediated cytotoxicity in three murine tumor systems, J. Natl. Cancer Inst. 66:1183 (1981).

45. E. Gorelik, B. Rosen and R. B. Herberman, Depression of NK reactivity in mice by leukemogenic doses of irradiation, in: "NK Cells and Other Natural Effector Cells," R. B. Herberman, ed., Academic Press, New York (1980).

46. E. Gorelik, R. H. Wiltrout, K. Okumura, S. Habu and R. B. Herberman, Role of NK cells in the control of metastatic spread and growth of tumor cells in mice, Int. J. Cancer 30:107 (1982).

47. T. Barlozzari, C. W. Reynold and R. B. Herberman, Reconstitution of NK activity and antitumor immunity in anti-asialo GM$_1$-treated rats by the adoptive transfer of LGL, in: "Natural Killer Activity and Its Regulation," T. Hoshino, H. S. Koren and A. Uchida, eds., Excerpta Medica Ltd. Tokyo (1984).

48. J. F. Warner and G. Dennert, In vivo function of a cloned cell line with NK activity: Effects on bone marrow transplants, tumor development and metastasis, Nature 300:31 (1982).

49. E. Gorelik and R. B. Herberman, Susceptibiltiy of various strains of mice to urethane-induced lung tumors and depressed natural killer cell activity, J. Natl. Cancer Inst. 67:1317 (1981).

50. E. Gorelik and R. B. Herberman, Role of natural cell-mediated immunity in urethane-induced lung carcinogenesis, in: "NK Cells and Other Natural Effector Cells," R. B. Herberman, ed., Academic Press New York (1982).

51. W. Heston and T. Dunn, Tumor development in susceptible strain A and resistant L lung transplants in LAFI host, J. Natl. Cancer Inst. 11:1057 (1951).

52. E. Gorelik, B. Rosen, D. Copland, B. Weatherly and R. B. Herberman, Evaluation of role of natural killer cells in radiation-induced leukemogenesis in mice, J. Natl. Cancer Inst. 72:1397 (1984).

53. G. R. Shellam, J. E. Grundy and J. E. Allan, The role of natural killer cells and interferon to resistance to murine cytomegalovirus, in: "NK Cells and Other Natural Effector Cells," R. B. Herberman, ed., Academic Press, New York (1982).

54. C. Lopez, D. Kirkpatrick and P. Fitzgerald, The role of NK (HSV-1) effector cells in resistance to herpes virus infection in man, in: "NK Cells and Other Natural Effector Cells," R. B. Herberman, ed., Academic Press, New York (1982).

55. J. F. Bukowski, B. A. Woda, S. Habu, K. Okumura and R. M. Welsh, Natural Killer cell depletion enhances virus synthesis and virus-induced hepatitis in vivo, J. Immunol. 131:1531 (1983).

56. J. Y. Djeu, T. Timonen and R. B. Herberman, Production of interferon by human natural killer cells in response to migotens, viruses and bacteria, in: "NK Cells and Other Natural Effector Cells," R. B. Herberman, ed., Adacemic Press, New York (1982).

57. W. Domzig and B. M. Stadler, The relation between human natural killer cells and interleukin 2, in: "NK Cells and Other Natural Effector Cells," R. B. Herberman, ed., Academic Press, New York (1982).

58. G. Scala, P. Allavena, J. Y. Djeu, T. Kasahara, J. R. Ortaldo, R. B. Herberman and J. J. Oppenheim, Human large granular lymphocytes are potent producers of interleukin-1, Nature, 309:56 (1984).

59. R. B. Herberman, P. Allavena, G. Scala, J. Djeu, T. Kasahara, W. Domiz, A. Procopio, I. Blanca, J. Ortaldo and J. J. Oppenheim, Cytokine production by human large granular lymphocytes (LGL), in: "Natural Killer Activity and Its Regulation," T. Hoshino, H. S. Koren and A. Uchida, eds., Excerpta Medica Ltd., Tokyo (1984).

IV. MECHANISMS OF VIRUS ASSOCIATED IMMUNODEREGULATION

VIRUSES, GENETICS AND AUTOIMMUNITY

Norman Talal, Michael Fischbach, and Richard Pope

The University of Texas Health Science Center and the
Audie L. Murphy Memorial Veterans Administration Hospital
San Antonio, Texas

INTRODUCTION

The many factors that contribute to the pathogenesis of autoimmune
disorders include: genetic (1), immunologic, viral, hormonal (2) and probably
neuropsychiatric (3). Patients with autoimmune disease are frequently characterized by an immunologic imbalance in which T cell activities are depressed and B cells are polyclonally activated (4).

Our laboratory has recently focused on interleukin-2 (IL-2) deficiency
which is a common feature of several human and murine autoimmune diseases
(5-7). MRL/lpr mice, for example, spontaneously develop a lupus-like illness
and massive lymphoproliferation due to an unusual T cell which we find to
be refractory to stimulation by mitogens and alloantigens. These mice are
defective in IL-2 production and in receptors for IL-2. This defect can be
overcome and functional in vivo immune response restored by the administration of the immunomodulating drug isoprinosine (8).

Similar IL-2 abnormalities occur in patients with systemic lupus erythematosus (SLE) and rheumatoid arthritis (RA) (7) in whom polyclonal B cell
activation is also present. The inflamed rheumatoid synovium develops ger-
minal centers and is actively producing immunoglobulins, rheumatoid factor
and immune complexes (9). RA patients have defective immune mechanisms for
regulation the expression of Epstein-Barr virus, an intrinsic polyclonal B
cell activator (10,11). We find natural killer (NK) cell activity to be
significantly depressed in RA patients, in the blood and particularly in
the joint fluid and tissue. We can increase NK activity by the addition of
IL-2, interferon inducers and synovial macrophages which are themselves
activated in RA (12).

These results in a murine model and in patients suggest that autoimmunity
represents a state of disordered immunoregulation in which IL-2 abnormalities
are a central focus and various other effector mechanisms are also deranged.

MATERIALS AND METHODS

IL-2 Production (mouse)

Spleen cells were cultured at a density of 1×10^7/ml in RPMI supplemented with 10% heat inactivated fetal bovine serum (FBS) and concanavalin

A (Con A) 10 μg/ml. The cells were cultured for 36 hr, supernatants removed and tested for IL-2.

IL-2 Production (human)

Peripheral blood mononuclear cells were suspended at 1×10^6 ml in 1% FBS, complete RPMI and incubated with and without phytohemagglutinin (PHA) for 24 hr at 37°C. Supernatants were harvested after centrifugation, filtered through Millipore filters (0.45 μm) then stored at -70°C until the time of assay.

IL-2 Assay (mouse and human)

Culture supernatants were serially diluted and each dilution assayed for IL-2 activity using an IL-2 dependent cell line, CTLL-2, a gift of Dr. Steven Gillis, Immunex Corporation of Seattle, Washington. Utilizing the method of Gillis et al., 5,000 IL-2 dependent T cells were incubated for 24 hr with culture supernatants in microtiter plates. The cells were pulsed with 1 μCi tritiated thymidine during the final 6 hr. Cultures were harvested onto glass fiber filters using a mini-MASH harvester. The quantity of IL-2 produced is expressed in units/ml calculated by the probit analysis method of Gillis et al. (13).

IL-2 Response (mouse)

Ten units of purified delectinated human IL-2 (Cellular Products, Buffalo, New York) was added to 5×10^3 spleen cells which had been previously activated with Con A. Cultures were supplemented with 10 mg/ml alpha-methyl-D-mannoside to block the possible mitogenic effects of Con A. Cultures were pulsed with tritiated thymidine during the last 18 hr of a 72 hr incubation.

IL-2 Response (human)

Lymphocyte blasts were obtained after stimulation with Con A and washed twice in α-methylmannoside (10 mg/ml). Ten thousand activated cells were cultured for 72 hr at 37°C with several dilutions of the standard IL-2 in complete media containing 10 mg/ml of α-methylmannoside. The cells were pulsed with ^{3}H for the last 6 hr.

Natural Killer (NK) Assay

Effector cells (5×10^6) were incubated for 16 hr at 37°C in 2 ml of 20% FBS-complete RPMI in culture plates (Costar #3506) with or without standard IL-2. The target for NK activity was K562, a myelogenous leukemia cell line. NK activity was quantitated in a 3 hr ^{51}Cr-release assay. Briefly, effector cells were mixed with labeled K562 target cells at concentrations which give effector:target ratios of 20:1, 10:1, and 5:1. Triplicate samples were prepared for each ratio. The supernatants were withdrawn after a 3 hr incubation period and the ^{51}Cr released from lysed targets was quantitated in a gamma counter (Packard Instrument Company). Incubation of targets with medium or saponin (7 mg/ml) and EDTA (0.1 mg/ml) determined spontaneous and maximum release. The percent cytotoxicity was calculated by the formula:

$$\frac{(\text{cpm of effector cells} - \text{cpm of spontaneous release}) \, (\times 100)}{(\text{cpm of maximum release} - \text{cpm of spontaneous release})}$$

Interferon (IFN) Assay

The supernatants of cells cultured to determine NK activity with and without added IL-2 were collected after centrifugation and tested for IFN activity. Total IFN was assayed for antiviral activity on microtiter plate cultures of human amnion WISH cells by using a 50% Sindbis virus yield reduction assay. Gamma (γ) IFN was determined by preincubation of samples at pH 3.0 and by treatment with an antibody specific for γ-IFN.

Antigen Presentation

Antigen presentation was performed by a modification of the method of Papoian and Talal (14). Trinitrophenyl (TNP) was coupled to keyhole limpet hemocyanin (KLH). Five mice were injected with 10 µg TNP$_{25}$ KLH in complete Freund's adjuvant at the base of the tail. Draining inguinal and para-aortic nodes were removed seven days later. T cells were enriched by nylon wool chromatography. Spleen cells from two naive mice were used as the source of antigen presenting cells. Ten million spleen cells were incubated with 10 µg TNP-KLH in the presence of 50 µg Mitocycin C for 1 hr at 37°C. The cells were extensively washed and 2×10^5 antigen pulsed presenting cells were cultured with 4×10^5 primed T cells at 37°C for five days. Cultures were pulsed with tritiated thymidine during the final 18 hr.

Ornithine Decarboxylase (ODC) Assay

Spleen cells were suspended at 2.5×10^6/ml and incubated with appropriate concentrations of mitogens. After incubation, cells were centrifuged. Cell pellets were sonicated in 0.5 ml of 50 mM Na$_2$HPO (pH 7.2) containing 0.1 mM EDTA, 2.0 mM dithiothreitol, 5 mM NaF, 2 mM phenylmethylsulfonyl-fluoride, and 60 µm pyridoxal phosphate, and centrifuged at 10,000 x g at 4°C for 5 min. Aliquots of 180 µl of the sonicated cell supernatant were incubated for 60 min at 37°C with 20 µl of ^{14}C-ornithine. The released ^{14}CO$_2$ was collected on filters and counted by standard liquid scintillation spectroscopy. Data are expressed as pmoles ^{14}Co$_2$ released/60 min/total cells assayed.

RESULTS

Interleukin-2 Abnormalities in Autoimmune Mice

The several autoimmune-susceptible strains of mice (NZB, NZB/NZW, BXSB, MRL/lpr) share in common a decreased ability to produce IL-2 (6). We have chosen to study this phenomenon in those strains of mice in which autoimmunity develops due to the presence of the gene lpr (for lymphoproliferation). The prototype strain, MRL/lpr, is thought to differ by a single autosomal recessive gene from its congenic partner MRL/++. As seen in Table 1, splenic IL-2 production in response to concanavalin A is impaired in MRL/lpr mice

Table 1. Decreased Splenic IL-2 Production by MRL/lpr Mice

Strain (Age)	Units IL-2 Produced
MRL/lpr (5 months)	< 0.1
MRL/++ (5 months)	50
MRL/lpr (2 months)	5
MRL/++ (2 months)	37
Media + Con A	0

Table 2. Decreased Spleen Cell Response to IL-2 in MRL/lpr Mice

Strain (Age)	^{3}H-Tdr Incorporation (cpm) (Mean ± S.E.M.)	
MRL/lpr (5 months)	3,452 ± 1,660	$p < 10^{-5}$
MRL/++ (5 months)	43,392 ± 4,417	
MRL/lpr (2 months)	25,075 ± 6,152	$p < .05$
MRL/++ (2 months)	45,454 ± 6,095	

as early as two months of age. A similar abnormality is also present in C57B16/lpr mice (5).

Mice bearing the lpr gene are also impaired in their ability to respond to IL-2 (Table 2). Again, this is present as early as two months of age and grows worse over time. These IL-2 abnormalities are not due to suppressor cells or inhibitory factors and cannot be corrected by altering mitogen concentration or incubation time (5). The decreased IL-2 production extends to stimulation with other mitogens, alloantigens and syngeneic stimulators. It cannot be overcome by exposure to interleukin 1 or to phorbol esters (5).

The decreased response to IL-2 is associated with diminished numbers of IL-2 receptors (Table 3) (15). Phorbol ester (PMA) in association with Con A can restore receptor number to normal in the C57B16/lpr mice which develop a milder autoimmune disease than do MRL/lpr mice. C57B16/lpr mice differ from MRL/lpr mice in their response to phorbol ester (16) as determined by activation of the enzyme ornithine decarboxylase (ODC) which serves as an early indicator to T cell activation (17). Both strains of lpr mice are incapable of ODC induction following mitogen stimulation (Table 4).

Table 3. IL-2 Receptors in C57B16 and C57B16/lpr Mice

Strain (Age)	PMA	Number of IL-2 Receptors/Cell
C57B1/6 (2 months)	0	530
	+	535
C57B16/lpr (6 weeks)	0	530
	+	420
C57B16/lpr (5 months)	0	220
	+	520

IL-2 receptors were measured after 18 hr in culture with or without the addition of PMA. IL-2 receptors were quantified by the binding of ^{35}S-methinonine labelled IL-2. Binding studies were performed in the laboratory of Dr. R. Robb, E. I. Dupont (15).

Table 4. Induction of Ornithine Decarboxylase Synthesis
Following Mitogen Stimulation

Strain	Age	Mitogen	ODC Induction[a]
MRL/++	3 months	PHA	26
		PHA + PMA	93
C57B16/1pr	2 months	PHA	93
		PHA + PMA	393
MRL/1pr	2 weeks	PHA	5
		PHA + PMA	4
MRL/1pr	2 months	PHA	2
		PHA + PMA	3

[a]Picomoles of $^{14}CO_2$ produced/60 min/10^7 cells.
Experiments performed in the laboratory of Dr. Rosanne
Fidelus-Gort, Veterans Administration Hospital, Houston, TX

PMA and Con A administered concurrently can restore ODC in C57B1/1pr mice
but not in the MRL/1pr strain (Table 4).

Functional Consequence of IL-2 Deficiency

We have studied the IL-2 dependent response to TNP-KLH in order to
determine the in vivo consequence of IL-2 deficiency on the ability to
mount an antigen-dependent T cell proliferative response. We find this
response markedly abnormal in MRL/1pr mice, C67B16/1pr mice and C3H/1pr
mice (19). Employing the normal C57B1/6 mouse as a congenic partner in
cell mixing experiments, we have studied whether the defect in response is

Table 5. The Defective Response to TNP-KLH in C57B1/1pr
Mice is Due to T Cells and Not to Antigen
Presenting Cells (APC)

Strain	APC	T Cells	^{3}H-Tdr Incorporation (cpm) (mean ± S.E.M.)
C57B1/6	+	+	41,300 ± 4,322
C57B16/1pr	+	+	322 ± 165
C57B1/6	+		
C57B16/1pr		+	1,402 ± 629
C57B1/6		+	38,039 ± 4,147
C57B16/1pr	+		

Controls: primed T cells, antigen presenting cells, unprimed
T cells alone or in any combination gave less than 900 cpm.

Table 6. Restoration of an IL-2 Dependent T Cell
Proliferative Response by Isoprinosine

Strain	Isoprinosine[a]	^{3}H-Tdr Incorporation (cpm) (Mean ± S.E.M.)
C57B1/6	0	25,075 ± 2,320
	+	38,321 ± 4,150
C57B16/1pr	0	1,185 ± 79
	+	28,545 ± 244

[a]Isoprinosine was administered daily at the base of the
tail.

a property of antigen-presenting macrophages or of responding T cells. As
shown in Table 5, antigen-presenting cells from 1pr mice function appropriately but 1pr T cells are unable to proliferate even when exposed to normal
C57B1/6 antigen-presenting cells. The in vivo or in vitro addition of IL-2
does not restore T cell responsiveness.

Restoration of IL-2 Response by Immunomodulation

The immunomodulating drug isoprinosine is able to restore a number of
defective T cell responses when added in vivo to human and murine lymphocytes
(20). We have studied its effect in vivo in C57B16/1pr mice using the antigen presentation system described above. Daily injection of 50 mg/kg for
one week starting immediately following immunization with TNP-KLH enabled
C57B16/1pr mice to mount an effective response (Table 6). T cell proliferation, as expected, was accompanied by the production of IL-2 (8).

IL-2 Abnormalities in Autoimmune Patients

PHA stimulated peripheral blood lymphocytes from patients with RA and

Table 7. Induction of IL-2 by PHA in Normal Controls
and Patients with Rheumatoid Arthritis

Subjects	IL-2 (units/ml)
Normal PB (n=15)	28.0 ± 17.4[a]
RA PB (n=13)	10.2 ± 11.9[b]
SF (n=13)	14.8 ± 26.3[c]
ST (n= 4)	2.6 ± 3.4
Gout SF (n= 4)	61.5 ± 32.8

[a]Mean ± SD
[b]Significantly reduced compared to normal PB (p<0.001).
[c]Significantly reduced compared to normal PB (p<0.02).

Table 8. Response to Exogenous IL-2 by Lymphocyte Blasts
From Patients with RA and Normal Controls.

| | Lymphocyte Proliferation | |
	No IL-2 (cpm)	Plus IL-2 (cpm)
Normal PB (n=10)	681 ± 547[a]	39,685 ± 13,759
RA PB (n=6)	604 ± 600	27,466 ± 6,447
RA SF (n=8)	561 ± 373	17,408 ± 6,700[b]

[a]Mean ± SD
[b]Significantly different from both normal PB ($p < 0.001$) and
RA PB ($p < 0.05$).

SLE showed an impaired ability to produce IL-2 (7). The response to IL-2
was also significantly diminished in RA (7).

Because of the inflamed rheumatoid synovium is accessible and is a
major site of immunopathology in RA, we have recently extended our human
IL-2 studies to RA synovial fluid (SF) and tissues (ST). Matched blood
(PB) and synovial fluid lymphocytes from 13 RA patients showed markedly
impaired IL-2 production following RHA stimulation (Table 7). Lymphocytes
recovered from RA synovial tissue specimens produced almost no IL-2 in response to PHA (21). Lymphocytes from the synovial fluid of control patients
with gout produced abundant quantities of IL-2 following PHA stimulation.
IL-2 production by RA-blood or synovial fluid did not correlate with therapeutic regimen, NK activity or clinical activity as measured by erythrocyte
sedimentation rate.

As in the autoimmune mice and in RA blood, the RA synovial lymphocytes
also showed a diminished ability to respond to IL-2 ($p < 0.001$) (Table 8).
Indeed, the proliferative response of synovial lymphoid cells to added IL-2
was even more impaired than that of blood ($p < 0.05$).

Decreased γ-IFN Induction After Treatment of RA Lymphocytes with IL-2

IL-2 has diverse effects on the immune response including the ability
to induce lymphocytes to produce γ-interferon (IFN). Since the proliferative response of RA blood and synovial lymphocytes to IL-2 is diminished,
we studied whether the IFN response to IL-2 would also be decreased (22).
The IFN activity released spontaneously by either RA or normal unstimulated
cells was negligible. Following exposure to IL-2, both blood ($p < 0.001$)
and synovial ($p < 0.02$) lymphocytes produced significantly less IFN than did
normal PB lymphocytes (Table 9). The IFN produced was primarily of the
gamma (γ) class, since incubation at pH 3.0—and treatment with an antibody
specific for γ-IFN either abolished or greatly reduced the IFN activity
compared to the pretreatment values.

Natural Killing and Interferon in RA

NK cell activity is significantly decreased in RA blood and synovial
fluid but is very responsive to augmentation by IL-2 and by poly I-poly C
(22). Table 10 demonstrates the effect of IL-2 on the enhancement of NK
activity. All increases were significant compared to baseline ($p < 0.005$).
IL-2 enhanced NK activity of RA synovial lymphocytes to a greater degree
than seen with normal or rheumatoid ($p < 0.02$) peripheral blood. The NK

Table 9. Induction of Interferon by Incubation of
Mononuclear Cells with IL-2

| | Interferon units/ml | |
	No IL-2	+IL-2
Normal PB (n=8)	1.3 ± 1.2[a]	62.5 ± 12.5
RA PB (n=8)	2.5 ± 2.5	16.1 ± 7.6[b]
RA SF (n=8)	2.5 ± 4.6	29.6 ± 11.5[c]

[a]Interferon in units/ml are presented as mean ± SE

[b]Decreased compared to normal PB (p <0.001)

[c]Decreased compared to normal PB (p <0.02)

activity of rheumatoid synovial fluid was enhanced to a level comparable to that seen in normal peripheral blood, even though the baseline values tended to be lower in the synovial fluid.

Despite the defective induction of IFN by IL-2, IL-2 increased the in vitro NK activity of RA blood and synovial lymphoid cells to a degree comparable to normals (Tables 9 and 10). Thus, there was a discordance between the poor ability of IL-2 to stimulate IFN production and its excellent ability to augment NK activity in RA. Removal of adherent cells did not restore but further decreased the IFN induced by IL-2 from 34.7 ± 10.1 units/ml (mean ± SE) to 3.3 ± 3.3 units/ml. Therefore, snynovial adherent cells, which have been shown in numerous studies to produce abundant quantities of suppressing prostaglandins, failed to suppress the IL-2 induction of interferon. In fact, adherent cells may promote this effect of IL-2.

Table 10. Effect of IL-2 on NK Activity in Rheumatoid
Arthritis and Normal Controls

| | Mean % of Cytotoxicity | | Percent |
	No IL-2	+IL-2	Increase
Normal PB (n=16)	47.1 ± 4.8[a]	64.0 ± 3.6	36%[b]
RA PB (n=9)	29.0 ± 4.6	42.3 ± 6.3	46%
RA SF (n=9)	37.9 ± 5.6	60.1 ± 4.3	59%

[a]Whole mononuclear cells were employed at an E:T ratio of 20:1 to measure NK activity (as percent of maximal ^{51}Cr released from K562).

[b]Percent increase over baseline by addition of IL-2.

DISCUSSION

Our current understanding of how autoimmune and malignant disease may develop out of a background of disordered immunoregulation is shown schematically in Figure 1. This concept of pathogenesis is very similar to one proposed fourteen years ago (4) and discussed more recently in relation to the impaired autologous mixed lymphocyte response that often accompanies these diseases (23).

The immune response gene predisposition is probably related to common structural products of DR and DS loci such as those recently found for HLA-DR4 in RA patients (24). Whether transposable genetic elements or structures similar to oncogenes (autogenes?) are also involved is a matter for speculation. Less speculative is the immunologic imbalance characteristic not only of autoimmunity but also seen in patients with AIDS (25) and those immunosuppressed with cyclosporine A (26). The essence of this imbalance is a depressed cellular immunity accompanied by IL-2 deficiency, and a polyclonal B cell activation with augmented and often inappropriate antibody responses. Several factors may account for this heightened humoral immunity including intrinsic mechanisms related to EB or other viruses (10,11), T-cell derived B cell growth and differentiation factors (27) or the recently described down-regulation of B cells by NK cells (28). Probably as a consequence of several mechanisms, "auto-antibodies" are produced which may be induced by viral antigens and/or nucleic acids and not truly be anti-self in that sense. Indeed, such reactivity might even derive from a physiologic basis as previously hypothesized (29).

The experimental focus in this report centers around the depressed IL-2 production and response to IL-2 which we feel to be hallmarks of immune dysregulation and autoimmunity. The functional consequences of this deficiency are presented here and also recently by Scott et al. who found a lack of IL-2 receptor sites on proliferating T cells in MRL/1pr mice but not on cytotoxic precursors (30).

We are able to overcome the IL-2 defect and restore IL-2 dependent responses by in vivo administration of isoprinosine. The mechanisms responsible for this modulation and possible therapeutic implications are currently under study.

We find that RA and SLE patients similarly manifest IL-2 abnormalities and have focused on the rheumatoid joint which is a site of intense B cell hyperactivity (9). Synovial lymphocytes from RA patients produce little IL-2 in response to mitogenic stimulation and respond poorly to exogenous

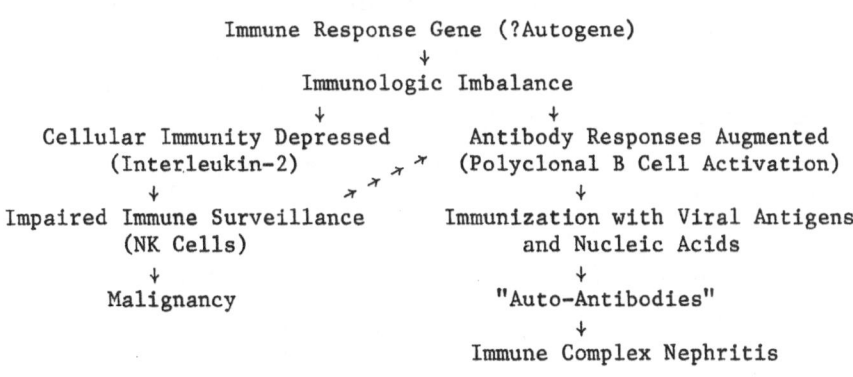

Figure 1. Schematic Representation of Immune Regulation

IL-2 as measured by proliferation and interferon production. Systemic as well as local production of interferon would be extremely important for the maintenance of NK cell activity as well as for more direct anti-viral defense.

We looked directly at NK cell activity in RA and found that it, like IL-2, is also diminished in blood and even more in the synovium. Several mechanisms in the RA synovium are present to bolster what little residual NK activity remains. For example, activated macrophages in the RA synovium are augmenters of NK (12) whereas RA blood macrophages suppress NK as do normal peripheral blood macrophages. IL-2, although it is a poor inducer of interferon in RA, is a good activator of NK both in RA blood and particularly in the synovium.

We are intrigued by the possibility that NK cells play a role in down-regulating B cells (28) and that the failure of this mechanism contributes to the persistent immunoglobulin, autoantibody and rheumatoid factor production seen in RA.

The mechanisms responsible for the IL-2 deficiency in autoimmune mice and patients need to be investigated. The inability of phorbol ester to induce ODC as well as IL-2 in MRL/1pr mice may be an important clue since much is now known about phorbol's mechanism of action which seems to involve a Ca-dependent kinase (31). The contrasting ability of phorbol ester to induce ODC in C57B16/1pr mice which develop a milder autoimmune disease may be a lead into non-H2 related genetic influences that contribute to immune dysregulation.

The IL-2 abnormalities in RA patients could develop for reasons different than those that pertain in 1pr mice. IL-2 deficiency may be a common final pathway through which multiple steps can contribute to creating a subsoil predisposing to autoimmunity. However, this is not to imply that IL-2 deficiency is either necessary or sufficient by itself for the emergence of frank autoimmune disease.

ACKNOWLEDGMENTS

This work was supported by General Medical Research Service of the Veterans Administration and grants from Newport Pharmaceutical and RGK Foundation.

REFERENCES

1. N. Talal, "Autoimmunity: Genetic, Immunologic, Virologic, and Clinical Aspects," Normal Talal, ed., Academic Press, New York (1977).
2. J. R. Roubinian, R. Papoian, and N. Talal, Androgenic hormones modulate autoantibody responses and improve survival in murine lupus, J. Clin. Invest. 59:1066 (1977).
3. G. F. Solomon, Emotional and personality factors in the onset and course of autoimmune disease, particularly rheumatoid arthritis, in: "Psychoneuroimmunology," Robert Ader, ed., Academic Press, New York (1981).
4. N. Talal, Immunologic and viral factors in the pathogenesis of systemic lupus erythematosus, Arthritis Rheum. 13:887 (1970).
5. D. Wofsy, J. B. Roths, E. D. Murphy, M. J. Dauphinee, S. B. Kipper, and N. Talal, Deficient interleukin-2 activity in MRL/Mp and C57B1/6J mice bearing the 1pr gene, J. Exp. Med. 154:1671 (1981).
6. M. J. Dauphinee, S. B. Kipper, D. Wofsy, and N. Talal, Interleukin-2 deficiency is a common feature of autoimmune mice, J. Immunol. 127(6):2483 (1981).

7. N. Miyasaka, T. Nakamura, I. J. Russell, and N. Talal, Interleukin-2 deficiencies in rheumatoid arthritis and systemic lupus erythematosus, Clin. Immunol. and Immunopathol. 31:109 (1984).

8. M. Fischbach, M. J. Dauphinee, and N. Talal, Ability of isoprinosine to restore interleukin-2 production and immune function in autoimmune mice (submitted).

9. R. Pope and N. Talal, Autoimmunity in rheumatoid arthritis, in: "Concepts in Immunopathology," Julius Cruse, ed., Karger Medical and Scientific Publishers, Basel and New York (1984).

10. J. Vaughan, D. Carson, and R. Fox, The Epstein-Barr virus and rheumatoid arthritis, Clin. and Exp. Rheum. 1:165 (1983).

11. J. M. Depper and N. J. Zvaifler, Epstein-Barr virus. Its relationship to the pathogenesis of rheumatoid arthritis, Arthritis Rheum. 24:755 (1981).

12. B. Combe, R. Pope, B. Darnell, W. Kincaid, and N. Talal, Regulation of natural killer cell activity by macrophages in the rheumatoid joint and peripheral blood, J. Immunol. (in press).

13. S. Gillis, M. M. Ferm, W. Ou, and K. Smith, T cell growth factor: parameters of production and a quantitative microassay for activity, J. Immunol. 120:2027 (1978).

14. R. Papoian and N. Talal, Ability of NZW but not NZB antigen-presenting cells to support T cell proliferative responses to DNA methylated albumin, J. Immunol. 174:525 (1980).

15. R. Robb, A. Munck, and K. A. Smith, T cell growth factor receptors: quantitation, specificity and biological significance, J. Exp. Med. 154:1455 (1981).

16. R. Fidelus, M. Fischbach, A. Laughter, and N. Talal, Defects in intracellular mechanisms of lymphocyte activation in autoimmune disease, Abstract, presented at meeting of American Association of Immunologists, St. Louis, Missouri (1984).

17. G. R. Klimpel, C. B. Byus, D. H. Russell, and D. O. Lucas, Cyclic AMP-dependent protein kinase activation and induction of ornithine decarboxylase during lymphocyte mitogenesis, J. Immunol. 123:817 (1979).

18. R. K. Fidelus, A. H. Laughter, and J. J. Twomey, Role of mitogens and lymphokines in the induction of ornithine decarboxylase in T lymphocytes, J. Immunol. 132:1462 (1984).

19. M. Fischbach, Defective T cell response to antigen presentation in autoimmune mice (submitted).

20. J. W. Hadden and J. Wybran, Immunopotentiators II: Isoprinosine, NPT 15392: Modulators of lymphocyte and macrophage development and function, Adv. Immunopharmacology 1:457 (1981).

21. B. Combe, R. M. Pope, M. Fischbach, B. Darnell, S. Baron and N. Talal, Interleukin-2 in rheumatoid arthritis: production of and response to interleukin-2 in rheumatoid synovial fluid, synovial tissue, and peripheral blood (submitted).

22. B. Combe, R. Pope, B. Darnell, and N. Talal, Modulation of natural killer cell activity in the rheumatoid joint and peripheral blood (submitted).

23. J. B. Smith and N. Talal, Significance of self-recognition and interleukin-2 for immunoregulation, autoimmunity and cancer, Scand. J. Immunol. (editorial) 16:269 (1982).

24. B. S. Nepom, G. T. Nepom, E. Mickelson, J. G. Schaller, P. Antonelli, and J. A. Hansen, Specific HLA-DR4-associated histocompatibility molecules characterize patients with juvenile rheumatoid arthritis, J. Clin. Invest. (in press, 1984).

25. N. Talal, A clinician and a scientist look at acquired immune-deficiency syndrome (AIDS). A validation of immunology's theoretical foundation, Immunology Today 4(7):180 (1983).

26. J. L. Touraine, S. E. Elyafi, E. Dosi, C. Cahpuis-Cellier, J. Ritter, N. Blanc, J. DuBernard, C. Pouteil-Noble, M. Chevalier, R. Creyssel,

and J. Traeger, Immunoglobulin abnormalities and infectious lympho-proliferative syndrome in cyclosporine-treated transplant patients, Trans. Proc. 15:2798 (1983).

27. G. J. Purd'homme, C. L. Park, T. M. Fieser, R. Kofler, F. J. Dixon, and A. N. Theofilopoulos, Identification of a B cell differentiation factor spontaneously produced by proliferating T cells in murine lupus strains of the lpr/lpr genotype, J. Exp. Med. 157:730 (1983).

28. L. V. Abruzzo and D. A. Rowley, Homeostasis of the antibody response: immunoregulation by NK cells, Science 222:581 (1983).

29. N. Talal, Autoimmunity and the immunologic network, Arthritis Rheum. 21(7):853 (1978).

30. C. F. Scott, Jr., M. Tsurufuji, C. Y. Lu, R. Finberg, and M.-S. Sy, Comparison of antigen-specific T cell responses in autoimmune MRL/Mp-1pr/1pr and MRL/Mp-++ mice, J. Immunol. 132:633 (1984).

31. A. S. Kraft and W. B. Anderson, Phorbol esters increase the amount of Ca^{2+}, phospholipid-dependent protein kinase associated with plasma membrane, Nature 301:621 (1983).

MOLECULAR MIMICRY AND AUTOIMMUNITY

Robert S. Fujinami and Michael B.A. Oldstone

Department of Immunology
Scripps Clinic and Research Foundation
La Jolla, California

There are several mechanisms by which viruses may initiate autoimmunity event. For example, a virus could interact directly with cells of the immune system and alter normal immune regulation. Inability to respond to self antigens is maintained, primarily in part, by tolerizing T cells (1). Such tolerant T cells cannot provide the appropriate signal for B cells to proliferate, differentiate and make antibodies. Many viruses are known to be polyclonal B cell activators and thus could induce production of antibodies including autoantibodies by bypassing these tolerized T cells and directly stimulating B lymphocytes (2). Epstein-Barr virus, other related herpesviruses and vesicular stomatitis virus are such B cell mitogens. Besides direct infection of lymphoid cells, the immune response generated against a virus may also cause autoimmunity. One way would be by the production of autoantibodies via anti-idiotype feedback controls (3). For example, regulation of immune responses is believed to take place through anti-idiotype networks. In the course of an immune response against a viral receptor for a cell surface component, antibodies could form and bind to the viral receptor whose combining site mirrors the cell surface component. Thus, antibodies produced in an anti-idiotype response against the anti-viral receptor antibody could bind to host cell receptors and thereby initiate autoimmunity. Further, interferon generated during virus infection may alter the expression of gene products important in regulating immune responses like HLA D, A, B, or C and IA, H-2$^{k \text{ or } d}$. An additional means by which an antiviral immune response may lead to autoimmunity is through antigenic or molecular mimicry. By molecular mimicry we mean the sharing of common immunodeterminants or epitopes between an invading microbe, i.e., virus, bacteria or parasite—and the host. Such common epitopes can be thought of as three-dimensional sites composed of an array of amino acids. Thus, the antiviral immune response recognizes both the virus determinant and the shared host "self antigen." These cross-reacting antibodies generated by molecular mimicry are the subject of this report and may, in large part, be responsible for the presence of autoantibodies found during many infections in man.

A few years ago we noted (4) during the process of raising monoclonal antibodies to measles virus, that three groups of reactants were produced. The first reacted only with measles virus specific proteins and these were the majority of antibodies generated. The second was directed against host cell components. The third and most interesting for this discussion reacted with both host cell components and viral proteins. When characterized, these monoclonal antibodies cross-reacted with both viral and self components.

One such cross-reactive monoclonal antibody (2A) reacted with an antigenic site shared by the phosphoprotein of measles virus and an intermediate filament protein found of normal cells. Two techniques were used to establish this observation. First, immunofluorescent staining with this cross-reactive monoclonal antibody of infected and uninfected cells was used to detect the separate patterns of viral and host protein localization. Infected cells showed globular staining typical of viral inclusion bodies in the cytoplasm (Figure 1A) and occasional staining within nuclei. Uninfected cells showed staining of the cytoplasm in a lacy network that is characteristic of intermediate filaments that reacted including primary human astrocytes, HeLa cells and Vero cells. Cell lines failing to react were those from hamster (BHK), mouse (L2), or rat kangaroo cells (PTK2). Not yet known is whether the protein(s) that reacted with monoclonal antibody 2A is absent from nonprimate cells, or the epitope in question is not conserved on these intermediate proteins.

The reactivity of monoclonal antibody 2A to infected cells was abrogated by absorbtion with an intermediate filament preparation derived from uninfected cells. In contrast, the reactivity of another monoclonal antibody specific for the measles virus phosphoprotein but not cross-reactive with intermediate filaments was not altered by an identical absorption procedure. Thus, absorption studies demonstrated specificity and showed the existence of a site on an intermediate filament protein in normal (uninfected) cells similar to a site on the phosphoprotein of measles virus.

Using western immunoblotting we demonstrated that monoclonal antibody 2A bound directly to measles virus phosphoprotein and to the intermediate filament protein. This technique avoids the nonspecific coprecipitation of proteins within the antibody-antigen complex. Further, proteins from infected or uninfected cytosols depleted of intermediate filaments, separated by polyacrylamide gel electrophoresis and electrophoretically transferred to nitrocellulose paper when reacted with monoclonal antibody 2A, demonstrated the 70,000 molecular weight phosphoprotein of measles virus. This viral protein is found only in cytosols of infected cells (Figure 2) not in the uninfected preparations. Thus, these data complement and support the results of the immunofluorescent assays, since the phosphoprotein is an integral part of the viral inclusion bodies visible in infected cells. When western

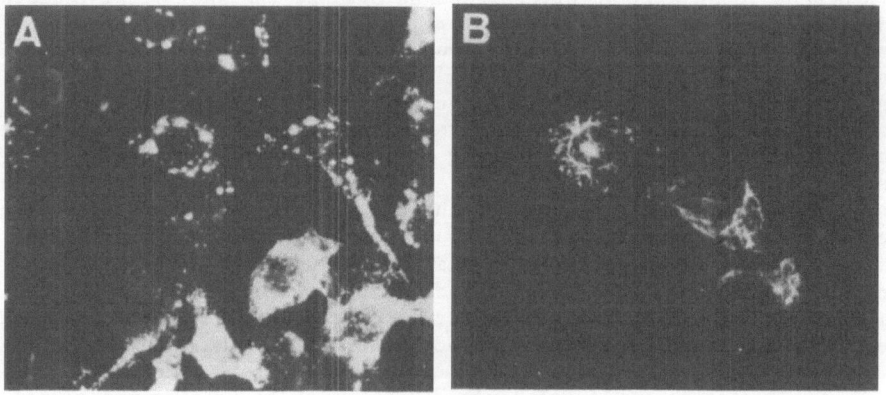

Figure 1. A. Measles virus infected HeLa cells reacted initially with monoclonal antibody 2A and secondarily with a rhodamine labeled goat antimouse Ig. A globular staining pattern is observed. B. Uninfected HeLa cells reacted with the same antibody reagents show a net-like pattern of staining.

blots were performed with purified virus monoclonal antibody 2A again bound only to the viral phosphoprotein (Figure 2). In toto, these results indicate that monoclonal antibody 2A reacts only with the measles phosphoprotein from infected cells or virions as well as intermediate filaments.

To characterize further the normal cell component reactive with monoclonal antibody 2A, intermediate filament protein prepared from uninfected cells were analyzed with the western blot technique. Monoclonal antibody 2A effectively binds to a protein whose molecular weight was approximately 54,000, similar to that of one of the cytokeratins and migrates slightly faster than vimentin (Figure 3).

Several other viruses were noted to be involved in molecular mimicry. We showed, in collaboration with Dr. Hilary Koprowski and his associates at the Wistar Institute (Philadelphia), that herpesvirus shares region in common with an intermediate filament protein (4). Further, with Dr. Sam Dales, we characterized a monoclonal antibody that recognized both the hemagglutinin of vaccinia virus and a normal cell component (6). Recently, other groups have noted molecular mimicry between other microbial agents and self antigens (7-9).

The binding of antibodies to self has several consequences. First, if the autoantibody is directed against a normal cell surface component, binding of the complex could activate the complement system leading to lysis of the cell. Additionally, surface bound antibody could bind non-immune lymphocytes by virtue of their Fc receptor and lead to host cell destruction. Events other than direct cell lysis may also be biologically relevant and disease

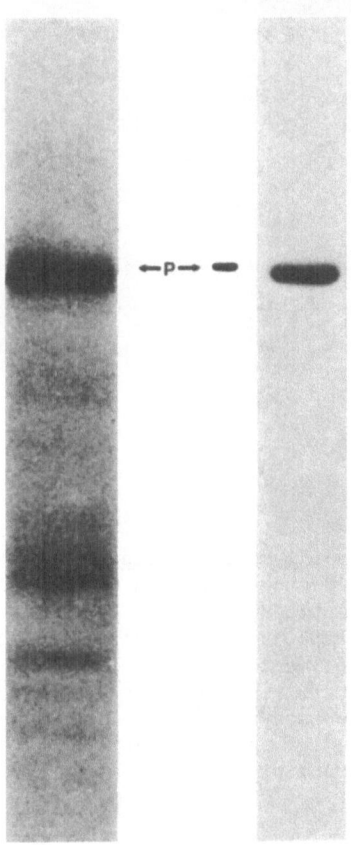

Figure 2.
Western Blot Analysis. Left lane illustrates the reaction of monoclonal antibody 2A with a measles virus infected cell cytosol preparation depleted of intermediate filament proteins. The phophoprotein (P) of measles virus is the prominent band. The lane on the right depicts the reaction of monoclonal antibody 2A with purified measles virus, again, with the phosphoprotein showing prominently. Both were visualized by using ^{125}I labeled goat anti-mouse Ig and autoradiography.

important. Autoantibody could modulate the expression of cell surface proteins. For example, binding of antibody to acetylcholine receptor might
lead to a marked decrease in receptor proteins and could cause myasthenia
gravis (10). Another possibility is that autoantibodies could play a role
in forming immune complexes that subsequently become trapped and cause disease (11). Binding to cell surface glycoproteins or to internal proteins
liberated after immune lysis or viral destruction of cells provide the antigen to which the antibody complexes. Accordingly, many of the immune complexes observed during infection may be composed not only of antibody-virus
aggregates but also of autoantibody-self proteins. This might explain, in
part, why the quantitative analyses of viral antibodies immune complexes in
many viral experimental models and natural infections do not account for
the total of the eluted antibody.

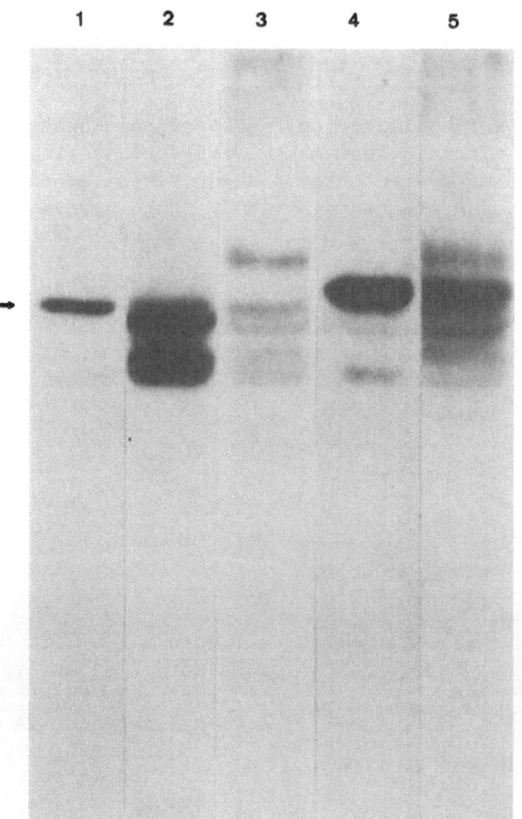

Figure 3. Western blot analysis of intermediate filament proteins
        (Triton-insoluble) bound to nitrocellulose strips and
        incubated with: lane 1, monoclonal antibody 2A; lane 2,
        monoclonal antibody to cytokeratin; lane 3, polyclonal
        antibody to keratin; lane 4, monoclonal antibody to
        vimentin; lane 5, polyclonal antibody to vimentin.
        The second antibody used on all strips was affinity
        purified ^{125}I labeled goat anti-mouse Ig. Arrow indi-
        cates migration of intermediate filament protein.

ACKNOWLEDGEMENTS

This is Publication Number 3666-IMM from the Department of Immunology, Scripps Clinic and Research Foundation, La Jolla, California 92037. We would like to thank Gay Wilkins for manuscript preparation and Phyllis Minick for editorial assistance.

This work was supported in part by U.S.P.H.S. grants NS-12428, AG-04342, AI-07007 and Biomedical Research Support Grant RRO-5514. RSF is a recipient of the Harry Weaver Scholarship (grant #NMS JF 2009A1) from the National Multiple Sclerosis Society.

REFERENCES

1. W. O. Weigle, Immunological unresponsiveness, Adv. Immunol. 16:61 (1973).
2. R. Ahmed and M. B. A. Oldstone, Mechanisms and biological implications of virus induced polyclonal B-cell activation, in: "Concepts in Viral Pathogenesis," A. L. Notkins and M. B. A. Oldstone, eds., Springer-Verlag, New York (1984).
3. P. H. Plotz, Autoantibodies are anti-idiotype antibodies to antiviral antibodies, Lancet ii:824 (1983).
4. R. S. Fujinami, M. B. A. Oldstone, Z. Wroblewska, M. E. Frankel, and H. Koprowski, Molecular mimicry in virus infection: cross-reaction of measles virus phosphoprotein or of herpes simplex virus protein with human intermediate filaments, Proc. Natl. Acad. Sci. USA 80:2346 (1983).
5. W. W. Franke, E. Schmid, C. Grund, and B. Geiger, Intermediate filament proteins in nonfilamentous structure: transient disintegration and inclusion of sub-unit proteins in granular aggregates, Cell 30:103 (1982).
6. S. Dales, R. S. Fujinami, and M. B. A. Oldstone, Infection with vaccinia favors the selection of hybridomas synthesizing autoantibodies against intermediate filaments, among them one cross-reacting with the virus hemagglutinin, J. Immunol. 131:1546 (1983).
7. J. N. Wood, L. Hudson. T. M. Jessell, and M. Yamamoto, A monoclonal antibody defining antigenic determinants on subpopulations of mammalian neurones and Trypanosoma cruzi parasites, Nature 296:34 (1982).
8. B. F. Haynes, M. Robert-Guroff, R. S. Metzgar, G. Franchini, V. S. Kalyanaraman, T. J. Palker, and R. C. Gallo, Monoclonal antibody against human T cell leukemia virus p19 defines a human thymic epithelial antigen acquired during ontogeny, J. Exp. Med. 157:907 (1983).
9. A. L. Notkins, Personal communications, Studies with coxsackie virus, Epstein-Barr virus, vaccinia virus and other RNA and DNA viruses (1984).
10. D. B. Drackman, C. W. Angus, R. N. Adams, and I. Kao, Effect of myasthenia patient's immunoglobulin on acetylcholine receptor turnover: selectivity of degradation process, Proc. Natl. Acad. Sci. USA 75:3422 (1978).
11. M. B. A. Oldstone, Virus-induced immune complex formation and disease: definition, regulation, and importance, in: "Concepts in Viral Pathogenesis, A. L. Notkins and M. B. A. Oldstone, eds., Springer-Verlag, New York (1984).

THE ACQUIRED IMMUNODEFICIENCY SYNDROME:

WHAT CAN IT TEACH US?*

Dale N. Lawrence

Centers for Disease Control
U. S. Department of Health and Human Services
Atlanta, Georgia 30333

The scientific presentations at this symposium have provided many clues
to the future direction of research in virology, immunobiological processes,
and AIDS. Exciting newscasts describing the identification of what appears
to be the AIDS agent have occurred concurrent with the symposium. It is
clear that much of the subject matter of this symposium is relevant to issues
of great interest to the general society. Against this scientific backdrop--
and at a historical moment--I would like to share some subjective reflections
about "what AIDS can teach us."

I will begin by describing an era in history and summarizing a series
of events with interesting parallels to the present.

In recent decades there has been a dramatic increase in travel
throughout the world. The most remote areas of the globe have
become accessible through modern methods of transportation. New
ideas are sweeping the Western world, resulting in the rapid evolution of many societal norms.

An epidemic of an unknown disease appears without clear
origins. Although initially confined geographically, it soon
spreads. When it is recognized on both sides of international
borders, prolonged arguments between countries arise as to which
one may have been the source. Within a short time the disease is
recognized to be transmitted sexually, the typical patient being
a very sexually promiscuous adult. Many later victims generally
lead lives of sexual moderation. Eventually, unborn or newborn
children of infected women are recognized to be at risk, as well
as recipients of blood from asymptomatic, infected persons. The
disease becomes linked with many famous names. Its tragic consequences are invoked by playwrights and others observing the human
condition.

After what seems an interminable wait, the causative agent
is identified, and screening tests are developed which can be
used to test blood for evidence of past or present infection.
The long-term significance of a person's being seropositive is

_____
*This chapter is based on the banquet address delivered by the author on
 April 24, 1984, at the Bay Harbor Inn, Tampa, Florida.

unclear until many years of observation of the disease's natural history have elapsed. The choice of therapy remains controversial--particularly for persons with long-standing, asymptomatic, latent infection. The persistent seropositivity--even after the patient has received appropriate therapy--frequently results in apprehension and stigmatization. If the agent cannot be demonstrated readily, it is difficult to distinguish between the contagious state and the infected but immune. However, the serological test eventually becomes a requirement of each state for the legally sanctioned sexual cohabitation of consenting adults. The serologic test is frequently a part of the prenatal testing of mothers-to-be.

As you recognize, I adapted the foregoing description from the history of syphilis, with some omissions and considerable compression. The scientific and medical advances that took several centuries to achieve in the history of syphilis have occurred in only three years of concentrated endeavor following the recognition of AIDS. Unfortunately, AIDS may be a public health problem for decades to come, in view of the well-known difficulty in controlling the spread of sexually transmitted diseases. Furthermore, the absence of an early cutaneous hallmark lesion and long incubation period of AIDS will compromise disease control efforts.

AIDS will continue to influence us in ways not directly related to our scientific hypotheses:

1. It prompts us to take special precautions in the laboratory, at the bedside, in the operating theater, and in the autopsy room. It can result in prolonged anxiety in health care personnel who have sustained an accidental needle stick or who have seroconverted and now await advice about what should be done. The unavailability of proper precautions and the general concern about accidentally acquiring infection from AIDS samples has kept some scientists out of the field. Their research aspirations and funding have been limited.

2. It has forced most of the people in this audience to consider issues related to allocating research funds and developing policy in areas of medical science and ethics that seemed quiescent only a short few years before.

3. It may strike a friend or associate.

WHAT CAN IT TEACH US ABOUT IMMUNOLOGY, VIROLOGY, GENETICS, AND ONCOLOGY?

The answers in these subjects are best found in the individual participants' presentations in the symposium. I shall not attempt to comment on subjects for which the original investigators have shown us impressive primary data. Certain related unmentioned points might be worth comment, however.

Since the work relating oncologic antigens and fetal antigens more than a decade ago, the boundary separating oncogenesis and developmental biology has become less discernible. Some viral gene sequences are now recognized as essentially identical to those found coding for molecules important to human immunoregulatory functions or coding for tissue growth factors. This hints at the antiquity of our human association with various integrated viral sequences. The global search for further families of retroviruses will raise fundamental questions about the origin of the gene sequences controlling the differentiation steps intrinsic to embryology. Perhaps we shall soon see a parallel to Lewis Thomas' popularization of the nature of the relationship between our own cells and the intracellular

mitochondria whose origins predate eukaryotic cells. How many regulatory
functions specified by the genetics of developmental biology are consequences
of a shared past with tame cousins of oncogenes? Are oncogenes fetal esca-
pees, or are some regulatory genes the products of an ancient domestication?

Fewer than one dozen different and somewhat unusual opportunistic infectious organisms have been the useful indices of AIDS. They have caused
infections that have been the precipitating cause of death in most cases.
All these organisms are known to us from clinical cases of opportunistic
disease occurring well before the era of chemotherapeutic immunosuppression
and before AIDS appeared in the United States. The immunologic shield which
has always protected the majority of the general population from overt
disease due to these organisms can probably now be attributed to a surprisingly select and potentially discretely identifiable cellular subpopulation.
What knowledge of host immune response and disease susceptibility will be
transferable from the accumulating information on AIDS-induced vulnerability
to these same organisms?

Of the extraordinary number of potentially available environmental
microorganisms, why have so few been capable of exploiting the AIDS-diseased
patient? One explanation, of course, is to acknowledge what we have known
for many years--that immunity to these opportunistic agents is dependent on
T-cell function. But maybe we should ask a more basic question: since it
seems that cell-mediated immune mechanisms evolved before humoral ones, why
have so few agents retained or evolved such a successful mode of quiescent
survival in the T-cell competent host? Does the nutritionally and immunologically sound host represent a dead end for these microbial parasites?
Perhaps they were not so innocuous during period of individual and collective
human history when depressed host responses prevailed: malnutrition, aging,
immaturity, or malignancy.

Toxoplasma gondii and Pneumocystis carinii are relatives in the para-
sitologic field; cytomegalovirus and herpes simplex virus have quite close
phylogeny. However, candida and Mycobacterium avium complex are not very
close kin to one another or to these and other opportunistic agents in AIDS.
Considering the disparate phylogenetic positions of these agents, is it
likely that they chanced independently upon a useful mechanism of survival?
Perhaps they uniquely retained a genetic relic coding for survival in this
immunological/ecological niche.

With the recent advent of novel culture techniques and the availability
of AIDS patients who have lost their host immunologic containment mechanisms,
we may speculate that new microorganisms may be identified. These organisms
may be found to be associated with previously poorly defined clinical condi-
tions--including some not hitherto considered infectious in origin. Of
special interest might be certain encephalopathies associated with AIDS
that were not attributable to other recognized pathogens.

With the continuing increase in cases, it should not be surprising
that among this large number there will be a few cases meeting the usual
criteria but with another, previously clinically inapparent congenital immunological deficiency. The concurrent clinical expression of this congenital deficiency will demonstrate that the now AIDS-affected lymphoid subpopulations had previously provided the host with an important coping mechanism.
Thus, we will learn about immunological defense redundancies and complementa-
tion from the recognition of disease due to unusual organisms.

If AIDS cases should occur in persons already affected by a serious
disease of disordered immunoregulation, the AIDS-induced alteration in the
immune system might be associated with an apparent clinical remission of
the antecedent disease. As the development of clinical AIDS intervenes,

the basis for the apparent, transient improvement may become tragically clear. Laboratory documentation of the sequence of changes could lead to better understanding of the fundamental processes of certain rheumatic diseases, for example.

WHAT CAN IT TEACH US ABOUT THE VALUE OF THE EPIDEMIOLOGIC METHOD?

Epidemiologists revere John Snow, the London physician who analyzed cholera cases in that city and found statistical association between drinking water from a particular pump and having cholera. He removed the handle to prevent subsequent infections. The cause of cholera was then unknown, therapy was ineffective, and pre-exposure prophylaxis (vaccine) was unimaginable--yet preventive measures followed the epidemiologic observations of the factor that significantly distinguished cases from unaffected community members. I think there are parallels to the prompt public health actions taken in the current AIDS epidemic.

The identification of risk groups--homosexual men, users of illicit intravenous drugs, recipients of certain blood products, and persons who had sexual contact with persons in these groups--provided the basis for public warnings and procedural changes in the blood banking industry. The inauguration of screening procedures by blood banks to eliminate donations by risk-group members probably significantly reduced the transmission of AIDS through blood products more than a year before the existence of the first serologic test to identify individual donors with serologic evidence of infection with the agent. Substantiation of this impression must await suitable analyses.

Another benefit of the employment of the epidemiologic method involved the identification of the generalized lymphadenopathy syndrome as a concurrent and new epidemic, occurring in the same at-risk populations and in the same communities as AIDS. Fortification for the impression of some immunologists that the two were interrelated came from epidemiologic studies. In retrospect, it is interesting that a successful isolation of the AIDS virus used lymph node tissue from patients with this AIDS-associated "syndrome" rather than overt disease. Laboratory progress was augmented by rapid epidemiological linkage of the syndromes. In fact, the entire epidemic has clearly highlighted the complementary roles of these disciplines.

WHAT CAN IT TEACH US ABOUT SOCIAL ISSUES?

It seems difficult to remember that only 24 months ago there were many who questioned that this disease existed at all or that it would ever come to their community. As the incidence of the disease has risen to a point where it strikes more than 1,000 persons every 90 days--and is generally perceived as doubling every six to eight months--the public has taken notice. Thus, we have all had a lesson in the rapidity with which completely new medical knowledge spreads and new perceptions gain transcendency. The effect of the scientific and lay press in the dissemination of new ideas is stunning. The use of established channels for preliminary scientific disclosures has been immensely beneficial in speeding the transmission of important information for protection of the public health. These channels have served a distinguishably different purpose from that of the traditional formal publication.

AIDS has provided us an opportunity to watch society and its institutions grapple with the concept of a new disease and with its ethical, social, and economic implications. Policy-oriented groups are now preparing to address various issues--for example, issues raised by the cost of medical care for AIDS patients. These issues affect individuals, hospitals, third-party insurance carriers, and communities. The staggering cost of the intensive care needs have been especially apparent in the cities with the largest numbers of cases.

Some provisions should be made to address some very practical problems. An example is the growing problem of placement of AIDS patients after their need for acute care for an opportunistic infection has concluded. Most patients will inevitably experience another complication necessitating repeated hospitalization, and some of these patients are not capable of self care in the periods between hospitalizations. Long-term care institutions are reluctant to take them because of the underlying infectious nature of their disease. What about the problem of the medical practitioner (e.g., surgeon, dentist) who develops clinical signs associated with AIDS-related complex? What benefits would be obtained by testing for evidence of infectivity? What can be done to reassure anxious patients and administrators of the effectiveness of the readily identifiable preventive procedures which might allow the practitioner's continued gainful employment?

WHAT CAN IT TEACH US ABOUT OUR FEDERAL, ACADEMIC, PRIVATE AND PUBLIC SECTORS?

We have an immense national resource in the collection of federal, state, and local public health agencies. They have demonstrated their respective abilities to catalyze national-level action through investigation and authentication of epidemics and the maintenance of standardized surveillance, to perform the basic research needed to understand the agent and develop vaccines, and to develop the regulatory guidelines for safe and effective therapeutic product usage. The close integration of federal endeavors in AIDS with activities of each of the states has prompted a collaborative spirit which will be of incalculable value as the epidemic grows.

The legislative branch has become crucially involved as the need for funding of both government and non-government endeavors become manifest. The effect of these congressional budgetary increases for AIDS research and control measures is already being felt nationally.

Not surprisingly, the judicial branch of the government will become progressively involved also as issues of infringement on personal liberties clash with demands for protection of the health of others. There will be the need for resolution of medicolegal disputes regarding liability, implied warranty of product, licensure, protection of patent rights, and prosecutions for fraudulent therapies and preventives.

The value of the work of many independent academicians has been apparent also in the course of the epidemic. As a group they have scientific credentials of the highest order. They are able to quickly initiate scientific investigations and build collaborations based on expected scientific productivity. Academic institutions are considered the origin of nascent ideas. Even if an academician presents some misbegotten ideas, the academic system typically demonstrates its inherent freedom and resilience by ascribing the error and associated discredit to the individual researcher. In contrast, the statements of officials must be carefully weighed for their consistency with other important, relevant policies and for possible damage to the credibility or legitimacy of the parent institution as a social structure.

WHAT CAN IT TEACH US ABOUT OUR AGE-OLD HEALTH PROFESSIONS?

Are the risks of personal disability and death that accompany our work as health professionals and biomedical scientists simply the price of having public respect, trust or reverence? Certainly, experience shows that remuneration is not the primary motivating force for the scientists among us. Are these personal health risks we may be taking simply like those taken in other occupations? Is there something more noble that motivates, for example, the nurse who must frequently perform venipuncture on the hemophilia patients under her supervision?

Our medical training--sometimes long dormant--has had to serve us under new circumstances. Society has expected no less. When some morticians wanted to refuse to embalm AIDS patients, their state licensing and accrediting body insisted they perform their professional duties responsibly or lose their licenses. The state effectively said that the morticians had received professional training in microbiology and contagion. These courses had not been meaningless exercises toward obtaining a license to practice but were designed to serve in the future as the basis for prudent professional conduct. Beset by the challenges and fears brought out by the emergence of a previously unknown, highly fatal, and seemingly infectious disease, institutions of our society have reviewed their reason for existence and have found direction to guide them.

We, too, have to search within ourselves to find a basis for our actions. Written into the ancient medical professional codes, such as the Oath of Hippocrates, are admonitions to the physician to assure confidentiality of what is learned about the private lives of patients. These issues are very current. The words from the prayer of the physician Maimonides seem very instructive: "Do not allow thirst for profit, for ambition, for renown and admiration to interfere with my profession, for these are the enemies of truth and of love for mankind--and they lead us astray in the great task of attending to the welfare of thy creatures."

CONCLUSION

The contributions of many of those attending this conference have brought us close to the end of the first phase of the AIDS epidemic: identification of the clinical disease patterns, the modes of spread, the nature of the likely agent, the immunologically complex disruptions induced by infection with the agent and suggestions for therapeutic interventions.

The second phase of the epidemic investigations will be characterized by improved tools to screen for evidence of inapparent or subclinical infection and the associated long-term study of the natural history of the infection. The influence of co-factors and innate host factors will attract more attention. There will be interesting research findings in leukemogenesis, the epidemiology of transmissible malignancies, and the host defense mechanisms heretofore traditionally associated with states of immunosuppression, nutritional deprivation, and aging.

The growing public realization of the magnitude of the involvement of the at-risk groups will necessitate greater attention to issues such as medical care costs and allocation of medical and public health resources in certain areas. The ability to identify the infective carrier state in many of the members of at-risk groups, including children, will require medical and social scientists to make sensitive and prudent judgments on a variety of issues.

The AIDS virus provides a previously unavailable, unique tool to dissect large parts of the immune system. We will be able to trace many previously obscured steps in the immunologic defense pathways. Just as the early tragedies associated with the history of radiation later led to the tools of roentgenography and radioisotopic tracers in the service of mankind, this disease should prove no less potent a stimulus to progress in understanding the mechanisms which intertwine infection, immunity, genetics, aging and malignancy.

As we work together to ameliorate this human tragedy, we can be sure that this disease will be used by historians as a case study to medically and sociologically characterize the last part of this century.

COXSACKIEVIRUS B, LIPIDS AND IMMUNITY AS SHARED

DETERMINANTS IN DIABETES AND ATHEROSCLEROSIS

Roger M. Loria

Department of Microbiology and Immunology and Pathology
The Medical College of Virginia
Richmond, Virginia

This report presents evidence to support the thesis that the human group B coxsackieviruses and hypercholesteremia function as common determinants in diabetes and atherosclerosis. Their independent and synergistic interactions result in suppression of host immunity leading to the initiation and exacerbation of the pathologic processes of diabetes and atherosclerosis.

The enteroviruses are among the most common infectious agents of man. They are frequently the cause of minor illness and inapparent infections, especially in childhood, although they may also cause more severe disease. The group B coxsackieviruses have been reported to be the most frequent causes of viral cardiomyopathies resulting in chronic vascular disease in humans. It has been estimated that five percent of all symptomatic infections with group B coxsackieviruses are followed by chronic heart disease. Manifestations of such infections range from myocarditis, pericarditis, and pancarditis to incompetence of the aortic and or mitral valves (1).

The epidemiological reports of Gamble et al. (2) confirmed the association between group B coxsackieviruses and juvenile onset diabetes mellitus and provided further incentive for these studies. Consequently, we have explored the diabetogenic properties of coxsackievirus B4, using the diabetic mutant mouse C57Bl/Ks db+/db+ as an experimental animal model system.

COXSACKIEVIRUS B4 AND DIABETES MELLITUS - EXPERIMENTAL ANIMAL MODEL STUDIES

The group B coxsackievirus have no envelope, and do not possess lipid in their capsid but have been known for their lipotropic qualities and their ability to cause fat necrosis (3). In tissue culture, these viruses can cause the formation of intracellular cholesterol crystals (4). Virus infection results in an increased cellular incorporation of choline in phospholipids (5), which is associated with virus-induced formation of membrane structures in the centrosphere region of the infected cells.

Coxsackievirus B4 used in these studies was isolated by Kibrick and Benirschke from the myocardial tissue of an infant with generalized disease including focal necrosis and inflammation of the pancreas; with both endocrine and exocrine involvement of the pancreas (6). A detailed passage history and preparation of these virus pools for experimentations has been reported (7).

The role of coxsackievirus B4 (CB4) infection as an initiating or contributing factor in diabetes mellitus was examined in mice with a known
genetic predisposition to this disease. This was achieved by the use of
the inbred C57B1/KsJ +/+ mouse strain and its genetic variants the homozygote diabetic mutant C57B1/KsJ db/db, which spontaneously develops diabetes,
and the heterozygote diabetic mutant C57B1/KsJ db/+ which remains normal.
Using dietary restriction, spontaneous onset of diabetes was prevented in
the inbred C57B1/KsJ db/db mouse.

Over a 56-week period glucose tolerance and radioimmunoinsulin assay
were performed on CB4 infected and uninfected heterozygote C57B1/KsJ db/+
mice, and the inbred controls, C57B1/KsJ +/+. Results revealed a diabetes-
like disease in CB4 infected heterozygote animals only. It was characterized
by periods of hypo- and hyperglycemia, hypoinsulinemia and glucose intoler-
ance. The uninfected heterozygote C57B1/KsJ db/+, or the CB4 infected inbred
C57B1/KsJ +/+ or the outbred virus-infected Swiss CD-1 (Crl:ICR/BR), Charles
River Breeding Laboratories, Wilmington, Massachusetts, mouse did not have
any alteration in glucose homeostasis (8).

In summary, a positive correlation between the genetic predisposition
to diabetes mellitus and susceptibility to CB4 was observed. In response
to CB4 challenge, the order of susceptibility of these diabetic genotypes
followed the pattern db/db >> db/+ > +/+, with the diabetic homozygote being
the most susceptible. In addition, pancreatic pathology in coxsackievirus
B infected mice was also dependent on the presence of the diabetic mutation.
In the homozygote C57B1/KsJ db/db mice both acinar and islet cell destruction
were observed; in the heterozygote db/+ only acinar cell damage was evident;
while in the normal C57B1/KsJ +/+ mice pancreatitis was the prominent histopathological observation (7). Since there were no significant differences
in CB4 titers in the pancreases, livers, hearts, or spleens of these genetic
variants, it was concluded that the virus-induced pathology most likely was
determined by host factors.

In an effort to determine the factors responsible for differences in
host strain susceptibility we have recently demonstrated that genetic predisposition to diabetes mellitus as characterized by the diabetes mutation was
associated with an impaired ability to produce neutralizing antibodies to
CB4. In these experiments, the diabetic mutant C57B1/KsJ db+/db+, the heterozygote C57B1/KsJ db+/+m and the inbred misty coat color mutant C57B1/KsJ
+m/+m were challenged with a previously determined 1/2 LD50 of CB4 for the
particular genotype. Assays for the level of neutralizing antibodies were
run by the constant-virus varying serum dilution procedure, and all sera
were heat inactivated at 56°C for 30 minutes. A 50% plaque reduction at a
1/40 dilution or more was taken as evidence of a positive antibody production. At seven days after infection, the animals homozygous for the diabetes
mutation did not produce any significant level of neutralizing antibodies.
The diabetic heterozygote and the misty coat color mutant controls, in contrast, did produce antibodies resulting in a 50% plaque reduction at antisera
dilutions of up to 1/1280 (9,10).

COXSACKIEVIRUS B AND ATHEROSCLEROSIS -

STUDIES IN HYPERCHOLESTEREMIC ANIMALS

Hyperlipidemia, and particularly hypercholesteremia has been reported
to be one of the complications of diabetes mellitus (11). hypercholesteremia has been associated with an increased risk of atherosclerosis (12)
while diabetes is an independent risk factor in cardiovascular disease,
particularly atherosclerosis (13).

Table 1. Plasma Total Cholesterol[1] and Free Fatty Acids Levels[2] in Outbred and Inbred Fasted Mice

Time on Diet in Weeks	Experimental Diet		Control Diet	
	T. Chol.	F.F.A.	T. Chol.	F.F.A.
----------------------------OUTBRED CD-1 (CR1:ICR/BR)----------------------				
0	--	--	133 ± 8	123 ± 11
2	303 ± 44	109 ± 8	174 ± 9	112 ± 6
4	309 ± 38	135 ± 12	163 ± 11	117 ± 10
8	393 ± 17	99 ± 9	137 ± 33	166 ± 65
16	424 ± 41	134 ± 42	142 ± 10	109 ± 8
34	589 ± 93	162 ± 29	103 ± 12	125 ± 19
52	229 ± 24	36 ± 6	69 ± 21	63 ± 12
----------------------------INBRED C57B1/6J +/+---------------------------				
0	--	--	152 ± 11	92 ± 8
2	147 ± 13	170 ± 23	142 ± 2	148 ± 12
4	243 ± 45	62 ± 2	162 ± 15	73 ± 6
8	413 ± 66	124 ± 26	131 ± 7	113 ± 14
16	346 ± 66	124 ± 23	118 ± 6	130 ± 6
34	440 ± 97	108 ± 26	106 ± 22	128 ± 23
52	199 ± 14	15 ± 6	96 ± 11	40 ± 1

[1] Total cholesterol = mg% free cholesterol + mg% esterified cholesterol.
[2] Values are expressed as averaged mg% ± S.D. of three animals. Triplicate measurements were done on each sample.

In addition, atherosclerosis is markedly accelerated in juvenile-onset and maturity-onset diabetic patients and recent surveys indicate that the risk of cardiovascular disease at any given age is two to five times higher for the diabetic individual than for the non-diabetic. Atherosclerosis has been implicated as the cause of death in 75% of all diabetics. Consequently, we have attempted to ascertain whether hypercholesteremia would influence the host response to infection by a diabetogenic or cardiotropic agent like CB, and to what extent the interactions would alter or modify the pathology.

Our initial experiments dealt with the modification of a diet developed for the rat which was high in cholesterol, cholic acid, lard and sucrose (14) for consumption by the outbred Swiss CD-1 mouse strain. This diet was tested over a 60-week period and found highly satisfactory. Within two weeks a four-fold increase in plasma total cholesterol, cholesterol esters, and free cholesterol was evident as compared with the control group fed a stock diet.

Mice plasma neutral lipid levels were quantitatively determined by a thin layer chromatography (TLC) procedure which allowed us to measure cholesterol, cholesterol ester, free fatty acids, and triglycerides using 0.002 ml plasma without prior extraction (14).

In contrast to plasma cholesterol elevation plasma triglyceride levels were less than half the control animals levels. After 28 weeks on the diet, free fatty acid levels were also lowered in the hypercholesteremic group (Table 1). This has been seen in other species as Fiser et al. (15) similarly showed that chronic hypercholesteremia in the Rhesus monkey, Macaca

<u>mulatta</u>, caused a 40% reduction in plasma triglyceride levels. This diet has had wide application and has been adapted for the inbred C57Bl/6J mouse (Jackson Laboratories, Bar Harbor, Maine), and its composition has been reported previously (14,16).

Pathological examination of animals on the hypercholesteremic diet showed greatly enlarged livers, more than twice the normal size with fatty changes around the portal veins. Prolonged hypercholesteremia, however, was not associated with either a shorter life span nor with atheromatous changes. In general, mice are resistant to dietary hypercholesteremia-induced atherogenesis (14,17) which has made this model of particular interest in the study of virus-induced pathogenesis and atherosclerosis.

The influence of hypercholesterolemia could be seen in that infection of hypercholesteremia mice with the human cardiotropic coxsackievirus B5 (CB5) resulted in a 97% mortality within two weeks while normocholesteremic mice infected with the same virus strain and dose survived. Coxsackievirus cardiopathy was markedly augmented in the hypercholesteremic host, as evident by a persistent cardiomyolysis which was not observed in virus infected normocholesteremic animals.

Histopathological studies demonstrated that cellular infiltrates were conspicuously absent from the tissues of virus infected hypercholesteremic mice. These findings suggested that dietary hypercholesteremia was associated with a suppression of the inflammatory response to viral infection (17). Subsequently, these observations were confirmed and extended by Campbell et al. (16) in both the outbred CD-1 and the inbred C57Bl/6J mice.

Following the development of a procedure to suppress the intense autofluorescence of the aortic tissueelastic (18) CB5 was localized in the aortic media and endothelial cells using anti-coxsackievirus B5 fluorescent antibody staining procedures (16).

Coxsackievirus B5 replicated in the mouse aorta, to high titers up to 10^5 plaque forming units/gram tissue. It was apparent that CB5 was actually replicating in the aorta and was not a blood contaminant since virus could not be isolated from the blood at that time. In general, dietary hypercholesteremia was associated with an increase in virus concentration in the liver, heart, and aorta.

Virus antigen persisted in the aortic tissue for the eight weeks of testing, however infectious CB5 could not be isolated from tissues or blood after 14 days. These findings did illustrate that the aortic blood vessel can serve as a target tissue for coxsackievirus replication and persistence. The latency of this effect is seen in that histopathological examination of aortic tissue of CB5 infected hypercholesteremic mice five months after infection revealed endothelial cell swelling and disruption of medial cells with lipid-like vacuolation. Classical atherosclerotic plaques were evident at seven to nine months after infection. Neither normocholesteremic mice infected with virus nor uninfected hypercholesteremic animals, or placebo-treated controls of the same sex and age developed any atherosclerotic lesions (Figure 1).

Kos et al. (19) demonstrated that dietary hypercholesteremia mediated a more generalized immunosuppressive effect that was not limited only to an increase in susceptibility to coxsackievirus infection. Susceptibility to the bacterial agent <u>Listeria</u> <u>monocytogenes</u> was also augmented since the LD50 response of hypercholesteremic mice was 3.7 x 10^5 CFU/mouse, 40.3 times lower than the LD50 for normocholesteremic animals challenged with the same organisms. In our laboratory we have shown an increase in tumor growth rate and a shorter mean survival time (MST) in hypercholesteremic animals inoculated with Lewis Lung Carcinoma cells. The MST was 28.6 ± 2.6 days as compared to 36 ± 2.7 days for the normocholesteremic animals inoculated with this tumor (p <0.05). Similar results were obtained with animals inoculated with methyl cholanthrene-induced syngeneic fibrosarcoma (MCA-2182) cells.

Injection of heat-activated Corynebacterium parvum, a macrophage attractant, into Lewis Lung Tumor, was associated with a 50% tumor regression in normal animals as compared to no regression of tumors in similar treated hypercholesteremic animals.

Dietary hypercholesteremia was also associated with a decreased antibody response to sheep erythrocytes in vivo where the number of antibody producing cells against sheep red blood cells, per 10^6 spleen cells were assayed. Normocholesteremic animals had 33% more antibody producing cells than hypercholesteremic animals, 294 ± 34.6 versus 182 ± 21.6, respectively (p <0.001, n = 8 per group).

Hypercholesteremic animals challenged with CB5 showed a ten-fold reduction of virus clearance from the blood or liver at one to four hours after challenge when compared with normocholesteremic animals, challenged with the same virus dose (20) suggesting that high cholesterol levels impede virus clearance thus prolonging the infections and the action of the virus in the tissue.

DISCUSSION AND SUMMARY

The results of our studies demonstrate that genetic predisposition to diabetes mellitus is associated with a greater susceptibility to infection with the human coxsackievirus B4. In this animal model, with the diabetes mutation db, coxsackievirus B4 infection leads to a more severe pancreopathy than in the host which does not have this mutation. Furthermore, diabetes heredity as defined by the mutation db, without overt disease, is also

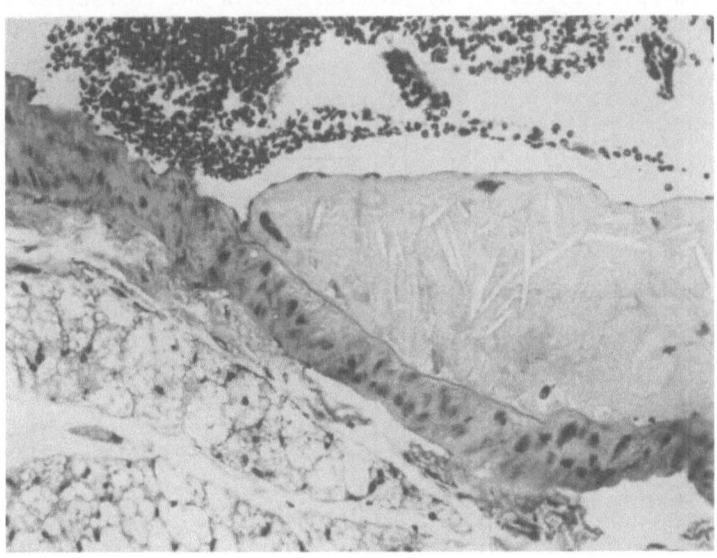

Fig. 1. Coxsackievirus B5 infected hypercholesteremic CD-1 mouse, ten months after infection. Note cholesterol clefts in atherosclerotic plaque adhering to aorta wall.

associated with an impairment in humoral immunity as evident from the inability of the host to produce neutralizing antibodies when challenged with coxsackievirus B4.

If applicable to man, these results suggest that coxsackievirus B could function as a selective agent in individuals with a genetic predisposition to this disease (Figure 2, left corner). The role of coxsackie B virus in the onset of mouse diabetes reinforces the need for clinical efforts to determine if similar genetic predispositions exist in man that would enable us to identify populations at risk for type I diabetes. If this could be shown, then an effective coxsackie B virus vaccine could be developed to protect this vulnerable population.

In another area, nutritionally-induced hypercholesteremia was shown to mediate an immune suppression. This immune impairment was characterized by an augmentation in host susceptibility to infection with coxsackievirus B and bacteria and as well an inability to reject tumors.

The increase in tissue-lipid deposition, resulted in an augmentation of virus replication and favored coxsackievirus B persistance. Consequently, in the hypercholesteremic host coxsackievirus B5 cardiopathy was aggravated and vascular infection lead to the development of atherosclerotic plaques (Figure 2, right corner). This suggests that hypercholesteremia can exert its atherosclerotic action, by suppression of the host resistance to a virus which induces the "initial vascular injury" leading to vasculitis. The deposition of cholesterol into this "injured" vessel would be augmented resulting in the onset of atherogenesis.

Both, i.e. coxsackievirus B and hypercholesteremia, independently caused immunosuppression which in turn promoted the particular pathological effect of each factor. Their synergistic interaction lead to a more severe cardiovascular disease and the development of atherosclerosis. This finding is pertinent to the association of high animal fat intake and its relationship to both atherosclerosis and tumor incidence.

As illustrated in Figure 2, hypercholesteremia and coxsackieviruses B appear to be common denominators in both diabetes and atherosclerosis.

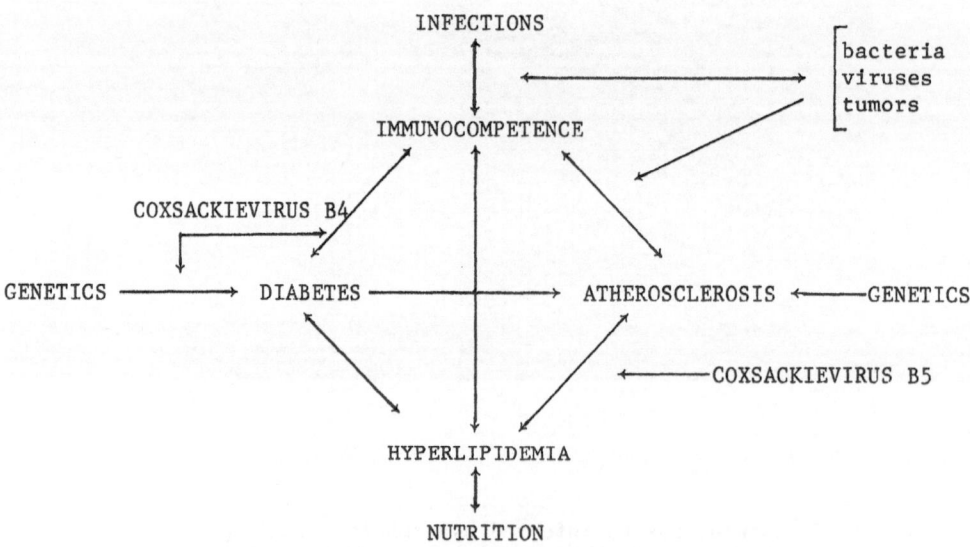

Figure 2. Hypercholesteremia and Coxsackieviruses B as Common Denominators in Diabetes and Atherosclerosis

Conceptually, these observations indicate that the group B coxsackieviruses which have a particular tropism for the pancreas and vascular tissues may have a role in the pathogenesis of diabetes and atherosclerosis. The severity of virus-induced lesions can be markedly aggravated by the level of cholesterol.

ACKNOWLEDGMENTS

This manuscript was supported in part by grants from NIADDK, AM21872 and AM24097, and the National Foundation for Cancer Research. The editorial assistance of Dr. William Regelson was greatly appreciated.

REFERENCES

1. J. F. Woodruff, Viral myocarditis, Am. J. Path. 101:426 (1980).
2. D. R. Gamble, The epidemiology of insulin-dependent diabetes with particular reference to the relationship of virus infection to its etiology, Epidemiol. Rev. 2:49 (1980).
3. G. Dalldorf, J. L. Melnick, and E. D. Curran, "The Coxsackie Group in Viral and Rickettsial Infections in Man," T. M. Rivers and F. L. Horsfall, Jr., eds., J. B. Lippincott Company, Philadelphia (1959).
4. C. G. Fabricant, L. Krook, and J. G. Gillespie, Virus induced cholesterol crystals, Science 181:556 (1973).
5. S. Penman, Stimulation of the incorporation of choline in poliovirus infected cells, Virology 25:148 (1965).
6. S. Kibrick and K. Benirschke, Severe generalized disease (encephalo-hepatomyocarditis) occurring in the newborn period and due to infection with coxsackievirus group B, Pediat. 22:857 (1958).
7. S. R. Webb, R. E. Loria, G. E. Madge, and S. Kibrick, Susceptibility of mice to group B coxsackievirus is influenced by the diabetic gene, J. Exp. Med. 143:1249 (1976).
8. S. R. Webb, R. M. Loria, G. E. Madge, and S. Kibrick, Coxsackievirus B infection in the mouse: effects associated with the diabetic gene, db, Current Microbiol. 3:15 (1979).
9. R. M. Loria and N. Tuttle-Fuller, Genetic predisposition to diabetes mellitus is associated with impaired humoral immunity to coxsackievirus B4, Amer. Soc. Microbiol. 62nd Annual Meeting, R65 E51 (1982).
10. R. M. Loria, L. B. Montgomery, and N. Tuttle-Fuller, The influence of heredity to diabetes mellitus and overt disease on the immunity to coxsackievirus B4 (in press, 1984).
11. L. J. Bennion and S. M. Grundy, Effects of diabetes mellitus on cholesterol metabolism in man, New Eng. J. Med. 246:1365 (1977).
12. J. L. Marx, Atherosclerosis: the cholesterol connection, Science 194:711 (1977).
13. G. M. Reaven and G. Steiner, eds., Proceedings of a conference on diabetes and atherosclerosis, Diabetes 30:Supp. 2 (1981).
14. R. M. Loria, S. Kibrick, D. Downing, G. Madge, and L. C. Fillios, Studies of hypercolesterolemia in the mouse, Nutrition Reports International 13:509 (1976).
15. R. H. Fiser, Jr., J. C. Dennington, V. G. McGann, J. Kaplan, W. H. Adler III, M. D. Kastello, and W. R. Biesel, Altered immune functions in hypercholesteremic monkeys, Infect. and Immunit. 8:105 (1973).
16. A. E. Campbell, R. M. Loria, and G. E. Madge, Coxsackievirus B cardiopathy and angiopathy in the hypercholesteremic host, Atherosclerosis 31:295 (1978).
17. R. M. Loria, S. Kibrick, G. Madge, Infection in hypercholesteremic mice with coxsackievirus B, J. Infec. Dis. 133:655 (1976).

18. R. M. Loria, W. L. Kos, A. E. Campbell, and G. E. Madge, Suppression of aortic elastic tissue autofluorescence for the detection of viral antigen, Histochem 61:151 (1979).
19. W. L. Kos, R. M. Loria, M. J. Snodgrass, D. Cohen, T. G. Thorpe, and A. M. Kaplan, Inhibition of host resistance by nutritional hypercholesteremia, Infec. Immun. 26:658 (1979).
20. A. E. Campbell, R. M. Loria, G. E. Madge, and A. M. Kaplan, Suppression of immunity to coxsackievirus by dietary hypercholesteremia, Infect. and Immunity 37:307 (1982).

MECHANISM OF "MODIFIED-SELF" INDUCED ANTI-HERPES SIMPLEX VIRUS

(HSV) ANTIBODY UNRESPONSIVENESS

Jerry M. Karabin and Lawrence A. Wilson

Department of Microbiology and Immunology
Louisiana State University Medical Center
New Orleans, Louisiana

It is apparent from recent reports that both antibody and cell-mediated immunity most likely participate in the immune response to primary herpes simplex virus (HSV) infections. Effective immune responses are evidently directed against elimination of infected cells through recognition of HSV glycoproteins of the cell surface. Neutralizing antibody apparently is not a factor in primary infection because of the cell to cell transfer of virus. Antibody-dependent cellular cytotoxicity (1) as well as T lymphocyte-mediated cytotoxicity (2) have been shown to be involved in the survival of mice challenged with lethal doses of virus. Delayed hypersensitivity is apparently involved in the elimination of HSV (3) and survival (4). However, the interaction between antibody and cell-mediated effector mechanism has not been completely explored. For example, antibody (at critical concentrations) may actually interfere with cell-mediated mechanisms thereby "enhancing" HSV infections. On the other hand, antibody may act in some manner to deregulate the induction of the cytotoxic T lymphocyte (CTL) response (5). Therefore, we have begun studies which will provide ways of "modulating" humoral and/or cell-mediated immune responses that would benefit the host's recovery from an HSV infection.

Hapten-modified syngeneic spleen cells have been shown by others to induce antibody unresponsiveness or tolerance when introduced intravenously prior to challenge (6). Under these conditions, the CTL response was either unaffected or slightly augmented. We have previously described similar results using an HSV "modified-self" system (7). Antibody response was suppressed, CTL was unaffected and a significant increase in survival of mice challenged with a LD_{50} was noted. Continuing these studies, we have investigated: 1) the effect of increased concentration of HSV antigen per modified cell; and 2) the mechanism of HSV modified-self induced antibody unresponsiveness.

The methods used in this study have been previously described (7). Briefly, detergent solubilized HSV virion envelope antigens were linked to C3H/HeJ splenocytes by $CrCl_3$. Mice were injected IV with up to 4×10^7 HSV modified-cells seven days prior to challenge IP with 1×10^6 PFU of virus. Antibody concentrations were determined by a complement-dependent microcytotoxicity assay using HSV infected, ^{51}Cr labeled L cells. To test for effects in the absence of T suppressor cells, mice received 100 mg/kg cyclophosphamide IP two days prior to modified-self pretreatment.

The typical result, which was previously reported (7), of HSV modified-self pretreatment on the antibody response fourteen days post challenge is shown in Figure 1A. The titer of antibody to HSV at 20% ^{51}Cr release in the HSV modified-self group is only 50% of the anti-HSV titer achieved in the BSA modified-self pretreated control (or 50% suppression). When we doubled the amount of HSV soluble antigen and $CrCl_3$ during linkage, even greater suppression occurred in the HSV modified-self group (Figure 1B). The titer at 20% ^{51}Cr release for the HSV pretreated group with this protocol was only 25% of the response observed with the control group (or 75% suppression). These results suggest that the extent of anti-HSV antibody unresponsiveness is dependent to some degree on the amount of HSV soluble antigen linked to spleen cells used for pretreatment.

Spleen cells (5 x 10^7) adoptively transferred from animals pretreated with HSV modified-self to naive animals six hours prior to infectious HSV challenge, were effective in producing an antibody unresponsiveness (Figure 2B). This transferred unresponsiveness was essentially just as effective as the unresponsiveness achieved with HSV pretreated animals challenged directly with HSV (Figure 2A). Both panels of Figure 2 indicate a greater than four-fold decrease in anti-HSV antibody (at 30% ^{51}Cr release) with HSV modified-self pretreated groups. The ability to transfer the anti-HSV

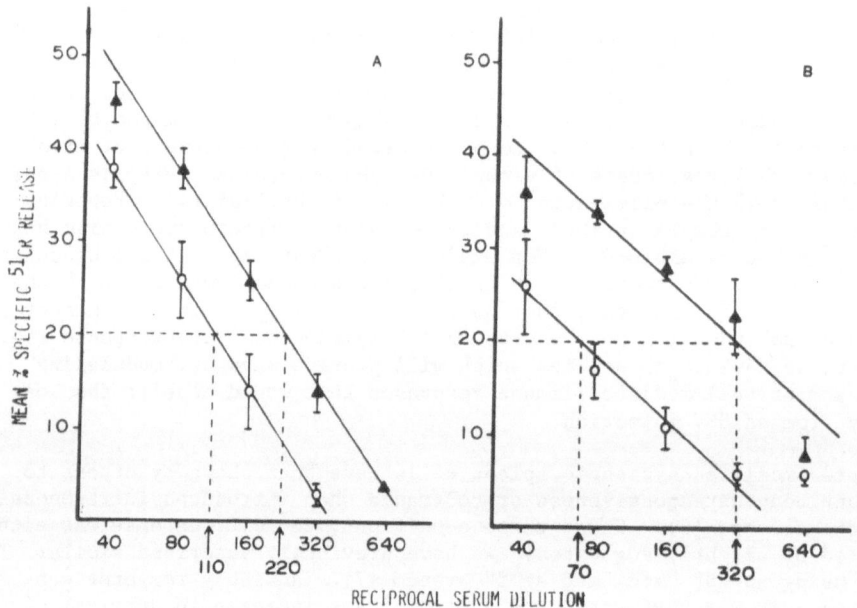

Fig. 1. Effect of increasing soluble HSV antigen during linkage to spleen cells. Anti-HSV antibody in serum from animals pretreated with HSV-modified splenocytes (O) or BSA-modified splenocytes (▲) was assayed. Points represent the means of four animals for each group at that particular dilution, with standard errors indicated. Panel A shows the results using the normal procedure for linking soluble HSV antigen to splenocytes previously reported (7). Calculated titers indicated that the HSV modified-self group was 50% suppressed. Panel B shows the effects of increasing soluble HSV antigen and $CrCl_3$ two fold while maintaining the same concentration of cells. Calculated titers indicated that the HSV modified-self group was 75% suppressed.

antibody unresponsiveness with spleen cells from HSV modified-self pretreated animals would indicate that some form of suppressor cell is involved, most likely T suppressor cells.

Cyclophosphamide has been shown by others to eliminate T suppressor induced tolerance (6). To determine if T suppressor cells were responsible for the observed modified-self induced unresponsiveness, we treated mice with cyclophosphamide prior to modified-self pretreatment. The results of this experiment are shown in Table 1. It is apparent from the P values that there was no difference between the cyclophosphamide treated and untreated HSV modified-self groups. However, a typical unresponsiveness was observed between HSV and BSA modified-self groups. These results would suggest that suppressor cells may not be the only mechanism of suppression involved in these experiments. Other investigators working with fowl gamma-globulin as antigen have found that both central T helper tolerance as well as T suppressor induction occurred with high doses of "modified-self;" whereas, only T suppressor induced unresponsiveness occurred at low doses of modified-self (8).

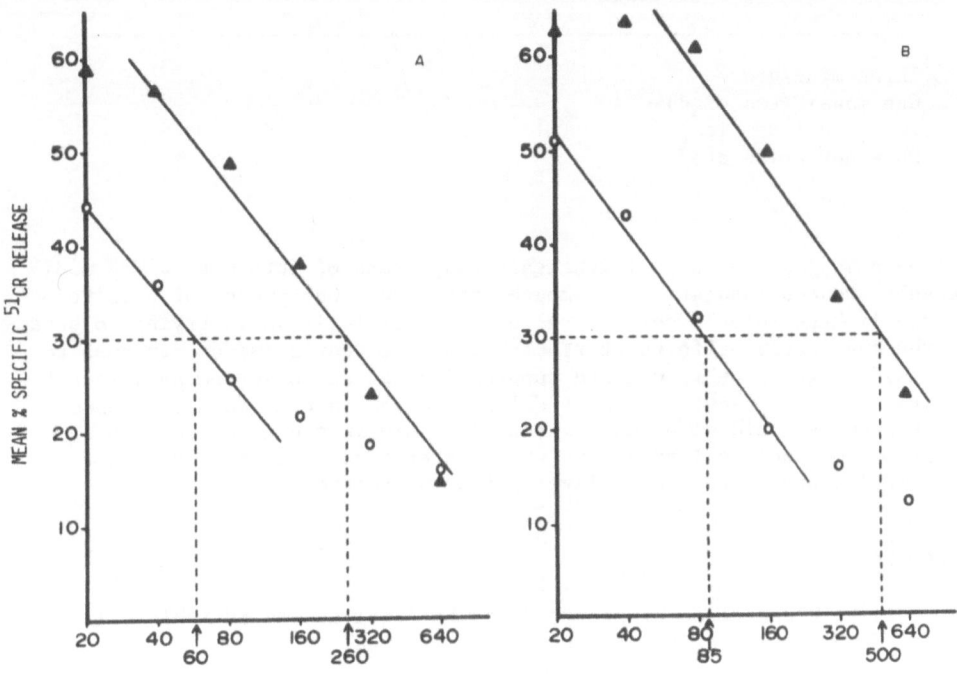

RECIPROCAL SERUM DILUTION

Fig 2. Adoptive transfer of HSV modified-self induced anti-HSV antibody unresponsiveness. Anti-HSV antibody was assayed from animals pretreated with or adoptively transferred from animals that were pretreated with HSV modified splenocytes (o). Panel A shows the typical unresponsiveness in the remaining animals not sacrificed for spleen cells used in adoptive transfer. Panel B shows that the anti-HSV unresponsiveness can be adoptively transferred with spleen cells from modified-self pretreated animals prior to HSV challenge. Calculated titers indicated that the adoptively transferred HSV modified-self group (Panel B) was suppressed to the same degree as the HSV modified-self group challenged directly (Panel A). Points represent the means of three animals for each group at that particular dilution.

Table 1. Effect of Cyclophosphamide on Anti-HSV Antibody
Unresponsiveness

Modified Spleen Cells	Serum Dilution	Mean % ^{51}Cr Release (S.E.)		P Values
		Cy+	Cy-	
HSV	1: 16	28^{1}(1.2)	31^{1}(2.9)	> 0.1
	1: 32	23 (1.2)	26 (1.7)	> 0.02
	1: 64	18 (3.5)	17 (2.3)	> 0.5
	1:128	7 (1.2)	7 (2.9)	> 0.5
	1:256	2 (0.6)	1 (0.6)	> 0.1
	1:512	1 (0.6)	1 (0.6)	> 0.5
BSA	1: 16	33^{2}	32^{3}	NC^{4}
	1: 32	36	29	
	1: 64	29	26	
	1:128	19	16	
	1:256	8	7	
	1:512	4	4	

[1] Three mice/group
[2] One mouse (two died)
[3] Two mice (one died)
[4] NC = not calculated

We have just begun to investigate many areas of interest in HSV modifiedself induced modulation of immune responses. Our system of passive antigen linkage to cell surfaces allows us some latitude in trying to separate the suppressive effects attributable to the host's immune response to cell surface antigens from those suppressive effects observed as a result of direct virus infection of host cells involved in the immune response. Future studies could have implications not only in the basic science of regulatory mechanisms involved in virus infections, but may also affect immunization procedures to achieve optimum protection.

ACKNOWLEDGMENTS

This work was aided by grants from the American Cancer Society (IN-150) and the Cancer Association of Greater New Orleans.

REFERENCES

1. S. Kohl and L. S. Loo, Protection of neonatal mice against herpes simplex virus infection: probable in vivo antibody-dependent cellular cytotoxicity, J. Immunol. 129:370 (1982).
2. H. S. Larsen, R. G. Russell, and B. T. Rouse, Recovery from lethal herpes simplex virus type 1 infection is mediated by cytotoxic T lymphocytes, Infect. and Immun. 129:370 (1982).
3. A. A. Nash, J. Phelan, and P. Wildy, Cell-mediated immunity in herpes simplex virus-infected mice: H-2 mapping of the delayed-type hypersensitive response and the antiviral T cell response, J. Immunol. 126:1260 (1981).
4. R. D. Schrier, L. I. Pizer, and J. W. Morehead, Type-specific delayed hypersensitivity and protective immunity induced by isolated herpes

simplex virus glycoproteins, J. Immunol. 130:1413 (1983).

5. K. K. Sethi, Effects of monoclonal antibodies directed against herpes simplex virus-specified glycoproteins on the generation of virus-specific and H-2 restricted cytotoxic T lymphocytes, J. Gen. Virology 64:2033 (1983).

6. D. W. Scott, C. Long, J. J. Jandinski, and J. T. C. Li, Role of self MHC carriers in tolerance and the immune response, Immunol. Rev. 50:275 (1980).

7. L. A. Wilson, J. M. Karabin, J. W. Smith, D. Dawson, and D. W. Scott, Modified self-induced modulation of the immune response to herpes simplex virus: effect on antibody formation, cytotoxic T lymphocyte induction, and survival, J. Immunol 132:1522 (1984).

8. P. H. Sherr, K. M. Heghinian, B. Benacerraf, and M. Dorf, Immune suppression in vivo with antigen-modified syngeneic cells. III. Distinction between T cell tolerance and T cell-mediated suppression, J. Immunol. 123:2682 (1979).

VIRUS ASSOCIATED IMMUNE AND PHARMACOLOGIC MECHANISMS IN

DISORDERS OF RESPIRATORY AND CUTANEOUS ATOPY

Judith Szentivanyi, Andor Szentivanyi, Joseph F. Williams
and Herman Friedman

University of South Florida College of Medicine
Tampa, Florida

INTRODUCTION

This chapter describes some immune and pharmacologic mechanisms associated with viral infections in certain immunologic diseases that belong
into the group of the so-called immediate hypersensitivities. The term
immediate hypersensitivity denotes an immunologic sensitivity to antigens
that manifests itself by tissue reactions occurring within minutes after
the antigen combines with its appropriate antibody. Such a reaction may
occur in any member of a species (nonatopic immediate hypersensitivity) or
only in certain predisposed or hyperreactive members (atopic immediate hypersensitivity).

The prototype of the nonatopic immediate hypersensitivity is local or
generalized anaphylaxis, whereas manifestations of atopic immediate hypersensitivity include bronchial asthma, hay fever, allergic rhinitis, chronic
urticaria, and atopic dermatitis.

The discussions that follow shall be confined to the atopic form of
immediate hypersensitivities in general, and to their respiratory and cutaneous manifestations, in particular. Of the latter, bronchial asthma, and
its cutaneous equivalent, atopic dermatitis, shall serve as the "model"
immunologic manifestations for our analysis below.

ATOPIC IMMEDIATE HYPERSENSITIVITIES (DISEASES OF ATOPIC ALLERGY)

Only a minority of the population shows some form of atopic disease in
spite of the fact that, by and large, identical conditions of antigen exposure must be presumed to exist for all members of the population. The nature
of the constitutional basis of atopy, that is, of the underlying determinant
for the development of atopic disease, is as yet unexplained.

Many theories of the constitutional basis of atopy have been proposed
since Coca and Cooke's original definition. Only two general ideas, however,
have survived: 1) the perception of atopy as a primary disorder of the
immune system with sequelae in the various effector tissues; and 2) a concept
of atopy as a primary autonomic imbalance, essentially beta-adrenergic in
character, with sequelae in effector cells including those engaged in the
production of antibodies. The autonomic imbalance is perceived as caused

not by some disorder of the autonomic nervous system itself but by a defective functioning of its effector cells.

These two concepts are not mutually exclusive. In fact, they may be interdependent. Although the immune features of atopic disease can be understood within the framework of a basic adrenergic disorder of various effector cells, many, if not most, of the nonimmune features of atopic conditions are not readily explicable on the basis of the primary immune abnormality.

The Original Concept of Atopy

At the time when the first concepts of atopy were being developed, it had long been known that hay fever and asthma often occurred together in the same individual and that both conditions showed a marked familial tendency. Similarly, it has been recognized that acute and chronic urticaria as well as gastrointestinal manifestations of idiosyncracy to a specific food were more common in patients with these diseases than in the general population, and a relation to infantile eczema (Besnier's prurigo, neurodermatitis) also was observed. Eczema was found to occur more frequently in the children of patients with hay fever or asthma, and individuals who had eczema in infancy showed an unusual incidence of hay fever and asthma later in life.

These diseases were, therefore, considered together by Cooke and Vander Veer as a special group of diseases of human sensitization with a hereditary background, and these authors concluded that such "sensitized individuals transmit to their offspring not their own specific sensitization, but an unusual capacity for developing bioplastic reactivities to any foreign proteins." With further progress in determining additional characteristics of "human sensitization" in contrast to those of experimental anaphylaxis in laboratory animals, Coca and Cooke concluded that a clear distinctions must be made between two types of hypersensitivity manifestations: 1) the anaphylactic type of allergic response to abnormal substances; and 2) the atopic type of response to substances that are generally innocuous. As they stated:

> "This latter sub-group evidently needs a special term by which it may be conveniently designated and this need is satisfactorily met with the word atopy, which was kindly suggested by Professor Edward D. Perry of Columbia University. The Greek word from which the term was derived, was used in the sense of a strange disease. However, it is not, on that account, necessary to include under the term all strange diseases; the use of the term can be restricted to the hay fever and asthma group."

To these, Wise and Sulzberger then added neurodermatitis under the new designation of "atopic dermatitis." Based on the close association of this condition with other atopic manifestations, Wise and Sulzberger concluded that the skin lesions of this disorder were the cutaneous analog of hay fever and asthma and suggested that the name atopic dermatitis replace disseminated neurodermatitis.

Several characteristics of the atopic state emerged from these early concepts: atopy was felt to be a hereditary manifestation, subject to a dominant gene, a peculiarly human disorder with a reacting serum element different from classic antibodies and reminiscent of the Wasserman reagin (hence the name, atopic reagin). Atopic antibodies, furthermore, seemed to occur only in humans, many times without any demonstrable prior exposure to incitant substances and induced by agents that often appeared to be nonantigenic (atopens of Grove and Coca).

Over the years, most of these postulated differences between atopy and anaphylaxis were gradually eliminated. Thus, antibody essentially identical with atopic reagin was found by Ishizaka in various animal species. Moreover, atopic disease was shown by Patterson to occur in animals. Some of the other distinctions between anaphylaxis and atopy also were amenable to various alternative explanations, indicating that these conditions may not be separated by wide and irreconcilable differences as it was believed by the originators of the concept of atopy. Nevertheless, some differences remained, and other important new differences emerged, making it imperative that a concept of atopy be reformulated.

The Reformulated Concept of Atopy

Since the 1960's, it has become increasingly evident that in addition to some of the remaining immunologic differences between anaphylaxis and atopic allergy, there are critically important nonimmune differences between the immediate hypersensitivities of the atopic and nonatopic type. Thus, it appears that in anaphylaxis we are dealing with a normal (physiologic) antibody response to an unnatural exposure to antigen, whereas in atopic allergy an "abnormal" antibody response to natural antigenic exposure seems to be involved. Anaphylactic reactivity of the sensitized individual depends on the release of an amount of pharmacologically active effector molecules sufficient to be toxic for most members of the same species. In contrast, individuals with atopic disease possess a quantitatively and qualitatively abnormal reactivity to otherwise nontoxic concentrations of endogenously released or exogenously administered pharmacologic mediators. Furthermore, the quantitative change consistently is in the direction of a decreased response when beta-adrenergic agents are the agonists and consistently in the direction of an increased response when any one of the other pharmacologically active effector molecules is involved.

Another essential difference between the atopic and nonatopic varieties of immediate hypersensitivities is the major contributory role played by infection in atopy, whereas infection has not been shown to be causally related to anaphylactic allergy--anaphylaxis, the Arthus reaction, or serum sickness. Moreover, atopic conditions can be precipitated by a number of totally unrelated stimuli, whereas anaphylaxis can be brought about only by the specific antigen. Finally, the latter conditions may be produced artificially, but atopic disease, with its spontaneous pattern of familial occurrence, cannot be induced at will. Acute human pulmonary anaphylaxis, which can include asthmatic features, for example, has never been reported to lead to the development of bronchial asthma or other atopic disease.

In the reformulation of the original concept of atopy by A. Szentivanyi, (1968) the essential difference between immediate hypersensitivities of the nonatopic and atopic varieties is that the former conditions are mediated by normal immune and pharmacologic mechanisms, whereas atopy is based on abnormal immune and pharmacologic mechanisms. This difference between anaphylaxis and atopy is regarded as fundamental. In this view, furthermore, it is the altered pharmacologic reactivity that is considered as the uniformly present, single atopic characteristic of pathognomonic significance.

Development of the Beta-Adrenergic Approach to the Study of the Constitutional Basis of Atopy

Authentic atopy cannot be produced at will in animals or humans--neither induced directly nor transferred passively. In addition to animal models of anaphylaxis, there are a number of experimental models simulating human atopy as well as isolated systems suitable for studying segmented areas of atopic reactivity. As such, they are useful for the analysis of some of the individual events (i.e., mediator release in the human reaction). Nevertheless, these in vivo and in vitro models are anaphylactic variants and represent immunologically and pharmacologically normal reactivities.

Therefore, they cannot be used for the study of the constitutional abnormality in atopy.

The Two Experimental Models for the Study of the Constitutional Basis of Atopy

The search for a laboratory model was guided by the premise that, if it is to be meaningful, the model must be able to imitate not only the immunologic but also the pharmacologic abnormality of the atopic state. The latter is manifested against substances that, in mammalian physiology, serve as the natural chemical organizers of autonomic action. It seemed likely, therefore, than an abnormal reactivity to these agents could be most effectively produced through some alteration of normal autonomic regulation significant enough to result in an autonomic imbalance.

The Hypothalamically "Imbalanced" Anaphylactic Guinea Pig

The first attempts to establish a more meaningful experimental counterpart of the atopic state were made by Filipp and Szentivanyi in the years from 1952 to 1958 during studies of hypothalamically "imbalanced" anaphylactic guinea pigs. Briefly, by electrolytic removal of one hypothalamic division or electric stimulation of the antagonistic division, it was possible to alter profoundly the anaphylactic reactivity of guinea pigs both immunologically and pharmacologically. From both the immunologic and pharmacologic standpoints, the conditions so produced more closely approximated those of the human atopic state than does anaphylaxis. Nevertheless, it was felt that the artificiality of such surgically induced hypothalamic imbalance is far removed from the natural setting (involving various inherited or acquired factors or both) that may surround the development of an atopic state. In their efforts to discover a more accurate representation of those naturally occurring conditions—some of which (i.e., infection) may conceivably serve as a developmental background for atopy—Szentivanyi and Fishel in the early 1960's found that the Bordetella pertussis-induced hypersensitive state served as a more appropriate model.

The Bordetella Pertussis-induced Hypersensitive State of Mice and Rats

Injection of live or killed Bordetella pertussis organisms into certain strains of mice and rats modifies the normal responses of these animals to a number of various stimuli. The possible applicability of the results of these investigations to atopy is implied by the following principal features of the B. pertussis-induced altered responsiveness: 1) hypersensitivity to endogenously released or exogenously administered histamine, serotonin, bradykinin, slow-reacting substance A, some prostaglandins, and, at least in two strains, to acetylcholine; 2) hypersensitivity to less specific stimuli, such as cold, changes in atmospheric pressure, and respiratory irritants; 3) in contrast with these increased sensitivities, a reduced beta-adrenergic sensitivity to catecholamines and, concerning some metabolic parameters, a reversal of normal beta-adrenergic activity; 4) enhanced antibody formation in general (adjuvant activity) and facilitated production in quantity of antibodies of the IgE class; and 5) presence of a marked eosinophilia.

As described by A. Szentivanyi, the major advance in these experiments that has paved the way for a meaningful analogy to atopic disorders has been the finding that hypersensitivity of the pertussis-sensitized mouse to pharmacologic mediators may be due to an acquired or genetically determined autonomic imbalance caused primarily by a reduced functioning of the adenylate cyclase coupled beta adrenergic receptors and the associated cyclic AMP system.

THE BETA ADRENERGIC THEORY OF ATOPIC DISORDERS:

UPDATED FORMULATION AND POSSIBLE EFFECTOR MECHANISMS

The previously discussed considerations and conclusions of the two consecutive series of animal experiments have culminated in the postulation of the original beta-adrenergic theory of atopic disorders as published by A. Szentivanyi in 1968. This theory regarded these disorders (i.e., perennial and seasonal allergic rhinitis, bronchial asthma, and atopic dermatitis) not as immunologic diseases but as unique patterns of altered reactivities to a broad spectrum of immunologic, psychic, infectious, chemical, and physical stimuli. This view gives to the antigen-antibody interaction the same role as that of a broad category of nonspecific stimuli that function only to trigger the same defective homeostatic mechanism in the various effector cells of the biochemical reaction sequence of immediate hypersensitivities.

Activation of the same defective mechanism by such a broad spectrum of unrelated stimuli is believed to be made possible by the unusual character of the pharmacologic mediators as a biologically distinct class of natural substances. These mediators, when viewed from the standpoint of their probable physiologic function, are the chemical organizers of autonomic action as well as of immunoregulation, that is, of homeostatic control. Consequently, regardless of the immunologic or nonimmunologic nature of the triggering event, its chemical realization would be expected to be brought about by essentially the same mediators.

Homeostatic adjustment to these influences requires, among other things, mobilization of the adrenergic neurotransmitters and their balanced (uninhibited) interaction with their effector systems. The theory postulated that the constitutional basis of atopy lies in the reduced functioning of the beta-adrenergic effector system, irrespective of what the triggering event may chemically be in a particular case (e.g., immunologic, infectious, or psychic). In this situation, the adrenergic neurotransmitters are released in the face of a relatively unresponsive beta-adrenergic effector system, and the resultant autonomic imbalance deprives the effector tissues of their normal counterregulatory adjustment. This constellation of mediators and effectors then leads to a unique pattern of quantitatively and qualitatively altered reactivity to the chemical organizers of autonomic action, mostly in response to trivial trauma.

When this theoretical scheme is applied to respiratory or cutaneous atopy, as least six levels of responses critical in these diseases are expected to be influenced by the beta adrenergic subsensitivity in question:

1. A reduction in the normal beta adrenergic inhibition of lysosomal enzyme release, chemotaxis, phagocytosis, antibody-dependent cellular cytotoxicity, increased expression of FcIgE receptors, and prostaglandin E snythesis to stimulation with histamine-induced suppressor factor, that is effector mechanisms that are known to play an important role in immunologic inflammation.

2. A reduction in lymphocytic beta adrenergic sensitivity resulting in abnormally decreased (lymphocyte transformation, E-rosette forming cells, T cells, suppressor cell function) and abnormally increased (IgE-producing B cells, Fc receptor-bearing lymphocytes) lymphocyte reactivities.

3. Mast cell mediator release to immunologic or nonimmunologic stimuli, ordinarily suppressed by beta adrenergic stimulation would become subsensitive to the same, while both cholinergic and alpha adrenergic enhancement of mediator release would be exaggerated.

4. Beta adrenergically mediated bronchial smooth muscle dilation is reduced, while cholinergically and alpha-adrenergically mediated constriction is augmented.

5. Increased mucous secretion in response to alpha-adrenergic and cholinergic stimulation would be increased, while sodium and water fluxes into tracheobronchial secretions in response to beta-adrenergic stimulation would be reduced.

6. The beta adrenergically mediated eosinopenia would be reduced and replaced by eosinophilia.

All these theoretically predictable manifestations do in fact exist, and represent the cardinal features of atopic disease. Similarly, they all point to the most critical component of this malfunctioning effector system that is to the adenylate cyclase-coupled beta adrenergic receptor and the associated cyclic nucleotide complex. It follows, therefore, that the fundamental abnormality common to all atopic persons may lie in an inherited or acquired lesion that causes defective functioning of this intracellular messenger system.

This reduced responsiveness to catecholamines could reflect alterations at any of a number of sites, including 1) changes in the affinity of catecholamines and their receptor sites; 2) decreases in the numbers or reactivities of beta receptors; 3) "interconversion" of adrenergic receptors from beta to alpha; 4) alterations in the efficiency of coupling of activated receptors to the catalytic units of adenylate cyclase; and 5) reductions in the concentration of adenylate cyclase. Alternatiavely, the postulated lesion may occur at a point beyond the cAMP generation step in the biochemical sequence leading to the adrenergic end response; in a cAMP-related pathway; in a complementary interacating or modulating system such as that provided by acetylcholine, histamine, the prostaglandins, leukotrienes, the interleukins, and a large group of lymphokines, monokines, and cytokines; or in an intracellular messenger system with counterregulatory potential, such as that connected with cyclic GMP. The currently available evidence seems to favor the possibility that there are inherited and/or acquired multiple abnormalities in the receptor-adenlyate cyclase-cyclic AMP system of esstentially all effector cells that are critical in the organization of immune reactivities.

Progression of the disease process from subclinical to a clinical form conceivably requires the operation of a preparatory and a triggering factor. The preparatory factor involves the postulated abnormality, and it may be familial (presumably hereditary) or acquired in nature; however, in either case, it must set the stage for the development of a functional imbalance. The triggering event must be appropriate to result in an increase in the rate of firing of adrenergic neurons, in the release of catecholamines from extraneuronal stores, or in any conceivable mediator constellations suitable to make the latent abnormality clincally manifest. However, the preparatory and triggering factors need not be separate or unrelated entities. Infection (probably viral), for example, could serve in both capacities.

With the exception of nonnucleated erythrocytes, the adenylate cyclase system has been found to be present in all animal cells examined to date. Its ubiquitious character suggests, therefore, that the ultimate clinical manifestation of the fundamentally same atopic abnormality will be determined by the type of cell primarily involved, that is, by the effector cell system that primarily harbors the postulated abnormality (cells of bronchial tissue versus those of nasal mucosa and skin and the circulating cells of blood).

For the extensive analyses of the experimental evidence supporting the validity of the beta adrenergic theory of atopic disorders, and its updated

216

formulation, the reader is referred to recent major reviews (Szentivanyi, 1980; Szentivanyi et al., 1980a; Szentivanyi and Fitzpatrick, 1980; Szentivanyi et al., 1980b; Szentivanyi et al., 1983; Szentivanyi and Szentivanyi, 1983; Krzanowski and Szentivanyi, 1983; Szentivanyi et al., 1984; Szentivanyi and Szentivanyi, 1985a; Szentivanyi and Szentivanyi, 1985b; Szentivanyi et al., 1985), whereas the discussion that follows will be addressed to the possible nature of the developmental mechanisms of the beta adrenergic subsensivity in respiratory and cutaneous atopy.

DEVELOPMENTAL MECHANISMS OF BETA ADRENERGIC SUBSENSIVITY IN

RESPIRATORY AND CUTANEOUS ATOPY

With respect to the apparent central feature of the atopic abnormality, that is the beta adrenergic subsensitivity of the effector cells that participate in the cellular organization of the atopic response, the question may be raised of how such an abnormality could develop. At present, at least three major developmental mechanisms can be envisaged. The abnormality may be 1) acquired by functional receptor regulatory shifts caused by hormonal changes, infection (viral, bacterial, etc.), allergic tissue injury, or other event; 2) genetically determined; or 3) caused by autoimmune disease. In case of a given atopic disorder, one, two or all three of these effector mechanisms may be operative. Because of the orientation of this chapter only the role of viral infection, the allergic tissue injury, and autoimmunity due to anti-receptor antibodies will be discussed below.

VIRAL INFECTIONS AS A DEVELOPMENTAL MECHANISM OF BETA-ADRENERGIC

SUBSENSITIVITY IN BRONCHIAL ASTHMA

Upper respiratory tract infection has frequently been shown to precipitate or exacerbate the asthmatic condition and to produce or increase airway hyperreactivity to bronchospastic agents (Szentivanyi et al., 1983). In an earlier era when whooping cough was common, Bordetella pertussis infection was considered a frequent cause of the development of asthma or of recurrent bronchospasm. Even today, there is evidence that Haemophilus influenzae infection is present in the deeper respiratory tract of asthmatic patients (Hirschmann and Everett, 1979), and since this bacterium was shown to produce in animal experiments (Schreurs et al., 1980a, 1980b; Terpstra, et al. 1979) beta adrenergic impairment and/or an increased cyclic GMP level, the relationship between H. influenzae infection and the pharmacologic abnormality in asthma may be an authentic one.

In the meantime, in contrast to bacterial pathogens, viral respiratory infection was shown to have a more significant role in the pathogenesis of asthma. During the Asian influenza pandemic in the late 1950's, severe exacerbations of bronchial asthma were found to be among the more frequently reported complications of this infection (Roldaan and Masural, 1982). Since then numerous reports have appeared describing an important relationship between asthma and viral respiratory infection. Recent refinements in epidemiologic methods, microbiologic isolation techniques, and pulmonary function testing have provided new opportunities to characterize this relationship more precisely (Hall and Hall, 1985).

A review of the available information indicates that 1) experiments in animal models (Katz, 1978), and observations in children (Frick et al., 1979), suggest that the expression of atopy occurs during a period termed "allergic breakthrough" which may follow viral infections; 2) a history of childhood viral respiratory illness is a risk factor for the development of chronic obstructive airway syndromes in later life; 3) if such infection does lead to obstructive airway disease, the resultant manifestation is likely to be a "wheezy" or asthmatic type of obstructive airway disease; 4) viral, as opposed to bacterial, respiratory pathogens commonly herald the onset of wheezing in childhood and predispose to the development of atopy, although bronchial pharmacologic hyperreactivity after viral illness may also proceed independent of immunologic mechanisms in bronchospasms; and finally 5) no matter what the ultimate effect of respiratory infection in infancy on the subsequent development of asthma may be, there is little doubt that respiratory viruses commonly induce acute exacerbations of bronchospasm in the older child, and adults with known asthma.

The significance of one or another respiratory virus in causing asthma or its exacerbations appears to depend on the age of the patient. Thus, in the preschool age (0-4 years) the predominant agent is respiratory syncytial virus followed by parainfluenza types 1-3, influenza, rhinovirus, and coronavirus. In the school age (5-16 years), rhinovirus leads the list followed in descending order of incidence by influenza, parainfluenza Types 1-3, and respiratory syncytial virus. In adults, the order of relative significance changes again with the dominance of influenza virus followed by rhinovirus and respiratory syncytial virus (Frick et al., 1979; Szentivanyi et al. 1983; Hall and Hall, 1985).

Another dimension of viral influences involves the problem of bronchial hyperreactivity or "lability" in asthma. It has been recognized for some time that normal subjects exhibit relatively short-lived bronchial hyperirritability to inhaled histamine when they have a viral respiratory infection (Empey et al., 1976) and as stated above asthma may worsen during and after viral respiratory infection. In some of these situations the documented increase in airway resistance could be partially or fully blocked by atropine aerosol prompting the hypothesis that damage to the epithelial surface of the upper airways by viral infection exposes and thereby sensitizes the rapidly adapting sensory irritant receptors in the upper airways to various inhaled irritants, causing reflex parasympathetic vagal bronchoconstriction (Nadel, 1980).

There are, however, several major considerations that discount the significance of a parasympathetically oriented interpretation of virus-induced asthmogenicity:

1) Not all viruses can be implicated in this phenomenon. For instance, adenoviruses, herpes virus hominis, influenza Type B virus, and enteroviruses do not show a relationship to episodes of asthma (McIntosh et al., 1973; Minor et al., 1974). Studies of rhinovirus infection suggest that only a few rhinovirus serotypes are associated with asthmogenicity. This is a finding that is difficult to reconcile with the damaged epithelium hypothesis (assuming equivalent severity of infection) and raises the question of other possible mechanisms related to the biochemical properties of the virus (Buckner et al., 1981; Busse et al., 1979).

2) Conversely, influenza Type A virus that is clearly associated with increased asthma (Minor et al., 1976), affects lung function largely through an effect on small airways (Szentivanyi et al. 1983), whereas the aforementioned rapidly adapting sensory irritant receptors are primarily distributed in the larger upper airways (Mills et al., 1970).

3) The hypothesis of a cholinergic hyperreactivity as a consequence of epithelial damage presupposes the de facto presence of an active viral infection which is the cause of the respiratory inflammation leading to the disruption of the airway epithelial barrier and activation of the subepithelial rapidly adapting sensory irritant receptors. Indeed, the characteristic

218

histologic marker of viral respiratory infection is epithelial destruction, and Welliver et al. (1980) has shown that IgE was bound to exfoliated nasopharyngeal epithelial cells in most patients during the acute phase of infection with respiratory syncytial virus. They also found that a continued presence of cell-bound IgE was more common in patients with bronchiolitis or asthma than in those with mild upper respiratory tract infection. In this regard, it has been established in avian species that experimentally induced viral laryngotracheitis results in disruption of airway epithelium, with resultant increased permeation of horseradish peroxidase (Richardson et al., 1981), and possibly increased uptake of inhaled antigens. Furthermore, Ida and associates (1977) have demonstrated that interferon elaborated during viral infections from leukocytes harvested from patients with ragweed allergy may induce histamine release suggesting that atopic patients may experience bronchial hyperreactivity if specific antigen exposure occurs at the time of viral infection.

Under these circumstances, it is important to mention that evidence is available that actual respiratory infection with influenza Type A virus is not a necessary condition for the development of increased airway irritability in patients with asthma. Thus, administration of killed influenza virus vaccine to asthmatic patients caused a significant increase in bronchial sensitivity to methacholine aerosol, reaching a maximum after one day and persisting for three days (Oulette and Reed, 1965). Normal subjects did not develop the heightened response to methacholine, and no evidence of allergy to the vaccine was detected. These investigators suggested that the effect might be explained by an endotoxin-like action of the influenza vaccine. Indeed, endotoxin sensitization of human bronchial smooth muscle to alpha-adrenergic agonists has been reported. Phenylephrine-induced contractions were enhanced two to ten times in normal lung and 1000 times in lung from a patient with chronic bronchitis. Endotoxin also caused a decrease in cyclic AMP of the tissue (Simonsson et al., 1972). These observations are complemented by recent findings obtained through vaccination with a purified LPS preparation from E. coli that resulted in a decreased number of beta-adrenergic receptors in guinea pig lung (Schreurs, Verhoef, and Nijkamp, 1983).

4) There are other observations calling into question the requirement of an active viral infection in the production of bronchial hyperactivity as mediated by cholinergically activated irritant receptors. Thus, pulmonary function abnormalities in adults with viral respiratory illness are generally more pronounced seven to ten days after the onset of symptoms--a time when the clinical manifestations and manifestations of viral inflammation are waning (Hall et al., 1976). Also, the abnormalities of pulmonary function are generally prolonged well beyond what we now recognize as the period of viral shedding. Furthermore, administration of the antiviral agent, amantadine hydrochloride, although clinically effective, has no effect on the magnitude or duration of airway hyperreactivity (Little et al., 1976).

5) In one longitudinal study, Minor et al. (1974) found that simple colonization of the respiratory tract by virus was not sufficient to provoke asthma: such attacks occurred only when the infection produced symptoms of fever, malaise, cough, or coryza. The dominant role of fever in these episodes immediately suggests the profound involvement of adrenergic effector mechanisms.

Additional support for the important effect of viral infections on adrenergic mechanisms in asthmatic patients came from the extensive studies of Busse and his associates. In their experiments human granulocytes served as a convenient in vitro model for the systematic study of virus incubation on the pharmacologic agonist response. At first, it was described (Busse, 1977) that an impairment of the inhibitory action of a beta adrenergic agonist (isoproterenol), normally observed on lysosomal enzyme release, occurred in granulocytes taken from asthmatic patients (control of release of lysosomal enzymes is known to play a major role in bronchial immunologic inflammation, Henson, 1971). The beta adrenergic impairment of lysosomal enzyme release was significantly greater if the cells were obtained during upper respiratory tract infection. Following these observations, Busse and colleagues have consistently reported virus-induced impairment of several neutrophil mechanisms which normally mediate inhibition of enzyme release. Impairment occurred after incubation in vitro with live influenza virus (Busse et al., 1979), and with live rhinovirus 16 (RV16) (Busse et al., 1980), a finding also observed following infection of normal subjects with RV16 (Bush et al., 1978). Both studies reported an impairment of the normal functioning of beta adrenergic, histamine H_2, and PGE, receptors, all responsible for inhibition of lysosomal enzyme release through stimulation of adenylate cyclase resulting in cyclic AMP formation (Ignarro and Colombo, 1973). Interference with granulocyte beta adrenergic receptor activity by influenza virus has subsequently been confirmed by Lee (1980), and extended to include lymphocytes, resulting in decreased inhibition of E-rosette formation to beta adrenergic stimulation by isoproterenol. Another important study by Buckner et al. (1981) showed that parainfluenza 3 virus infection in vivo causes a selective blockade of the beta adrenergic inhibition of antigen-induced contraction of isolated airway smooth muscle. These abnormalities moreover are not limited to those with known atopy but may also be demonstrated in cell systems from normal subjects. Viral infections, therefore, may have important inhibitory effects on beta adrenergic responsiveness in the course of bronchoconstriction. This area has recently been extensively reviewed by Norris and Eyre (1982).

6) Up to this point an analysis of the evidence against a parasympathetically (cholinergically) oriented virus induced asthmogenicity included arguments based on information obtained from the current state of our understanding of some aspects of virology, immunology, immunologic inflammation, and the cyclic nucleotide system. In the discussion below, these arguments will be extended to include some basic principles of neurophysiology and neuropharmacology which also contradict the basic validity of the hypothesis of Nadel and his associates (1980).

For the purpose of establishing the appropriate framework for this discussion, the basic tenets of this hypothesis will be restated as follows. In the past two decades, Nadel, Boushey, Holtzman, and their associates have accumulated evidence indicating that stimulation of rapidly adapting epithelial nerve receptors of the airways by mechanical, chemical, and pharmacologic stimuli, reflexly increases the output of acetylcholine by the vagus nerves, causing a reflex bronchoconstriction. In particular, it was shown that although histamine is capable of constricting airway smooth muscles directly, most of its bronchoconstrictor effect in vivo is indirect, and due to this reflex mechanism. This is accomplished both by direct stimulation of these epithelial receptors and also by decreasing their firing threshold to other introduced stimuli. Thus, when histamine is injected into dog bronchial arteries, most of the airway constriction can be abolished by atropine. In otherwise healthy subjects, viral upper respiratory tract infections, through damage to the bronchial epithelium, cause transient bronchial hyperreactivity to inhaled histamine and citric acid, a phenomenon that also is abolished by anticholinergic drugs. On the basis of these and similar observations as well as the fact that bronchial hyperreactivity is associated with a decrease in cough threshold, these workers suggested that airway epithelial damage with sensitization of airway nerve endings causes exaggerated cough and bronchomotor responses. With this background, Nadel, Boushey, Holtzman, and their associates, further postulated that bronchial asthma is a constellation involving two ingredients: release of pharmacologic mediators, and sensitization of airway epithelial nerve receptors providing a positive feedback system for increasing bronchomotor tone.

220

This mechanism in fact probably contributes to the bronchial obstructive process in asthma. The altered pharmacologic reactivity in atopy, however, is not restricted to airway epithelial effectors, but it is a universal atopic trait. In fact, as explained earlier, the altered pharmacologic reactivity is the uniformly present, single atopic characteristic, which by its very nature must be explained by any theory attempting to elucidate the constitutional basis of atopy (Szentivanyi and Williams, 1980; Szentivanyi and Fitzpatrick, 1980; Szentivanyi et al., 1985; and discussion later on atopic dermatitis). For the reasons below, cholinergic overactivity cannot serve in this capacity.

Using spontaneously breathing, unanesthetized guinea pigs, it has been found that the vagal reflex component in histamine bronchoconstriction is small and probably a consequence rather than a cause of the constriction. In histamine-sensitive and histamine-insensitive strains of guinea pigs it has been demonstrated that the ease of in vivo histamine-induced reduction in lung compliance in the guinea pig is inversely related to its in vitro tracheal sensitivity to isoproterenol, revealing the primary homeostatic importance of the tracheobronchial beta adrenergic receptors rather than that of cholinergic control, in determining the sensitivity of this effector tissue to histamine (Holgate and Warner, 1960; Douglas et al., 1973, 1976). In harmony with these findings are the extensive studies carried out in humans in the past 20 years (Altounyan, 1964; Chen-Yeung et al., 1971; Casterline et al., 1976; Fish et al., 1977; Deal et al., 1978; Woenne et al., 1978; Rosenthal et al., 1977; Bandouvakis et al., 1981; O'Byrne et al., 1983; Boulet et al., 1984). The most recent findings by O'Byrne et al. (1985) further support the conclusions of these long series of observations indicating not only that blockade of the muscarinic cholinergic receptors has only a small effect on the response to inhaled histamine but also the observations that such a blockade elicits only a minor degree of protection against the response to inhaled allergen (Rosenthal et al., 1977), exercise (Deal et al., 1978), and inhalation of cold air (O'Byrne et al., 1983) in subjects with asthma. Taken together, these experiences indicate that the bronchial effect of histamine is exerted not by reflex bronchoconstriction but through stimulation of H_1-receptors on airway smooth muscle. Therefore, hyperresponsiveness to histamine in asthma is not primarily caused by a defect in the parasympathetic nervous supply to the airway.

Futhermore, no reproducible evidence of elevated levels of acetylcholine in tissues or body fluids of atopic individuals is available. This, in fact, is not surprising when the issue of cholinergic overactivity is examined in the broader biologic context of the general nature of cholinergic versus adrenergic control. Thus, the sympathetic system is distributed to effectors throughout the body, whereas the parasympathetic distribution is much more limited. For instance, sympathetic postganglionic fibers also innervate smooth muscles and glands of somatic (nonvisceral) regions; no comparable distribution has been established for the parasympathetic division. Moreover, the sympathetic fibers ramify to a much greater extent, and their preganglionic terminals make contact with a large number of postganglionic neurons. In general, the ratio of preganglionic to postganglionic axons may be about 1:20 or more. In addition, there is an overlapping of synaptic innervation so that one ganglion cell is supplied by several preganglionic fibers. By contrast, the parasympathetics are more discrete in their action, i.e., there is a closer to a 1:1 relation between pre- and postganglionic neurons (Szentivanyi, Krzanowski, and Polson, 1983). Also the parasympathetic nervous system has no reinforcing mechanism comparable to that of the adrenal medulla for the sympathetic division.

Usually, when any part of the sympathetic nervous system is stimulated, the entire system, or at least major portions of it, are stimulated at the same time, a phenomenon called mass discharge. Norepinephrine and epinephrine, therefore, are almost always released by the adrenal medulla at the same time that the different tissues are being stimulated directly by the sympathetic nerves. The two means of stimulation support each other and either can actually substitute for the other. Without any stimulation, however, the normal resting rate of secretion by the adrenal medulla is sufficient to maintain blood pressure almost to normal even if all direct sympathetic pathways to the cardiovascular system are removed. Another important value of the adrenal medulla is the capability of catecholamines to stimulate structures of the body that are not innervated by sympathetic fibers. In contrast, the characteristics of parasympathetic reflexes are discrete. For instance, they usually act only on the heart to increase or decrease its activity, or frequently cause secretion only in the mouth or, in other instances, secretion only by the stomach glands.

Acetylcholine (ACh), i.e, the cholinergic transmitter released by para-sympathetic fibers, is almost instantaneously destroyed in the junctional clefts by an unusual enzyme, acetylcholinesterase (true cholinesterase, AChE). The principal evidence for this is the decay time of the end-plate current, which is more rapid than diffusion of ACh out of a synaptic cleft would allow. Also, the most recent preparation of AChE hydrolyzed 960 nmoles ACh per mg of protein per hour, thus placing it among the enzymes having the highest turnover number that is known (Szentivanyi, Krzanowski, and Polson, 1983). This powerful destructive capacity is reinforced by a battery of butyryl cholinesterases ("pseudo" or nonspecific cholinesterases) which destroy most of whatever acetylcholine may have escaped into the blood stream. Thus, it is doubtful whether acetylcholine can reach noninnervated cells or is present in the extracellular space in regulatory concentrations for cells with immunologic significance such as the antigen-sensitive lymphocytes. There is no comparable system of rapid destruction for the catecholamines, a fact which accounts in part for the widespread nature of sympathetic action.

Another way to determine whether we are dealing with a primary choliner-gic overactivity in atopy is to examine whether there is any evidence for an enhanced guanylate cyclase activity in cells obtained from patients with atopic disease. This is all the more necessary, since as mentioned earlier, cholinergic and alpha adrenergic agents activate guanylate cyclase, and markedly reduced adenylate cyclase-cyclic AMP responses to beta adrenergic stimulation have been shown to be present in atopic individuals.

Under these circumstances, it is highly significant that the available evidence shows not an enhanced but a reduced cholinergic responsiveness in lymphocytes of atopic individuals. Thus, it was found that in normal sub-jects alpha adrenergic stimulations with norepinephrine plus propranolol, and cholinergic stimulation with acetylcholine evoked significant increases in cyclic GMP formation. In contrast, the lymphocytic guanylate cyclase activity did not show a significant response to the same agents in patients with acute asthma, but the normal guanylate cyclase responsiveness was found to be partially restored in patients in remission (Haddock, Patel, Alston and Kerr, 1975). Similarly, Lang, Goel and Grieco (1978), in their study on adrenergic and cholinergic responses of peripheral lymphocytes in the "active" E rosette assay, demonstrated not only a subsensitivity of T lympho-cytes to beta adrenergic but also to cholinergic stimulation in patients with bronchial asthma. In the same experiments, phenylephrine, an alpha adrenergic agonist, showed no difference between the normal and asthmatic groups in enhancing the "active" E rosette formation. A subsensitive beta adrenergic and cholinergic system with a normal alpha adrenergic effector system may produce a state of relatively enhanced alpha adrenergic activity, a circumstance which may explain some of the findings showing that by giving alpha receptor blockers one can restore beta adrenergic responsiveness toward normal in lymphocytes of asthmatics (Logsdon et al., 1973; Alston, Patel, and Kerr, 1974). There are additionally at least three major arguments against cholinergic overactivity as the primary mechanism of atopy.

First, neither pulmonary sympathectomy nor pulmonary vagotomy produces any lasting improvement in bronchial asthma. Second, as discussed in detail elsewhere (Szentivanyi and Williams, 1980; Szentivanyi and Fitzpatrick, 1980; Szentivanyi et al., 1983; Szentivanyi et al. 1985), it is never the excessive presence of a neurohumor, but if anything, it is its prolonged lack that is likely to result in the development of chronic effector hypersensitivities. Consequently, it is inconceivable that cholinergic overactivity could produce a hypersensitivity to acetylcholine or similar mediators of immediate hypersensitivities. On the contrary, cholinergic overactivity would be expected to lead to desensitization of the cholinergic receptors, as has been extensively demonstrated in numerous preparations such as the skeletal muscles of the frog, the hearts of vertebrates and invertebrates, the Renshaw cells, the neurons of molluscks, etc. (Michelson and Danilov, 1971). This is in harmony with more recent findings obtained in non-obstructed, non-reversibly obstructed, and reversibly obstructed (asthma) patients. Using H^3-quinuclidinyl benzilate, a stereospecific radioligand for muscarinic cholinergic receptors a significant reduction in receptor density was found in the lung preparations of asthmatics, and no difference in the numbers of such receptors in lung specimens derived from the non-reversibly obstructed and non-obstructed groups (Szentivanyi, 1982). An important question of course is how can one possibly find a reduction in the number of muscarinic cholinergic receptors in lung membranes derived from patients with reversible obstruction (asthma) in the simultaneous presence of an exquisite bronchial hyperreactivity to cholinergic agents? At the time of this writing, we can only offer two possible interpretations. One is that the bronchial hyperreactivity to cholinergic agents in asthma is not mediated through cholinergic mechanisms, but is basically due to the beta adrenergic abnormality, which is also responsible for the atopic feature of the disease. The second possibility is that the reduction in muscarinic receptor densities is caused by a heightened vagus activity resulting in a cholinergic "downturn" and ultimately producing a pharmacological "denervation supersensitivity" to cholinergic agents (Szentivanyi, 1971; Szentivanyi, Krzanowski and Polson, 1983). Whether one or the other, or both of these interpretations will prove to be correct, it is evident that they represent important evidence against the validity of Nadel's (1980) reflex hypothesis of the virally induced mechanisms of bronchoconstriction in asthma. Finally, if the atopic state were to be due to cholinergic overactivity produced by viruses through the postulated reflex mechanisms, then anticholinergic agents should have a far more demonstrable therapeutic effect than what we are able to observe in asthma (Altounyan, 1964; Chen-Yeung et al., 1971; Casterline et al., 1976; Fish et al., 1977; Deal et al., 1978; Woenne et al., 1978; Rosenthal et al., 1977; Bandouvakis et al., 1981; Boulet et al. 1984; O'Byrne et al., 1983, 1985), let alone the other atopic conditions where they are useless.

VIRAL INFECTION AS A DEVELOPMENTAL MECHANISM OF BETA ADRENERGIC SUBSENSITIVITY IN ATOPIC DERMATITIS

The most typical viral infection that affects children with atopic dermatitis is Kaposi's herpetic eruption. It is caused by herpes simplex, type 1 or 2, and also the virus coxsackie A16 can mimic perfectly the eruption caused by a herpetic virus. Other viruses associated with this disease include herpes zoster, vaccinia, warts, and molluscum contagiosum. While it has long been known that recurrent viral cutaneous infections are more prevalent in atopic dermatitis, there is now growing evidence for recurrent cold sores and upper respiratory infections in this condition. Serological studies have also revealed that atopic dermatitis patients display significantly higher serum levels of antibodies against Epstein-Barr virus (EBV) than their non-atopic controls. It appears therefore, that the increased susceptibility to viral infections is not restricted to dermatotropic viruses but rather reflects an abnormal host response to viral infections in general (Bonifazi et al., 1985; Strannegård et al. 1985).

Host defense against most viral infections is dependent to a large extent on cell-mediated immune mechanisms, and there is abundant clinical and experimental evidence of defective cell-mediated immunity in atopic dermatitis. In early studies, a reduction in the number of T cells was found which correlated with the severity of the disease, and these findings were later complemented by the demonstration of a defective functioning of these cells. Soon it was also shown that the T cell defect is particularly evident in suppressor/cytotoxic T cell subsets (Strannegård and Strannegård, 1978; Schuster et al., 1979; Jensen et al., 1981; Strannegård et al., 1982; Kang et al., 1983).

Defective cytotoxic T cells and also the association of abnormally functioning macrophages (Kragballe et al., 1980) and natural killer cells (Jensen et al., 1984), appear to have an important role in the impaired host defense against viral infections in atopic dermatitis. Since these cell types produce, or are capable of producing interferon, a deficient production of this agent may at least be partly responsible for the increased susceptibility to viral infections in atopic dermatitis. A reduced production of interferon-alpha in children with atopic dermatitis (Strannegård and Strannegård, 1980) as well as of interferon-gamma in atopic patients with food allergy has recently been demonstrated (Bengston et al.: cited by Strannegård et al., 1985).

Central to the immunologic and other abnormalities (discussed later) is the T cell defect which to many workers in this field appears to be a primary, inherited feature of atopic disease. In the context of the T cell, therefore, it is important to focus our interest on the gene products, primarily enzymes, that affect T cell maturation or function in atopic dermatitis. For the first time in 1982, it has been reported that the activity of lymphocytic cyclic AMP-phosphodiesterase (that is the enzyme that destroys cyclic AMP) is increased in atopic dermatitis as well as allergic respiratory disease of adults (Grewe et al., 1982), and that this increased activity correlated closely with histamine release from basophils (Butler et al., 1983). When the same enzymatic activity together with histamine release was investigated in the newborn using umbilical cord blood, the significant elevation of phosphodiesterase activity was reconfirmed in newborns with a positive atopic history in first degree relatives, compared to newborns with a negative history. In contrast to adults, however, there was no correlation between phosphodiesterase activity and histamine release (McMillan et al., 1985). Elevation of cyclic AMP phosphodiesterase activity in cord blood leukocytes before the development of clinical manifestations of atopy strongly suggests that increased cyclic AMP phosphodiesterase activity plays a primary role in the pathogenesis of atopic disease. The lack of correlation between phosphodiesterase activity and histamine release in neonates further suggests that elevated cyclic AMP phosphodiesterase activity is a primary, genetically linked defect rather than secondary to in vivo desensitization by inflammatory mediators such as histamine and prostaglandin E_1 (Safco et al., 1981).

These considerations complete the full circle of the core argument of this chapter and guide us back to the primary nature of the constitutional basis of respiratory and cutaneous atopic disease. Following the publication of the original beta adrenergic theory (Szentivanyi, 1968), a series of experiments have been carried out to examine the applicability of this theory to atopic dermatitis. Studies of peripheral blood leukocytes and lymphocytes in atopic dermatitis have frequently demonstrated impaired beta adrenergic reactivity as revealed by a loss of regulatory effects on lysosomal enzyme secretion (Busse and Lee, 1976; Reed et al., 1976), by reduced formation of cyclic AMP to beta adrenergic stimulation (Parker and Eisen, 1972; Reed et al., 1976; Parker et al., 1977), by decreased affinity of binding for radio-labeled beta-adrenoceptor agonists (Pochet et al., 1980), and by a shift in the numbers of beta adrenergic receptors to alpha adrenergic receptors resulting in an increased ratio of alpha to beta binding sites (Szentivanyi et al.,, 1980; Szentivanyi and Szentivanyi, 1983). More recently, an extensive effort has been made by Hanifin and his group to determine the lymphocyte and monocyte localization of altered adrenergic receptors, cyclic AMP responses, and cyclic AMP phosphodiesterase in atopic dermatitis (Cooper et al., 1981, 1982, and 1985; Holden et al., 1984, 1985; Giustina et al, 1984).

In these experiments, the numbers and affinities of beta adrenergic surface receptors on mononuclear leukocyte subpopulations were measured by the binding of propranolol-displaceable [^{3}H] dihydroalprenolol to cell surfaces. Unfractionated atopic mononuclear-leukocytes showed reduced numbers of beta adrenergic receptors per cell together with the absence of a normal, lower affinity subpopulation of high affinity beta receptors, resulting in a linear Scatchard plot of beta adrenergic binding to mononuclear-leukocytes from atopic patients, instead of the biphasic plot seen in normal control cells. These alterations of surface receptors for cyclic AMP-elevating ligands were localized to T cells and monocytes of patients with atopic dermatitis, whereas atopic B-cell receptor numbers and affinities were identical to those of normal B-cells (Cooper et al., 1981 and 1982). Of the various subpopulations of T-cells, a lymphocyte subset which is activatable by self Ia-bearing antigen presenting monocytic cells, has been identified as a radiosensitive (functionally dependent upon a proliferative step) OKT4$^+$, T29$^+$ helper/inducer T cell (Rheinherz et al., 1981; Uchiyama et al., 1981; Leung et al., 1983). A primary abnormality in the numbers and/or in the intracellular regulation of the cyclic AMP system of the radiosensitive, T29$^+$, helper/inducer T-cells generated by the interaction with autologus Ia$^+$ antigen presenting macrophages may explain many of the characteristic features of immune dysfunction in atopic dermatitis (Cooper et al., 1985).

For instance, soluble mitogen-stimulated proliferation is critically dependent on successful macrophage/T-cell interaction, and can be reduced in patients with atopic dermatitis (Lobitz et al., 1972; Elliott and Hanifin, 1979). Development of the pool of blood PWM-recruitable B-cells for in vitro antibody production requires induction by a radiosensitive T-cell inducer (Rheinherz et al., 1979, 1981; Stevens et al., 1980), and indeed, B-cells from patients with atopic dermatitis demonstrate decreased mitogen-stimulated antibody secretion, even when corrected for number or when normal T-cells are used to provide helper function (Leung et al., 1981). T-cells associated with suppressor and cytotoxic functions, such as T-cells with FcIgG receptors, OKT8 cells and histamine H$_2$-receptor-bearing T-cells often show significantly reduced values in patients with atopic dermatitis (Schuster et al., 1980; Cooper et al., 1983; Leung et al., 1981, 1983; Beer et al., 1982; Kang et al., 1983) which is in accord with findings indicating that the development of mature suppressor and cytotoxic effector T cells requires induction by the aforementioned radiosensitive T-helper cells (Henney and Gillis, 1984; Rheinherz and Schlossman, 1980; Broder et al., 1981). It may be added that development of cytoxic T lymphocytes is known to be dependent upon Ia$^+$ monocyte stimulation of helper T-cell factors such as Interleukin-2 (Henney and Gillis, 1984), and a decrease in the production of Interleukin 2 as well as interferon by these abnormal helper/inducer T-cells, or their altered ability to respond to these signals may explain the reduced natural killer activity in atopic dermatitis (Jensen et al., 1984; Kuscimi et al., 1982). Thus, the aforementioned multiple abnormalities of the cyclic AMP system in the helper/inducer T-cells in question may account for the immune dysfunction in atopic dermatitis. Alternatively, each of the immune abnormalities listed could be due to altered immune signal processing by distal effector cells with their own malfunctioning intracellular cyclic AMP systems as will be further pointed out below.

In closing the discussion of viral infection as one of the major developmental mechanisms of beta adrenergic subsensitivity in cutaneous atopy, we need to briefly revisit the issue of whether the atopic diathesis increases the susceptibility to viral infections, or the viruses themselves may produce the atopic disposition. As stated above, the demonstration of higher serum levels of antibodies against EBV in atopic dermatitis were interpreted in support of the assumption that defective immune mechanisms rather than cutaneous alterations predispose for increased susceptibility to viral infections. Although the findings of raised EBV antibody titers in atopic dermatitis may in fact reflect on abnormal host response to the virus, it cannot be excluded that the cause and effect relationship is the reverse, so that EBV may play a causative role for the development of atopic dermatitis. Thus, EBV is a B cell mitogen, which may stimulate IgE antibody formation, and infectious mononucleosis, which is caused by EBV, is associated with raised serum levels of IgE (Nordbring et al., 1972). The recent report of a case of atopic dermatitis developing soon after an episode of infectious mononucleosis suggests that EBV may in fact occasionally precipitate atopic disease (Barnetson et al., 1981). Essentially the same causative role of viral agents has been described for respiratory atopy above.

THE ALLERGIC TISSUE INJURY AS A DEVELOPMENTAL MECHANISM OF

BETA ADRENERGIC SUBSENSITIVITY

The allergic tissue injury is another major developmental mechanism of beta adrenergic subsensitivity. Advances in knowledge of the immune response and immune reactivity achieved since the early 1960's have been accompanied by a more complete understanding of the different pathways of immune tissue injury. Based on this new understanding, the various types of immunopathologic processes have been subdivided by the classification by Coombs and Gell (1962) into the following four basic types:

Type I: Immediate hypersensitivities
Type II: Cytotoxic tissue injury
Type III: Immune complex tissue injury
Type IV: Cell-mediated immune tissue injuries

This classification is oversimplified because of the complex interrelationships that exist between the several events that constitute an inflammatory response. Nevertheless, this view represents the closest approximation of the various basic patterns of immune tissue injury, and the classification does not depend on the host species or on the method of antigen exposure. Another valuable feature of the classification is its integrated emphasis on the important central point that in these various patterns of immune injury the tissue damage results from the immune activation of cellular and biochemical mediator systems of the host. The combination of the immune reactants produces only minimal direct effects, but as a trigger mechanism it sets the destructive factors into play.

Because of the subject of this chapter only the general pattern of immunologic tissue injury that occurs in immediate hypersensitivities will be discussed. Furthermore, no distinction will be made between the atopic and nonatopic varieties of immediate hypersensitivities since in both cases the pattern of tissue injury follows the characteristic triphasic reaction sequence of these manifestations.

In these reactivities, following the initiation of antibody production, the cytotropic antibodies (primarily IgE) that are formed disseminate throughout the circulation to become almost selectively and uniquely attached to the cell membranes of basophils in the circulation and mast cells in the tissues. The attachment occurs through a structural area in the Fc part of the antibody molecule to a specific receptor on the basophil or mast cell membrane. Although evidence indicates that subpopulations of monocytes, macrophages, and lymphocytes also express Fc receptors for IgE antibody, of all mammalian cells only basophils and mast cells exhibit an extraordinary binding affinity for this antibody. There is a relative abundance of these IgE molecules bound along the membrane, and they are located close to each other physically. When the IgE becomes attached, the cells are said to be sensitized, and the individual is now in a sensitive state for reactivity on subsequent exposure to the antigen (Szentivanyi and Szentivanyi, 1985b).

A second, or subsequent, exposure can occur via many routes, such as inhalation, ingestion, or injection. The antigen must move across membrane and tissue barriers in order to come to the surface of the sensitized cells. When this close encounter occurs with an antigen of sufficient size to react with the antigen-binding sites of two closely adjacent IgE molecules, it produces a "bridging" effect. In this molecular interaction, one antigen molecule combines with two antibody molecules to form a bridge. This bridging brings together two IgE receptor molecules, which results in distortion of the cell membrane, triggering an enzymatic cascade that causes the release of pharmacologically active effector molecules responsible for the clinical symptomatology of immediate hypersensitivities. Accounting only for those pharmacologic mediators where the cell-type has been identified, the spectrum of mediator-storing, synthesizing, or transporting cells, includes the neutrophil leucocyte [slow-reacting substance of anaphylaxis (SRS-A), eosinophil chemotactic factor of anaphylaxis (ECF-A), enzymes, vascular permeability factors, kinin-generating substances, a complement-activating factor, histamine-releasers, and a neutrophil inhibitory factor (NIF)], basophilic leucocyte [histamine, SRS-A, ECF-A, neutrophil chemotactic factor (NCF) and platelet-activating factor (PAF)], the murine basophilic leucocyte (histamine, SRS-A, ECF-A, PAF, and serotonin), the eosinophilic leucocyte (histamine, PAF, and possibly SRS-A), the mast cell (histamine, SRS-A, ECF-A, NCF and PAF), the murine mast cell (histamine, SRS-A, ECF-A, PAF, NCF and serotonin), the "chromaffin-positive" mast cell (dopamine in ruminants; in other mammals possibly norepinephrine), the enterochromaffin cell (serotonin), the chromaffin cell (catecholamines), the platelet (depending on species: histamine, serotonin, catecholamines, and prostaglandins), the neurosecretory cell (histamine, serotonin, catecholamines, acetylcholine, and prostaglandins), and the nerve cell (potentially all amine-mediators as well as prostaglandins and kinins, Szentivanyi and Szentivanyi, 1985a). Collectively, these pharmacologically active agents produce an increase in blood flow, capillary permeability, constriction of smooth muscles, and secretion of mucous glands, that is manifestations that dominate the clinical picture of immediate hypersensitivities and the associated inflammatory responses.

Reactivities of the Mediator-storing Cells to Antigenic and Pharmacologic Influences and their Relations to Cyclic Nucleotides

Depending on concentrations and other experimental conditions, pharmacologically active adrenergic agents can both release as well as inhibit the release of allergic mediators. Thus, amphetamine, phenylethylamine, tyramine, and the like--substances that induce sympathomimetic activity indirectly through the endogenous release of catecholamines--are capable of liberating histamine. The same can be accomplished by the exogenous administration of catecholamines and of their specific blocking agents. While nonimmunologic histamine release is elicited by all these agents, they render sensitized mast cells incapable of responding to antigen challenge with histamine release (Schild, 1936; Tabachnick et al., 1965; Lichtenstein and Margolis, 1968).

Analysis of these seemingly contradictory findings suggests that 1) adrenergic agents interfere with binding or release of histamine because of their catecholamine-like intrinsic activity, and 2) they operate on a cellular system that is antigen activated and thus central to the mechanism of the allergic reaction.

The first conclusion is supported by the residual agonistic activity of the blocking agents employed, since the only common feature of these directly acting adrenergic compounds is their basic catecholamine structure. The second conclusion is based on the observation that methylxanthines also inhibit immunologic release of histamine (Lichtenstein and Margolis, 1968). Thus, when ragweed antigen was made to interact in vitro with IgE antibody on the surface of leukocytes from ragweed-sensitive human donors, both methylxanthines and catecholamines inhibited histamine release. The significance of these findings is seen in the fact that methylxanthines are competitive inhibitors of the specific phosphodiesterase that inactivates cyclic 3',5'AMP, and thereby they may induce "adrenergic action" by increasing the intracellular concentration of the compound. Indeed, catecholamines and methylxanthines were found to act synergistically in inhibiting histamine release, and the phosphodiesterase-inhibitory potencies of the various methylxanthines correlated well with their inhibitory effects on histamine release (Szentivanyi and Fitzpatrick, 1980). Of further significance is the fact that the methylxanthines and catecholamines were shown to inhibit only if added to the cells when antigen was present; they had no effect if removed from the environment of the sensitized cells before antigen exposure (Lichtenstein and Margolis, 1968). The adenylate cyclase system therefore must be considered as a critical regulatory system in allergic histamine release.

In addition to beta-adrenergic agents, allergic release of histamine or of other pharmacologic mediators of immediate hypersensitivity is also inhibited by prostaglandins of the E series, prostacycline, adenosine, and histamine (i.e., by substances that interact with cell membrane receptors that activate adenylate cyclase)(Bourne et al., 1974; Orange et al., 1971). Inhibition of allergic mediator release by these agents is generally paralleled by an increase in the intracellular concentration of cyclic AMP in the respective cell preparations. Furthermore, since the release-inhibitory activities of these agents are blocked by their specific antagonists, it is presumed that these agents increase cyclic AMP by acting on receptors linked to adenylate cyclase. The mechanism by which cyclic AMP blocks mediator release is not known, but current evidence suggests that cyclic AMP acts early in the release process, that it is linked to the obligatory inward flux of calcium, and that it related to microtubule function (Plaut et al., 1980). There are, however, exceptions when changes in cyclic nucleotide levels do not correlate with inhibition of immunologic mediator release (Marone et al., 1979; Schreurs et al., 1980). The nature of such dissociation between cyclic AMP elevation and inhibition is unclear but may be explained if there are functionally separate intracellular cyclic AMP pools (Szentivanyi and Fishel, 1974) and if a product of the lipoxygenase or some other pathway can block selectively a biochemical sequence linking adenylate cyclase activation to inhibition of mediator release (Plaut et al., 1980).

The effect of changes in intracellular cyclic GMP levels on allergic mediator release has been less extensively studied. In lung tissue, alpha-adrenergic and cholinergic stimulation increase cyclic GMP levels (Krzanowski et al., 1976; Polson et al., 1976), and such effects as well as extracellular cyclic GMP derivatives potentiate antigen-induced mediator release (Kaliner, et al., 1972). However, cyclic GMP does not enhance release from rat mast cells and has minimal or no effect on immunologic mediator release from basophils (Gillespie and Lichtenstein, 1975). Furthermore, it is not known whether cyclic GMP-induced enhancement of pulmonary mediator release is a direct effect of alpha-adrenergic or cholinergic agents on the mast cells or whether it reflects their actions on other cell types (Szentivanyi, 1982). Nevertheless, in this context it may be added that pertussis or pharmacologically established beta-adrenergic blockade has been reported to cause peritoneal mast cell degranulation in rats and mice, whereas beta-adrenergic stimulation protects these cells against propranolol-induced degranulation (Guirgis and Townley, 1976). As judged by the PCA reaction in guinea pigs, propranolol has the same enhancing effect on immunologic mediator release (Nakazawa and Townley, 1976).

The Allergic Tissue Injury, Beta Adrenergic Subsensitivity and Bronchial Asthma

Recent studies in patients with extrinsic asthma (deVries et al., 1982; Koeter et al., 1982) and in animal models of experimental asthma (Barnes et al., 1980; Rinard et al., 1979 and 1983) raised the possibility that the allergic tissue injury itself may result in the development of some forms of beta-adrenergic subsensitivity. In the studies of deVries et al. (1982), and Koeter et al. (1982), patients with complaints of episodic wheezing after exposure to allergens, specific IgE and skin tests, and an increased bronchial response to histamine inhalation were included. Symptoms of these seven patients were mild and well controlled without a history of respiratory tract infections or acute asthmatic attacks two months prior to the study. No patient was on beta-adrenergic or corticosteroid therapy.

These studies were designed with the assumption that there might be a relationship between the allergic tissue injury and the adrenergic system. Therefore, the latter was studied before and after an inhalational allergen challenge. Two parameters were measured: 1) in vivo propranolol threshold to assess bronchial beta adrenergic reactivities; and 2) in vitro lymphocytic cAMP production in response to beta-agonist stimulation. The propranolol threshold changed from 1.32 percent before challenge to 0.86 percent the day after. In the same patients the maximal cAMP response of lymphocytes changed from 339 percent above basal level before the challenge to 194 percent after the challenge.

Recently, the development of beta subsensitivity of airways smooth muscle was studied in greyhound dogs in order to determine its relationship to the hyperreactivity of the same airways to aerosols of Ascaris suum antigen (Rinard et al., 1979 and 1983). Using thoracic trachealis smooth muscle, it was found that the airways hyperreactivity was statistically significantly inversely correlated with 1) beta-adrenoceptor density; 2) isoproterenol-stimulated cAMP production; and 3) isoproterenol-stimulated relaxation. These authors concluded that the beta-adrenergic subsensitivity of airway smooth muscle that is associated with airways hyperreactivity in this canine asthma model is due to a deficiency of beta-adrenoceptors, since all postreceptor beta adrenergic responses that were measured (cAMP, protein kinase, relaxation) tended to be depressed in animals with airways hyperreactivity.

These studies clearly indicate that the allergic tissue injury may be one of the contributory factors in the development of beta-adrenergic subsensitivity in some forms of human asthma, or alternatively the sole factor in some subsets of human asthma. They may not, however, support the interpretations of deVries (1982) and Koeter et al. (1982) that these findings suggest that 1) in the seven asthmatics they studied the beta-adrenergic subsensitivity was due to endogenous desensitization by catecholamines released in response to the allergic tissue injury; and 2) in all forms of asthma, this same mechanism is responsible for the manifestation of beta-adrenergic subsensitivity.

Several lines of evidence argue against the general applicability of these interpretations to human asthma and other manifestations of atopy.

First of all endogenous catecholamines released from neuronal and adrenal medullary catechol stores would be expected to desensitize both alpha- and beta-adrenoceptors more or less evenly. In the foregoing studies alpha-adrenoceptor concentrations or their sensitivities were not measured, but in those studies where they were, this was not the case. Thus, pulmonary homogenates of sensitized guinea pigs that had been exposed chronically to antigen aerosol showed significant increase in alpha-adrenoceptors and a decrease in beta-adrenoceptors (Barnes et al., 1980) reminiscent of the reciprocal adenoceptor changes observed in a number of other human and animal studies described in the literature (Kunos and Szentivanyi, 1968; Szentivanyi et al., 1970; Szentivanyi and Pek, 1973; Ahlquist, 1977; Nickerson and Kunos, 1977; Kunos, 1978 and 1980; Sharma and Banerjee, 1978; Popovich et al, 1979; Szentivanyi, 1979a, 1979b; Szentivanyi, 1980; Szentivanyi et al, 1979 and 1980). This alpha dominance is also reflected by the demonstration that alpha-adrenergic agonists produce bronchoconstriction in asthmatic patients but not in normal subjects (Anthracite et al., 1977; Snashall et al., 1978). Similarly, in vitro studies show alpha-receptor mediated constriction of bronchial smooth muscle from patients with increased airways resistance but not from normal controls (Kneussl and Richardson, 1978; Simonsson, 1972). In addition, increased alpha-adrenergic receptor mediated responses in vascular and pupillary smooth muscle have been reported in asthmatics (Henderson, 1970).

Furthermore, beta-adrenergic subsensitivity in asthma can be shown to occur in the absence of allergic symptoms or beta adrenergic medication, and under circumstances in which prior or concurrent beta adrenergic medication can be only one contributing factor to defective beta adrenergic function. This is also reflected by the presence of beta adrenergic subsensitivity in atopic dermatitis in which beta adrenergic medication is not used as a therapeutic modality. Nevertheless, endogenous release of catecholamines in response to the allergic tissue injury may contribute to the development of beta-adrenergic subsensitivity through homologous desensitization of the beta adrenergic receptors. At the same time the endogenous release of other pharmacologic mediators (i.e., histamine) in response to the allergic tissue injury may contribute to the beta adrenergic subsensitivity through heterologous desensitization (Szentivanyi et al., 1985). The differences between these two mechanisms are explained below.

The Allergic Tissue Injury, Beta Adrenergic Subsensitivity, and Atopic Dermatitis

Differences between homologous and heterologous desensitization resulting in beta-adrenergic subsensitivity could be most conveniently explained through the model of DeLean and associates (1980) originally used for the interpretation of adrenoceptor-adenylate cyclase interactions and based to a large extent on ligand binding experiments. This model envisions three principal components of the system in the plasma membrane, i.e., the receptor (R), a nucleotide-binding regulatory protein (N), and adenylate cyclase (C). The binding of an agonist (A) to the receptor is believed to bring about a change that either promotes or stabilizes the formation of a ternary complex, ARN (Figure 13-1 in Szentivanyi, Polson, and Szentivanyi, 1985). The formation of the complex promotes the dislodging of a tightly bound guanosine diphosphage (GDP) molecule from N and its replacement with guanosine triphosphate (GTP), which enables N to activate C, thus stimulating the formation of cAMP. The GTP is subsequently hydrolyzed to GDP by guanosine triphospatase (GTPase) associated with N, and this leads to inactivation of the cyclase. All three components of the system are then capable of being reactivated by renewed interactions of R with agonist molecules. The formation of the ternary complex ARN is of crucial importance to the functional coupling of the receptor to the cyclase in this hypothetical model. Antagonists occupy the receptor but do not promote or stabilize the formation of the ternary complex and thus do not activate the catalytic moiety of adenylase cyclase. Biochemical experiments indicate that the free form of the receptor (R) has a low affinity for agonists, while the complex of the receptor plus the nucleotide protein (RN) has a high affinity for agonists. Changes in receptor binding properties showing a lack of high affinity of R for agonists are thus believed to indicate that the crucial ARN complex is not formed. Not surprisingly, there is no activation of the cyclase under these circumstances. This phenomenon resulting in the inability of agonist-stimulated beta-receptors to activate adenylate cyclase is referred to as uncoupling. As discussed below, uncoupling is one of the mechanisms by which agonist-induced desensitization of beta-adrenergic receptors takes place (Davies and Lefkowitz, 1981).

The loss of a tissue's responsiveness to an agonist caused by repeated exposure to the agonist has been described using a variety of terms including desensitization, tolerance, refractoriness, and tachyphylaxis. Su and colleagues (1976) have divided these phenomena into two major categories, heterologous and homologous desensitization. Heterologous desensitization refers to the desensitization that occurs after exposure of cells to a biologically active agent that produces tissue refractoriness to itself and to a variety of other pharmacologically different agonists. By contrast, homologous or agonist-specific desensitization is a loss of responsiveness to only the particular agonist that induced the desensitization (or to a specific group of pharmacologically related agonists, all acting at the same tissue receptor site, e.g., the catecholamines).

The mechanisms by which desensitization is produced are complex and variable depending on the tissue. Isoproterenol-induced desensitization of turkey erythrocytes appears to fall into the category of heterologous desensitization because loss of sensitivity to fluoride ion and 5'guanylylimidodiphosphate* (Gpp(NH)p) (a less hydrolyzable analog that can substitute for GTP) is also produced in this situation. There is no decrease in receptor number in the isoproterenol-desensitized turkey erythrocyte, but rather an apparent uncoupling of the beta-adrenergic receptor from adenylate cyclase takes place due to impairment of the ability of occupied receptors to form a stable high-affinity ARN complex (Stadel et al., 1981). Similar refractoriness can be produced by exposure of the cells to 8-bromo-adenosine 3',5'-cyclic monophosphate, a cAMP analog, suggesting that the desensitization to isoproterenol is caused by the agonist-stimulated levels of cAMP within cells. Stadel and coworkers (1981) suggested that cAMP-dependent phosphorylation of the nucleotide regulatory protein (N) may be the mechanism of desensitization in this system, and thus no alteration in the receptor per se but rather uncoupling of the receptor from adenylate cyclase due to modification of the nucleotide regulatory protein takes place in this example of heterologous desensitization.

Homologous desensitization of beta-receptors has been observed in a number of different types of cells including frog erythrocytes and astrocytoma cells and is produced by agonists but is blocked by antagonists (Hoffman and Lefkowitz, 1980). Experiments on astrocytoma cells have shown that beta-adrenoceptor desensitization produced by isoproterenol involves at least two steps. The earliest change to occur is uncoupling of the receptor from the cyclase, followed by the second step which involves a loss of 80 to 95 percent of the assayable beta-receptors on the cell surface (Su et al., 1980). More recent studies on catecholamine-desensitized frog erythrocytes have shown that the down-regulated (unavailable) beta-receptors are sequestered in cytosolic vesicles apart from the guanine regulatory protein and catalytic moiety of the adenylate cyclase which remain in the plasma

---

*5'Guanylylimidodiphosphate is an analog of GTP that contains an imidodiphosphate rather than a pyrophosphate linkage.

membrane (Stadel et al., 1983). The sequestered receptors appear not to be rapidly degraded and, therefore, may be recycled later during recovery of the tissue from desensitization (Doss et al., 1981; Stadel et al., 1983). Human neutrophils have been found to undergo desensitization involving both an uncoupling, which is highly analogous to that demonstrated in frog erythrocytes, and also a 40 percent reduction in number of receptors (Davies and Lefkowitz, 1983).

Drawing on the information available at the present time, one might formulate the following view: heterologous desensitization of beta-adrenoceptors involves uncoupling due to impairment of the ability of receptors to form the high-affinity ARN complex and consequently to activate adenylate cyclase; this impairment is produced by the agonist-stimulated accumulation of cAMP within cells. By contrast, homologous regulation is a multistep process involving early uncoupling of the receptor from the cyclase followed by later internalization of the uncoupled receptors in vesicles.

With this understanding we can return to the foregoing section on the reactivities of the mediator-storing cells to antigenic and pharmacologic influences and their relations to cyclic nucleotides. As stated earlier, in addition to beta adrenergic agents, allergic release of histamine or of many, if not most of other pharmacologic mediators of immediate hypersensitivities, is also inhibited by prostaglandins of the E series, prostacycline, adenosine, and histamine (i.e., by substances that interact with cell membrane receptors that activate adenylate cyclase). Normal physiologic inhibition of allergic mediator release by these agents is kept in check by their feedback effect on their respective receptors through the mechanisms of homologous and heterologous desensitization. In atopic disease, however, where there are multiple abnormalities in the receptor-adenylate cyclase- and cyclic AMP systems, this physiologic balance between inhibition versus enhancement of mediator release would be expected to lead to an exaggerated release reaction to the allergic tissue injury.

Indeed, enhanced "releasability" of histamine from basophils and mast cells has been shown to occur in atopic dermatitis. "Releasability" is defined in this context as the capacity of mediator secreting cells to release preformed or newly synthesized mediators (Conroy et al., 1977; Lichtenstein et al., 1983; Ring, 1984). Among the pharmacologic mediators, histamine is the best studied substance, and the best established mechanism is the IgE-mediated release reaction. The first study to show enhanced anti-IgE induced histamine releasability from basophils was performed by Lebel et al. (1960) which was confirmed by Ring and his associates (1980). During the last few years numerous, more extensive investigations have been carried out that further confirmed the de facto existence of altered releasability in atopic dermatitis (Ring and Dorsch, 1985; McMillan et al., 1985; Butler et al., 1983 and 1985). Similarly, increased releasability of histamine was also found to occur in bronchial asthma (Findlay and Lichtenstein, 1978; Assem and Attallah, 1981).

In a way, in vitro IgE-secretion by peripheral lymphocytes might also be viewed as a form of "releasability" too. Therefore, it is important to mention that several authors have provided evidence of increased spontaneous in vitro IgE-secretion in patients with atopic dermatitis (Fisher and Buckley, 1979; Ishizaka, 1983; Ring and Senner, 1983). A significant positive correlation between serum IgE and in vitro IgE secretion has also been demonstrated (Ring and Dorsch, 1985). In this connection, it should be noted that although much is known about IgE regulation in rodents (Ishizaka, 1983), the mechanisms involved in the regulation of IgE-synthesis in man are not well established. It is generally assumed that isotype specific suppressor and helper T-cells play an important role, but the relevant subpopulation (perhaps FcE-receptor bearing lymphocytes, Spiegelberg, 1983), is not known

at present. Furthermore, the exact pathogenetic role of IgE-reactions is
atopic dermatitis is still controversial (Hanifin, 1983; Rajka, 1980;
Wutrich, 1975).

AUTOIMMUNITY AS A DEVELOPMENTAL MECHANISM OF BETA-ADRENERGIC SUBSENSITIVITY

The concept that an autoantibody interacting with a cell membrane receptor of a hormone or neurotransmitter could cause functional derangements
and subsequent disease is now becoming widely accepted, and the number of
diseases that may be mediated by antireceptor antibodies is rapidly growing
(Rose, 1978; Svejga-Ard et al., 1978).

The leading examples of such diseases include myasthenia gravis, involving autoantibodies directed at nicotinic acetylcholine receptors at the
neuromuscular end-plates (Abramsky et al., 1975; Drachman et al., 1978;
Lindstrom et al., 1976), Graves' disease involving autoantibodies to the
thyrotropin receptor (Manley et al., 1974; Smith and Hall, 1974), and the
severe insulin resistance in Type B insulin-resistant diabetes that has
been ascribed to autoantibodies to the insulin receptor (Flier et al., 1975;
Harrison et al., 1978; Kahn et al., 1976).

Thus, the foregoing diseases may be viewed as receptor diseases, and
some subsets of asthma and other atopic diseases may ultimately be recognized
as legitimate members of this group. Indeed, it has been recently described
that autoantibodies to $beta_2$ adrenoceptors can be identified in the plasma
of some subjects with atopic allergy (Fraser et al., 1981; Kaliner et al.,
1982; Venter et al., 1980). Although these antibodies appear to be heterogeneous, they share the ability to affect binding of I^{125} protein A to calf
lung membranes, to inhibit stereospecific beta-adrenergic radioligand binding
to calf lung $beta_2$ adrenoceptors, and to precipitate solubilized calf lung
beta-adrenergic receptors in an indirect immunoprecipitation assay. Furthermore, the presence of autoantibodies to $beta_2$ adrenoceptors in these subjects
correlates well with a reduced $beta_2$- and an increased alpha-adrenergic
responsiveness. It may be added that from the currently available material
even the three of the 19 apparently normal subjects with circulating antibodies were significantly less responsive to beta-adrenergic stimulation
than the remainder of the normal controls (Halonen and Kaliner, 1983).

The precise frequency and distribution of these autoantibodies in various subsets of patients with asthma and other atopic disease are currently
under investigation in several American and European laboratories, as is
the molecular mechanism by which they produce beta-adrenergic subsensitivi-
ties. For a general account of the molecular mechanisms that are involved
in the development of autoimmunities in general, the reader is referred to
a most recent analysis by Szentivanyi and Szentivanyi (1985b). In the orientation of this chapter, however, we shall only mention the role of virus
infections as a developmental mechanism of autoimmunity produced by anti-
receptor antibodies specifically directed to $beta_2$ adrenoceptors. Thus,
virus infections can elicit autoantibody formation by two mechanisms. First,
the viral antigens and autoantigens may become associated to form immunogenic
units. Viral antigens stimulating host T-lymphocytes could then function
as helper determinants, thereby stimulating B-lymphocyte responses to autoantigens. Second, some viruses such as the Epstein-Barr virus (EBV) stimulate proliferation of the B-lymphocyte cell line with autoantibody production.
There are two ways in which viral and host antigens can form immunogenic
units. Host antigens can be incorporated in the envelopes of some viruses,
and viral antigens can appear on the surfaces of infected host cells (Figures
5-9 in Szentivanyi and Szentivanyi, 1985b). The viral antigens also may
form complexes with and modify histocompatibility antigens or other membrane
constituents such as the contractile protein, actin. The modified viral

antigens could stimulate T-cell helper effect and elicit autoantibody formation (Figures 5-10 in Szentivanyi and Szentivanyi, 1985b).

In humans, infection with viruses such as influenza, measles, varicella, and herpes simplex has often resulted in autoimmune manifestations such as platelet and red cell autoantibodies. The development of cold autoagglutinins after Mycoplasma pneumoniae infection probably occurs by a T-cell bypass mechanism. Following infectious mononucleosis, many patients' sera often react against several autoantigens. These include autoantibodies against nuclei, lymphocytes, erythrocytes, and smooth muscle. In addition, cross-reactive heterophile antibodies may be noted following infectious mononucleosis and other infections. The autoantibody is produced by a mechanism similar to that observed in altered self component with virus or bacteria.

There has been much speculation about the possible involvement of an oncornavirus in the pathogenesis of human systemic lupus erythematosus (Theofilopoulos, 1984).

REFERENCES

1. O. Abramsky, A. Aharonov, C. Webb, and S. Fuchs, Cellular immune response to acetylcholine receptor-rich fraction in patients with myasthenia gravis, Clin. Exp. Immunol. 19:11 (1975).
2. R. P. Ahlquist, Adrenoceptor sensitivity in disease as assessed through response to temperature alteration, Fed. Proc. 36:2572 (1977).
3. W. C. Alston, K. R. Patel and J. W. Kerr, Response of leukocyte adenyl cyclase to isoprenaline and effect of alpha-blocking drugs in extrinsic bronchial asthma, Br. Med. J. 1:90 (1974).
4. R. E. C. Altounyan, Variation of drug action on airway obstruction in man, Thorax 19:406 (1964).
5. R. F. Anthracite, L. Vachon, and P. H. Knapp, Alpha-adrenergic receptors in the human lung, Psychosom. Med. 33:481 (1977).
6. E.S.K. Assem and N. A. Altallah, Increased release of histamine by anti-IgE from leucocytes of asthmatic patients and possible heterogenicity, Clin. Allergy 11:367 (1981).
7. J. Bandouvakis, A. Cartier, R. Roberts, G. Ryan, and F. E. Hargreave, The effect of ipratropium and fenoterol on methacholine- and histamine-induced bronchoconstriction, Br. J. Dis. Chest. 75:295 (1981).
8. P. J. Barnes, C. T. Dollery, and J. MacDermot, Increased pulmonary alpha-adrenergic and reduced beta-adrenergic receptors in experimental asthma, Nature 285:569 (1980).
9. R. Barnetson, R. A. Hardie, and T. G. Merret, Late onset atopic eczema and multiple food allergies after infectious mononucleosis, Br. Med. J. 283:1086 (1981).
10. D. J. Beer, M. E. Osband, R. P. McCaffrey, et al., Abnormal histamine induced suppressor cell function in atopic individuals, N. Eng. J. Med. 306:454 (1982).
11. E. Bonifazi, L. Garofalo, V. Pisani, and C. L. Meneghini, Role of some infectious agents in atopic dermatitis, Acta. Derm. Venereol. (Stockh.) Suppl. 114:98 (1985).
12. L.-P. Boulet, K. M. Latimer, R. S. Roberts, E. F. Juniper, D. W. Cockroft, N. C. Thomson, E. Daniels, and F. E. Hargreave, The effect of atropine on allergen-induced increases in bronchial responsiveness to histamine, Am. Rev. Respir. Dis. 130:368 (1984).
13. H. R. Bourne, L. M. Lichtenstein, K. L. Melmon et al., Modulation of inflammation and immunity by cyclic AMP, Science 184:19 (1974).
14. S. Broder, T. T. Uchiyama, L. Muul, C. Goldman, S. Sharrow, D.

Poplack, and T., Waldman, Activation of leukemic pre-suppressor cells to become suppressor effector cells, $\underline{N}$. $\underline{Eng}$. $\underline{J}$. $\underline{Med}$. 304:1382 (1981).

15. C. K. Buckner, D. E. Clayton, A. A. Ain-Shoka, et al., Parainfluenza 3 infection blocks the ability of a beta-adrenergic receptor agonist to inhibit antigen induced contraction of guinea pig isolated airway smooth muscle, $\underline{J}$. $\underline{Clin}$. $\underline{Invest}$. 67:376 (1981).

16. R. K. Bush, W. W. Busse, D. K. Flaherty, D. Warshaver, E. C. Dick, and C. E. Reed, Effects of experimental rhinovirus 16 infection on airways and leukocyte function in normal subjects, $\underline{J}$. $\underline{Allergy}$ $\underline{Clin}$. $\underline{Immunol}$. 61:80 (1978).

17. W. W. Busse, Decreased granulocyte response to isoproterenol in asthma during upper respiratory infections, $\underline{Am}$. $\underline{Rev}$. $\underline{Respir}$. $\underline{Dis}$. 115:783 (1977).

18. W. W. Busse and T. P. Lee, Decreased adrenergic responses in lymphocytes and granulocytes in atopic eczema, $\underline{J}$. $\underline{Allergy}$ $\underline{Clin}$. $\underline{Immunol}$. 58:586 (1976).

19. W. W. Busse, W. Cooper, D. M. Warshaver, E. C. Dick, I. H. L. Wallow, and R. Albrecht, Impairment of isoproterenol, H_2 histamine, and prostaglandin E_1 response of human granulocytes after incubation in vitro with live influenza vaccines, $\underline{Am}$. $\underline{Rev}$. $\underline{Respir}$. $\underline{Dis}$. 119:561 (1979).

20. W. W. Busse, C. L. Anderson, E. C. Dick, and D. M. Warshaver, Reduced granulocyte response to isoproterenol, histamine and prostaglandin E_1 after in vitro incubation with rhinovirus 16, $\underline{Am}$. $\underline{Rev}$. $\underline{Respir}$. $\underline{Dis}$. 122:641 (1980).

21. J. M. Butler, S. C. Chan, S. R. Stevens, and J. M. Hanifin, Increased leukocyte histamine release with elevated cyclic AMP-phosphodiesterase activity in atopic dermatitis, $\underline{J}$. $\underline{Allergy}$ $\underline{Clin}$. $\underline{Immunol}$. 71:490 (1983).

22. J. M. Butler, M. Ebertz, S. C. Chan, S. R. Stevens, D. Sobieszczuk, and J. M. Hanifin, Basophil histamine release in atopic dermatitis--its relationship to disordered cyclic nucleotide metabolism, $\underline{Acta}$. $\underline{Derm}$. $\underline{Venereol}$. (Stockh.) Suppl. 114:55 (1985).

23. C. L. Casterline, R. Evans, III, and G. W. Ward, Jr., The effect of atropine and albuterol aerosols on the human bronchial response to histamine, $\underline{J}$. $\underline{Allergy}$ $\underline{Clin}$. $\underline{Immunol}$. 58:607 (1976).

24. M. M. W. Chan-Yeung, M. N. Vyas, and S. Grzybowski, Exercise-induced asthma, $\underline{Am}$. $\underline{Rev}$. $\underline{Respir}$. $\underline{Dis}$. 104:915 (1971).

25. M. C. Conroy, N. F. Adkinson, and L. M. Lichtenstein, Measurement of IgE on human basophils: relation to serum IgE and anti-IgE-induced histamine release, $\underline{J}$. $\underline{Immunol}$. 118:1317 (1977).

26. K. D. Cooper, S. C. Chan, and J. M. Hanifin, Differential T and B cell beta adrenergic responsiveness implies alternative regulatory mechanisms in atopy, $\underline{Clin}$. $\underline{Res}$. 29:281A (1981).

27. K. D. Cooper, S. C. Chan, and J. M. Hanifin, Absence of low affinity beta adrenergic receptors in atopic dermatitis and histamine desensitized normal leukocytes, $\underline{Clin}$. $\underline{Res}$. 30:27A (1982).

28. K. D. Cooper, J. A. Kazmierowski, K. D. Wuepper, and J. M. Hanifin, Immunoregulation in atopic dermatitis: functional analysis of T-B cell interactions and the enumeration of Fc receptor bearing T cells, $\underline{J}$. $\underline{Invest}$. $\underline{Dermatol}$. 80:139 (1983).

29. K. D. Cooper, S. C. Chan, and J. M. Hanifin, Lymphocyte and monocyte localization of altered adrenergic receptors, cAMP responses, and cAMP phosphodiesterase in atopic dermatitis. A possible mechanism for abnormal radiosensitive helper T cells in atopic dermatitis, $\underline{Acta}$. $\underline{Derm}$. $\underline{Venereol}$. (Stockh.) Suppl. 114:41 (1985).

30. A. O. Davies and R. J. Lefkowitz, Agonist-promoted high affinity state of the beta-adrenergic receptor in human neutrophils: modulation by corticosteroids, $\underline{J}$. $\underline{Clin}$. $\underline{Endocrinol}$. $\underline{Metabol}$. 53:703 (1981).

31. A. O. Davies and R. J. Lefkowitz, In vitro desensitization of beta

adrenergic receptors in human neutrophils: attenuation by
corticosteroids, J. Clin. Invest. 71:565 (1983).

32. E. C. Deal, Jr., E. R. McFadden, Jr., R. H. Ingram, Jr., and J. J.
Jaeger, Effects of atropine on potentiation of exercise-induced
bronchospasm by cold air, J. Appl. Physiol. 45:238 (1978).

33. A. DeLean, J. M. Stadel, and R. J. Lefkowitz, A ternary complex model
explains the agonist-specific binding properties of the adenylate
cyclase-coupled beta-adrenergic receptor, J. Biol. Chem. 255:7108
(1980).

34. K. deVries, G. H. Koeter, and J. D. M. Gokemeyer, Some aspects of the
regulation of the bronchial tree in obstructive lung disease, Eur.
J. Respir. Dis. 63(Supp. 121):60 (1982).

35. R. C. Doss, J. P. Perkins, and T. K. Harden, Recovery of beta-adrenergic receptors following long-term exposure of astrocytoma cells to
catecholamine: role of protein synthesis, J. Biol. Chem. 256:12281
(1981).

36. J. S. Douglas, M. W. Dennia, P. Ridgway, and A. Bouhuys, Airway
constriction in guinea pigs: interactions of histamine and
autonomic drugs, J. Pharmacol. Exp. Ther. 184:169 (1973).

37. J. S. Douglas, C. Brink, and A. Bouhuys, Actions of histamine and
other drugs on guinea pig airway smooth muscle, in: "Lung Cells in
Disease," A. Bouhuys, ed., Elsevier/North Holland Biomedical Press,
Amsterdam (1976).

38. D. B. Drachman, C. W. Angus, R. N. Adams, J. D. Michelson, and G. J.
Hoffman, Myasthenic antibodies cross-link acetylcholine receptors
to accelerate degradation, N. Eng. J. Med. 298:1116 (1978).

39. S. T. Elliott, and J. M. Hanifin, Lymphocyte response to phytohemagglutinin in atopic dermatitis, Arch. Dermatol. 115:1424 (1979).

40. D. W. Empey, L. A. Laitinen, L. Jacobs et al., Mechanisms of bronchial
hyperreactivity in normal subjects after upper respiratory tract
infection, Am. Rev. Respir. Dis. 113:131 (1976).

41. S. R. Findlay and L. M. Lichtenstein, Basophil "releasibility" in
patients with intrinsic asthma, J. Allergy Clin. Immunol. 61:157
(1978).

42. P. M. Fiser and R. H. Buckley, Human IgE biosynthesis; in vitro
studies with atopic and normal blood mononuclear cells and
subpopulations, J. Immunol. 122:1799 (1979)

43. J. E. Fish, R. R. Rosenthal, W. R. Summer, H. Menkes, P. S. Norman,
and S. Permutt, The effect of atropine on acute antigen-mediated
airway constriction in subjects with allergic asthma, Am. Rev.
Respir. Dis. 115:371 (1977).

44. J. S. Flier, C. R. Kahn, J. Roth, and R. S. Bar, Antibodies that
impair insulin receptor binding in an unusual diabetic syndrome
with severe insulin resistance, Science 190:63 (1975).

45. J. Fraser, J. Nadeau, D. Robertson, and A. J. J. Wood, Regulation of
human leukocyte beta receptors by endogenous catecholamines:
relationship of leukocyte beta receptor density to the cardiac
sensitivity to isoproterenol, J. Clin. Invest. 67:1777 (1981).

46. O. L. Frick, D. F. German, and J. Mills, Development of allergy in
children. I. Association with virus infections, J. Allergy Clin.
Immunol. 63:228 (1979).

47. P. G. H. Gell and R. R. A. Coombs, "Clinical Aspects of Immunology,"
F. A. Davis Company, Philadelphia (1963).

48. E. Gillespie and L. M. Lichtenstein, Histamine release from human
leukocytes: relationships between cyclic nucleotide, calcium, and
antigen concentrations, J. Immunol. 115:1572 (1975).

49. T. A. Giustina, S. C. Chan, M. L. Thiel, J. W. Baker, and J. M.
Hanifin, Increased leukocyte sensitivity to PDE inhibitors in
atopic dermatitis: tachyphylaxis after theophylline therapy, J.
Allergy Clin. Immunol. 74:252 (1984).

50. S. Grewe, S. Chan, and J. M. Hanifin, Elevated leukocyte cyclic AMP

phosphodiesterase in atopic disease: a possible mechanism for cAMP agonist hyporesponsiveness, J. Allergy Clin. Immunol. 70:452 (1982).

51. H. M. Guirgis and R. G. Townley, The effect of pertussis and beta adrenergic blocking agent on mast cells, J. Allergy Clin. Immunol. 58:241 (1976).

52. A. M. Haddock, K. R. Patel, W. C. Alston and J. W. Kerr, Response of lymphocyte guanyl cyclase to propranolol, noradrenaline, thymoxamine, and acetylcholine in extrinsic bronchial asthma, Br. Med. J. 2:357 (1975).

53. W. J. Hall and C. B. Hall, Bacterial and viral infections in etiology and therapy, in: "Bronchial Asthma: Mechanisms and Therapeutics," Second Edition, E. B. Weiss, M. Segal, and M. Stein, eds., Little, Brown and Company, Boston and Toronto (1985).

54. W. J. Hall, R. G. Douglas, Jr., R. W. Hyde, F. K. Roth, A. S. Cross, and D. M. Speers, Pulmonary mechanics after uncomplicated influenza A infection, Amer. Rev. Respir. Dis. 113:141 (1976).

55. M. Halonen and M. Kaliner, Determinants of autonomic abnormalities in atopy, in: "Proceedings of Invited Symposia XI International Congress on Allergy and Immunology," J. W. Kerr and M. A. Ganderton, eds., MacMillan Press, New York (1983).

56. J. M. Hanifin, Clinical and basic aspects of atopic dermatitis, Semin. Dermatol. 2:5 (1983).

57. L. E. Harrison, J. S. Flier, C. R. Kahn, D. B. Jarrett, M. Muggeo, and J. Roth, in: "Genetic Control of Autoimmune Disease," N. R. Rose, P. E. Bigazzi and N. L. Warner, eds., North Holland Biomedical Press, New York (1978).

58. W. R. Henderson, J. H. Shelhamer, D. B. Reingold, L. J. Smith, R. Evans, and M. Kaliner, Alpha adrenergic hyperreactivity in asthma. Analysis of vascular and pupillary responses, N. Eng. J. Med. 300:642 (1970).

59. C. S. Henney and S. Gillis, Cell mediated cytotoxicity, in: "Fundamental Immunology," W. Paul, ed., Raven Press, New York (1984).

60. P. M. Henson, The immunologic release of constituents from neutrophil leukocytes. I. The role of antibody and complement on nonphagocy-tosable surfaces or phagocytosable particles, J. Immunol. 107:1525 (1971).

61. J. V. Hirschman and E. D. Everett, Haemophilus influenze infections in adults: report of nine cases and a review of the literature, Medicine 58:80 (1979).

62. B. B. Hoffmann and R. J. Lefkowitz, Radioligand binding studies of adrenergic receptors: new insights into molecular and physiological regulation, Ann. Rev. Pharmacol. Toxicol. 20:581 (1980).

63. C. A. Holden, D. R. Austen, S. C. Chan, and J. M. Hanifin, Defective cyclic nucleotide metabolism in atopic monocytes, Clin. Res. 32:591A (1984).

64. C. A. Holden, S. C. Chan, and J. M. Hanifin, Adenylate cyclase activity in mononuclear leukocytes from patients with atopic dermatitis, Acta. Derm. Venereol. (Stockh.) Suppl. 114:149 (1985).

65. J. A. Holgate and B. T. Warner, Evaluation of antagonists of histamine, 5-hydroxytryptamine, and acetylcholine in the guinea pig, Br. J. Pharmacol. 15:561 (1960).

66. S. Ida, Enhancement of IgE mediated histamine release from human basophils by viruses: role of interferon, J. Exp. Med. 145:892 (1977).

67. L. J. Ignarro, and C. Colombo, C., Enzyme release from polymorpho-nuclear leukocyte lysosomes: regulation by autonomic drugs and cyclic nucleotides, Science 180:1181 (1973).

68. K. Ishizaka, Regulation of IgE response by IgE-binding factors, Monogr. Allergy 18:52 (1983).

69. J. R. Jensen, M. Cramers, and K. Thestrup-Pedersen, Subpopulations of T-lymphocytes and non-specific suppressor cell activity in patients with atopic dermatitis, Clin. Exp. Immunol. 45:118 (1981).

70. J. R. Jensen, T. T. Sard, A. S. Jorgensen, and K. Thestrup-Pedersen, Modulation of natural killer cell activity in patients with atopic dermatitis, J. Invest. Dermatol. 82:30 (1984).

71. C. R. Kahn, G. S. Flier, R. S. Bar, et al., The syndromes of insulin resistance and acanthosis nigricans: insulin-receptor disorders in man, N. Eng. J. Med. 294:739 (1976).

72. M. Kaliner, R. P. Orange, and K. F. Austen, Immunologic release of histamine and slow reacting substance of anaphylaxis from human lung. IV. Enhancement by cholinergic and alpha adrenergic stimulation, J. Exp. Med. 136:556 (1972).

73. M. Kaliner, J. H. Shelhamer, P. B. Davis, L. J. Smith, and J. E. Venter, Autonomic nervous system abnormalities and allergy, Ann. Intern. Med. 96:349 (1982).

74. K. Kang, K. D. Cooper, A. Vanderbark, I. L. Strannegård, O. Strannegård, and J. M. Hanifin, Immunoregulation in atopic dermatitis: T-lymphocyte subsets defined by monoclonal antibodies, Semin. Dermatol. 2:59 (1983).

75. D. H. Katz, The allergic phenotype: manifestation of "allergic breakthrough" and imbalance in normal "damping" of IgE antibody production, Immunol. Rev. 41:77 (1978).

76. M. P. Kneussl and J. B. Richardson, Alpha-adrenergic receptors in human and canine tracheal and bronchial smooth muscle, J. Appl. Physiol. 45:307 (1978).

77. G. H. Koeter, H. Meurs, H. F. Kauffman, and K. deVries, The role of the adrenergic system in allergy and bronchial hyperreactivity, Eur. J. Respir. Dis. 63 (Suppl. 121):72 (1982).

78. K. Kragballe, T. Herlin, and J. R. Jensen, Impaired monocyte cytotoxicity in atopic dermatitis, Arch. Dermatol. Res. 269:21 (1980).

79. N. T. Kuscimi, and J. J. Trentin, Natural cell mediated cytotoxic activity in the peripheral blood of patients with atopic dermatitis, Arch. Dermatol. 118:568 (1982).

80. J. J. Krzanowski and A. Szentivanyi, Invited Editorial: Reflections on some aspects of current research in asthma, J. Allergy Clin. Immunol. 72:433 (1983).

81. J. J. Krzanowski, J. B. Polson, and A. Szentivanyi, Pulmonary patterns of adenosine-3',5'-cyclic monophosphate accumulations in response to adrenergic or histamine stimulation in Bordetella pertussis-sensitized mice, Biochem. Pharmacol. 25:1631 (1976).

82. G. Kunos, Adrenoceptors, Ann. Rev. Pharmacol. 18:291 (1978).

83. G. Kunos, Reciprocal changes in alpha and beta adrenoreceptor reactivity - myth or reality? Trends in Pharmac. Sci. 1:282 (1980).

84. G. Kunos and A. Szentivanyi, Evidence favoring the existence of a single adrenergic receptor, Nature 217:1077 (1968).

85. P. Lang, Z. Goel, and M. H. Grieco, Subsensitivity of T lymphocytes to sympathomimetic and cholinergic stimulation in bronchial asthma, J. Allergy Clin. Immunol. 61:248 (1978).

86. G. Lebel, P. Y. Venencie, J. H. Saurat, C. Soubrane, and J. P. Paupe, Anti-IgE induced histamine release from basophils in children with atopic dermatitis, Acta. Dermato. Venerol. Suppl. 92:57 (1980).

87. T. P. Lee, Virus exposure diminishes beta-adrenergic response in human leukocytes, Res. Comm. Chem. Path. Pharmac. 30:469 (1980).

88. D. Y. M. Leung, A. R. Rhodes, and R. S. Geha, Enumeration of T cell

subsets in atopic dermatitis using monoclonal antibodies, J. Allergy Immunol. 67:450 (1981).

89. D. Y. M. Leung, N. Wood, D. Dubey, A. R. Rhodes, and R. S. Geha, Cellular basis of defective cell mediated lympholysis in atopic dermatitis, J. Immunol. 130:1678 (1983).

90. L. M. Lichtenstein and S. Margolis, Histamine release in vitro: inhibition by catecholamines and methylxanthines, Science 161:902 (1968).

91. L. M. Lichtenstein, R. P. Schleimer, S. P. Peters, A. Kagey-Sobotka, N. F. Adkinson, G. K. Adam, E. S. Schulman, and D. W. MacGlashan, Studies with purified human basophils and mast cells, Monogr. Allergy 18:259 (1983).

92. J. A. Lindstrom, M. E. Seybold, V. A. Lennon, S. Whittingham, and D. D. Duane, Antibody to acetylcholine receptor in myasthenia gravis: prevalence, clinical correlates, and diagnostic value, Neurology 26:1054 (1976).

93. J. W. Little, W. J. Hall, R. G. Douglas, Jr., R. W. Hyde, and D. M. Speers, Amantadine effect on peripheral airways abnormalities in influenza, Ann. Intern. Med. 85:177 (1976).

94. W. C. Lobitz, J. F. Honeyman, and M. W. Winkler, Suppressed cell mediated immunity in two adults with atopic dermatitis, Br. J. Dermatol. 86:317 (1972).

95. P. J. Logsdon, D. V. Carnright, E. Middleton, and R. G. Coffey, The effect of phentolamine on adenylate cyclase and on isoproterenol stimulation in leukocytes from asthmatic and nonasthmatic subjects, J. Allergy Clin. Immunol. 52:148 (1973).

96. S. W. Manley, G. R. Bourke, and R. W. Hawker, The thyrotrophin receptor in guinea pig thyroid homogenate: interaction with the long-acting thyroid stimulator, J. Endocrinol. 61:437 (1974).

97. G. Marone, A. K. Sobotka, and L. M. Lichtenstein, Effects of arachidonic acid and its metabolites on antigen-induced histamine release from human basophils in vitro, J. Immunol. 123:1669 (1979).

98. K. McIntosh, E. F. Ellis, L. S. Hoffman, et al., The association of viral and bacterial respiratory infections with exacerbations of wheezing in young asthmatic children, J. Pediatr. 82:578 (1973).

99. J. C. McMillan, N. S. Heskel, and J. M. Hanifin, Cyclic AMP-phospho-diesterase activity and histamine release in cord blood leukocyte preparations. Acta. Derm. Venereol. (Stockh.) Suppl. 114:24 (1985).

100. M. J. Michelson and A. F. Danilov, Cholinergic transmissions, in: "Fundamentals of Biochemical Pharmacology," Z. M. Bacq, ed., Pergamon Press, Oxford (1971).

101. J. E. Mills, M. Sellick, and J. C. Widdicombe, Epithelial irritant receptors in the lung in breathing, in: "Breathing: Herring-Breuer Centenary Symposium," R. Porter, ed., Churchill Livingstone, London (1970).

102. T. E. Minor, E. C. Dick, J. W. Baker, et al., Rhinoviruses and influenza type A infections as precipitants of asthma, Am. Rev. Respir. Dis. 113:149 (1976).

103. T. E. Minor, E. C. Dick, A. N. DeMeo, et al., Viruses as precipitants of asthmatic attacks in children, J. A. M. A. 227:292 (1974).

104. J. A. Nadel, Pathophysiology of asthma: neural effects on airway smooth muscle, submucosal glands, breathing and cough, Prog. Respir. Res. 14:1 (1980).

105. H. Nakazawa and R. G. Townley, The effects of propranolol on the bronchoconstriction by histamine, acetyl-beta-methylcholine, and anaphylaxis in inbred guinea pigs in vivo, Ann. Allergy 36:77 (1976).

106. M. Nickerson and G. Kunos, Discussion of evidence regarding induced changes in adrenoceptors, Fed. Proc. 36:2580 (1977).

107. F. Nordbring, S. G. O. Johansson, and A. Espmark, Raised serum levels of IgE in infectious mononucleosis, Scand. J. Infect. Dis. 4:119 (1972).

108. A. A. Norris and P. Eyre, Pharmacological abnormality in bronchial asthma and the role of respiratory pathogens, Medical Hypotheses 8:199 (1982).

109. P. M. O'Bryne, N. C. Thomson, M. Morris, R. S. Roberts, E. E. Daniel, and F. E. Hargreave, The protective effect of inhaled chlorpheniramine and atropine on bronchoconstriction stimulated by airway cooling, Am. Rev. Respir. Dis. 128:611 (1983).

110. P. M. O'Bryne, N. C. Thomson, K. M. Latimer, R. S. Roberts, M. M. Morris, E. E. Daniel, and F. E. Hargreave, The effect of inhaled hexamethonium bromide and atropine sulphate on airway responsiveness to histamine, J. Allergy Clin. Immunol. 76:97 (1985).

111. R. P. Orange, W. G. Austen, and K. F. Austen, Immunological release of histamine and slow-reacting substance of anaphylaxis from human lung. I. Modulation by agents influencing cellular levels of cyclic 3',5'-monophosphate, J. Exp. Med. 134:136 (1971).

112. J. J. Ouellette and C. E. Reed, Increased response of asthmatic subjects after influenza vaccine, J. Allergy 38:558 (1965).

113. C. W. Parker and A. Z. Eisen, Altered cyclic AMP metabolism in atopic eczema, Clin. Res. 20:418 (1972).

114. C. W. Parker, S. Kennedy, and A. Z. Eisen, Leukocyte and lymphocyte cyclic AMP response in atopic eczema, J. Invest. Dermatol. 68:302 (1977).

115. M. Plaut, G. Marone, L. L. Thomas, and L. M. Lichtenstein, Cyclic nucleotides in immune responses and allergy, Adv. Cyclic Nucleotide Res. 12:161 (1980).

116. R. Pochet, G. Delepesse, and J. DeMaubeuge, Characterization of beta adrenoreceptors on intact circulating lymphocytes from patients with atopic dermatitis, Acta. Derm. Venereol. (Stockholm) 92:26 (1980).

117. J. B. Polson, J. J. Krzanowski, and A. Szentivanyi, Pulmonary guanosine-3',5'-monophosphate in sensitized mice: accumulations produced by H-1 receptor activation and evidence of altered phosphodiesterase activity, J. Allergy. Clin. Immunol. 57:265 (1976).

118. W. J. Popovich, J. E. Brown, and J. W. Adamson, Modulation of in vitro erythropoiesis. Studies with euthyroid and hypothyroid dogs, J. Clin. Invest. 64:56 (1979).

119. G. Rajka, Itch and IgE in atopic dermatitis, Acta. Derm. Venereol. (Stockholm) 92:38 (1980).

120. C. E. Reed, W. W. Busse, and T.-P. Lee, Adrenergic mechanisms and the adenyl cyclase system in atopic dermatitis, J. Invest. Dermatol. 67:333 (1976).

121. E. L. Rheinherz and S. Schlossman, Regulation of the immune response-inducer and suppressor T lymphocyte subsets in human beings, N. Eng. J. Med. 303:370 (1980).

122. E. L. Rheinherz, P. Kung, G. Goldstein, and S. Schlossman, Further characterization of helper/inducer T cell subsets defined by monoclonal antibody, J. Immunol. 123:2894 (1979)

123. E. L. Rheinherz, C. Morimoto, J. A. Penta, and S. Schlossman, Subpopulations of the T4 positive inducer cell subset in man, J. Immunol. 126:67 (1981).

124. J. B. Richardson, A. DeNotariis, C. C. Ferguson, and R. C. Boucher, Effect of a viral laryngotracheitis on the epithelial barrier of chicken airways, Lab. Invest. 44:144 (1981).

125. G. A. Rinard, A. D. Jensen, A. M. Puckett, T. J. Torphy, K. P. Minneman, and S. E. Mayer, Depressed beta-adrenergic response (cyclic AMP, protein kinase, relaxation) and receptor density in

tracheal smooth muscle of allergic-asthmatic dogs, 5th
International Conference on Cyclic Nucleotides and Protein
Phosphorylation, Milan, Italy (1983).

126. G. A. Rinard, A. R. Rubinfeld, L. L. Burnston, and S. E. Mayer,
Depressed cyclic AMP levels in airway smooth muscle from asthmatic
dogs, Proc. Natl. Acad. Sci. USA 76:1472 (1979).

127. J. Ring, Reaktionsbereitschaft ("Releasability"): Veranderte reaktion-
smuster in der freisetzung vasoaktiver mediatoren. Untersuchungen
am beispiel der histamin-freisetzung aus menschlichen basophilen
leukozyten, Allergologie 7:41 (1984).

128. J. Ring and W. Dorsch, Altered releasability of vasoactive mediator
secreting cells in atopic eczema, Acta. Dermato. Venereol.
(Stockh.) Suppl. 114:9 (1985).

129. J. Ring, and H. Senner, In vitro IgE synthesis in patients with atopic
eczema, Monogr. Allergy 18:242 (1983).

130. J. Ring, D. H. Allen, D. A. Mathison, and H. L. Spiegelberg, In vitro
releasability of histamine and serotonin: studies of atopic
patients, J. Clin. Lab. Immunol. 3:85 (1980).

131. A. C. Roldaan, and N. Masural, Viral respiratory infections in
asthmatic children staying in a mountain resort, Eur. J. Respir.
Dis. 63:140 (1982).

132. N. Rose, The autoimmune diseases, in: "Principles of Immunology," N.
Rose, F. Milgrom and C. Van Oss, eds., MacMillan Publishing
Company, New York (1978).

133. R. R. Rosenthal, P. S. Norman, W. K. Sumner, and S. Permutt, Role
of the parasympathetic system in the antigen-induced bronchospasm,
J. Appl. Physiol. 42:600 (1977).

134. M. J. Safko, S. C. Chan, K. D. Cooper, and J. M. Hanifin, Heterologous
densensitization of leukocytes: a possible mechanism of beta
adrenergic blockade in atopic dermatitis, J. Allergy Clin. Immunol.
68:218 (1981).

135. H. O. Schild, Histamine release and anaphylactic shock in isolated
lungs of guinea pigs, Q. J. Exp. Physiol. 26:165 (1936).

136. A. J. M. Schreurs, G. K. Terpstra, J. A. M. Raaijamkers, and F. P.
Nijkamp, The effects of Haemophilus influenzae vaccination on
anaphylatic mediator release and isoprenaline induced inhibition of
mediator release, Eur. J. Pharmacol. 62:261 (1980).

137. A. J. M. Schreurs, G. K. Terpstra, J. A. M. Raaijmakers, and F. P.
Nijkamp, Effects of vaccination with Haemophilus influenzae on
adrenoceptor function of tracheal and parenchymal strips, J.
Pharmac. Exp. Ther. 215:691 (1980).

138. A. J. M. Schreurs, J. Verhoef and F. P. Nijkamp, Bacterial endotoxins
decrease the number of respiratory beta-adrenergic receptors in
guinea pig lung, Agents Actions 13:449 (1983).

139. D. L. Schuster, D. Pierson, B. Bongiovanni, and A. F. Levinson,
Suppressor cell function in atopic dermatitis associated with
elevated immunoglobulin E, J. Allergy Clin. Immunol 64:139 (1979).

140. D. L. Schuster, B. A. Bongiovanni, D. L. Pierson, J. F. Barbaro, D. T.
Wong, and A. I. Levinson, Selective deficiency of a T cell
subpopulation in active atopic dermatitis, J. Immunol. 124:1662
(1980).

141. V. K. Sharma and S. P. Banerjee, Alpha-adrenergic receptors in rat
heart. Effects of thyroidectomy, J. Biol. Chem. 253:5277 (1978).

142. B. G. Simonsson, N. Svedmyr, B. E. Skoogh, R. Andersson, and N. P.
Bergh, In vivo and in vitro studies of alpha-receptors in human
airways. Potentiation with bacterial endotoxin, Scan. J. Resp. Dis.
53:227 (1972).

143. B. R. Smith and R. Hall, Thyroid-stimulating immunoglobulins in
Grave's disease, Lancet 2:427 (1974).

144. P. D. Snashall, F. A. Boother, and G. M. Sterling, The effect of

alpha-adrenergic stimulation on the airways of normal and asthmatic man, Clin. Sci. Mol. Med. 54:283 (1978).

145. H. L. Spiegelberg, Fc receptors for IgE on macrophages and lymphocytes: IgE synthesis, Fed. Proc. 42:122 (1983).

146. J. M. Stadel, A. DeLean, D. Mullikin-Kilpatrick, D. D. Sawyer, and R. J. Lefkowitz, Catecholamine-induced desensitization in turkey erythrocytes: cAMP mediated impairment of high affinity agonist binding without alteration in receptor number, J. Cyc. Nucl. Res. 7:37 (1981).

147. J. M. Stadel, B. Strulovici, P. Nambi, T. N. Lavin, M. M. Briggs, M. G. Caron, and R. J. Lefkowitz, Desensitization of the beta-adrenergic receptor of frog erythrocytes: recovery and characterization of the down-regulated receptors in sequestered vesicles, J. Biol. Chem. 258:3032 (1983).

148. R. Stevens, E. Macy, C. Morrow, and A. Saxon, Characterization of a circulating subpopulation of spontaneous antitetanus toxoid antibody production, J. Immunol. 122:2498 (1980).

149. O. Strannegård and I.-L. Strannegård, T-lymphocyte numbers and function in human IgE-mediated allergy, Immunol. Rev. 41:149 (1978).

150. I.-L. Strannegård and O. Strannegård, Natural killer cells and interferon production in atopic dermatitis, Acta. Derm. Venereol. (Stockh.) Suppl. 92:48 (1980).

151. O. Strannegård, I.-L. Strannegård, K. Kang, K. D. Cooper, and J. M. Hanifin, FcIgG receptor-bearing lymphocytes and monoclonal antibody defined T-cell subsets in atopic dermatitis. Effect of treatment with thymopoietin pentapeptide (TP-5), Int. Arch. Allergy Appl. Immunol. 69:328 (1982).

152. O. Strannegård, I.-L. Strannegård, and I. Rystedt, Viral infections in atopic dermatitis, Acta. Derm. Venereol. (Stockh.) Suppl. 114:121 (1985).

153. Y.-F. Su, L. Cubeddu-Ximenez, and J. P. Perkins, Regulation of adenosine-3',5'-monophosphate content of human astrocytoma cells: desensitization to catecholamines and prostaglandins, J. Cyclic Nucleotide Res. 2:257 (1976).

154. Y.-F. Su, T. K. Harden, and J. P. Perkins, Catecholamine-specific desensitization of adenylate cyclase: evidence for a multistep process, J. Biol. Chem. 255:7410 (1980).

155. A. Svejgaard, M. Christy, J. Nerup, et al., HLA and autoimmune diseases with special reference to the genetics of insulin-dependent diabetes, in: "Genetics Control of Autoimmune Diseases," N. Rose, P. Bigazzi, and N. Warner, eds., Elsevier/North Holland, New York (1978).

156. A. Szentivanyi, The beta adrenergic theory of the atopic abnormality in bronchial asthma, J. Allergy 42:203 (1968).

157. A. Szentivanyi, Effect of bacterial products and adrenergic blocking agents on allergic reactions, in: "Textbook of Immunological Diseases," M. Samter et al., eds., Little, Brown and Company, Boston (1971).

158. A. Szentivanyi, La flexibilite de conformation des adrenorecepteurs et la base constitutionelle du terrain allergique, Rev. Franc. Allergol. 19:205 (1979a).

159. A. Szentivanyi, The conformational flexibility of adrenoceptors and the constitutional basis of atopy, Triangle 18:109 (1979b).

160. A. Szentivanyi, Invited Editorial: The radioligand binding approach in the study of lymphocytic adrenoceptors and the constitutional basis of atopy, J. Allergy Clin. Immunol. 65:5 (1980).

161. A. Szentivanyi, "Adrenergic and Cholinergic Receptor Studies in Human Lung and Lymphocytic Membranes and their Relations to Bronchial Hyperreactivity in Asthma," Patient Care Publications, Inc., Darien (1982).

162. A. Szentivanyi and C. W. Fishel, Neuro-humoral concepts of bronchial asthma, <u>Acta</u>. <u>Allergologica</u> 29 (Suppl.11):26 (1974).

163. A. Szentivanyi and D. F. Fitzpatrick, The altered reactivity of the effector cells to antigenic and pharmacological influences and its relation to cyclic nucleotides. II. Effector reactivities in the efferent loop of the immune response, <u>in</u>: "Grafelfing bei Munchen," G. Fillip, ed., Werk-Verlag (1980).

164. A. Szentivanyi and L. Pek, Characteristic changes of vascular adrenergic reactions in diabetes mellitus, <u>Nature New Biol</u>. 243:276 (1973).

165. A. Szentivanyi and J. Szentivanyi, Some selected aspects of the immunopharmacology of adrenoceptors, <u>Advances in Immunopharmacol</u>. 2:269 (1983).

166. A. Szentivanyi and J. Szentivanyi, Cellular and molecular foundation of immunity, immunologic inflammation, and hypersensitivity. Component parts and their relation to neurohumoral control mechanisms, <u>in</u>: "Sodeman's Pathologic Physiology - Mechanisms of Disease," Seventh Edition, W. A. Sodeman and T. M. Sodeman, eds., W. B. Saunders Company, Philadelphia and London (1985a).

167. A. Szentivanyi and J. Szentivanyi, The pathophysiology of immunologic and related diseases, <u>in</u>: "Sodeman's Pathologic Physiology - Mechanisms of Disease," Seventh Edition, W. A. Sodeman and T. M. Sodeman, eds., W. B. Saunders Company, Philadelphia and London (1985b).

168. A. Szentivanyi and J. F. Williams, The constitutional basis of atopic disease. Chapter 14, <u>in</u>: "Allergic Diseases of Infancy, Childhood, and Adolescence," C. W. Bierman and D. S. Pearlman, eds., W. B. Saunders Company, Philadelphia and London (1980).

169. A. Szentivanyi, G. Kunos, and A. Juhasz-Nagy, Modulator theory of adrenergic receptor mechanism: vessels of the dog hind limb, <u>Amer</u>. <u>J. Physiol</u>. 218:869 (1970).

170. A. Szentivanyi, O. Heim, and P. Schultze, Changes in adrenoceptor densities in membranes of lung tissue and lymphocytes from patients with atopic disease, <u>Ann</u>. <u>N.Y</u>. <u>Acad</u>. <u>Sci</u>. 332:295 (1979).

171. A. Szentivanyi, J. Krzanowski, J. Polson, and W. Anderson, Evolution of research strategy in the experimental analysis of the beta adrenergic approach to the constitutional basis of atopy, <u>in</u>: "Advances in Allergology and Clinical Immunology, A. Oehling, E. Mathov, I. Glazer, and C. Arbesman, eds., Pergamon Press, Oxford (1980).

172. A. Szentivanyi, O. Heim, P. Schultze, and J. Szentivanyi, Adrenoceptor binding studies with [^{3}H]dihydroalprenolol and [^{3}H]dihydroergocryptine on membranes of lymphocytes from patients with atopic disease, <u>Acta</u>. <u>Dermato</u>. <u>Venereol</u>. Suppl. 92:19 (1980).

173. A. Szentivanyi, J. B. Polson, and J. J. Krzanowski, The altered reactivity of the effector cells to antigenic and pharmacological influences and its relation to cyclic nucleotides. I. Effector reactivities in the efferent loop of the immune response, <u>in</u>: "Pathomechanismus and Pathogenese Allergischer Reaktionen," G. Filipp, ed., Banachewski Verlag, Grafelfing bei Munchen (1980).

174. A. Szentivanyi, E. Middleton, J. F. Williams, and H. Friedman, Effect of microbial agents on the immune network and associated pharmacologic reactivities, <u>in</u>: "Allergy: Principles and Practice," Second Edition, E. Middleton, C. E. Reed, and E. F. Ellis, eds., The C. V. Mosby Company, St. Louis (1983).

175. A. Szentivanyi, J. B. Polson, and J. Szentivanyi, Issues of adrenoceptor behavior in respiratory and cutaneous disorders of atopic allergy, <u>Trends in Pharmac</u>. <u>Sci</u>. 5:280 (1984).

176. A. Szentivanyi, J. J. Krzanowski, and J. B. Polson, The autonomic nervous system, <u>in</u>: "Allergy: Principles and Practice," Second Edition, E. Middleton, C. E. Reed, and E. F. Ellis, eds., The C. V.

Mosby Company, St. Louis (1983).

177. A. Szentivanyi, J. B. Polson and J. Szentivanyi, Adrenergic regulation, in: "Bronchial Asthma: Mechanisms and Therapeutics," E. B. Weiss, M. S. Segal, and M. Stein, eds., Little, Brown and Company, Boston (1985).

178. I. I. Tabachnick, A. Gulbenkian, and L. J. Schobert, Effects of a beta adrenergic blocking agent and isopropylmethylamine on the release of histamine from guinea pig lung during anaphylaxis in vitro, Biochem. Pharmacol. 14:1283 (1965).

179. G. K. Terpstra, J. A. M. Raaijmakers, and J. Kreukniet, Comparison of vaccination of mice and rats with Haemophilus influenzae and Bordetella pertussis as models of atopy, Clin. Exp. Pharmac. Physiol. 6:139 (1979).

180. A. N. Theofilopoulos, Autoimmunity, in: "Basic and Clinical Immunology," Fifth Edition, D. P. Stites, J. D. Stobo, H. H. Fudenberg, and J. W. Wells, eds., Lange Medical Publications, California (1984).

181. T. Uchiyama, D. Nelson, T. Fleisher, and T. Waldmann, A monoclonal antibody (Anti-T) reactive with activated and functionally mature human T cells. II. Expression of Tac antigen on activated cytoxic killer T cells, J. Immunol. 126:1398 (1981).

182. J. C. Venter, C. M. Fraser, and L. C. Harrison, Auto-antibodies to beta$_2$-adrenergic receptors: a possible cause of adrenergic hyporesponsiveness in asthma and allergic rhinitis, Science 207:1316 (1980).

183. R. C. Welliver, T. N. Kaul, and P. L. Ogra, The appearance of cell-bound IgE in respiratory-tract epithelium after respiratory syncytial virus infection, N. Eng. J. Med. 303:1198 (1980).

184. R. Woenne, M. Kattan, R. P. Orange and H. Levison, Bronchial hyperreactivity to histamine and methacholine in asthmatic children after inhalation of SCH 1000 and chlorpheniramine maleate, J. Allergy Clin. Immunol. 62:119 (1978).

185. B. Wutrich, "Zur Immunopathologie der Neurodermitis Constitutionalis," Hans Huber, Bern (1975).

SCRAPIE INFECTION IN ATHYMIC AND GERM-FREE MICE

W. F. Wade, C. Dees, T. L. German and R. F. Marsh

Department of Veterinary Science
University of Wisconsin - Madison
Madison, Wisconsin

INTRODUCTION

Scrapie, a slow virus disease of sheep and goats, is unusual in that there is no detectable scrapie-specific immune response. Using the mouse model, investigators have studied the early involvement of the reticuloendo-thelial system (RES) and/or immune response cells in extraneural scrapie pathogenesis. The results of these studies have revealed a paradox with regard to immune modulation. Treatments that are immunostimulatory, e.g. BCG (1) or interferon (2) treatment, reduce the incubation period compared to the non-treated controls, whereas immunodepressive (3) treatments such as splenectomy, prednisone, or arachis oil tend to lengthen the incubation period.

The purpose of this experiment was to evaluate the role of the RES and immune response cells in murine scrapie pathogenesis by studying the effect of bacterial flora, the presence or absence of a thymus, and the route of inoculation on the length of the incubation period and scrapie agent titer in spleen and brain.

MATERIALS AND METHODS

Female BALB/c mice eight to eleven weeks old were maintained in either a germfree (GF) or defined flora (DF) state using flexible-film isolators at the University of Wisconsin Gnotobiotic Laboratory. Mice were handled the same throughout the course of the study. Ten euthymic (H) and ten athymic (N) mice were inoculated intraperitoneally (IP) with a five percent infected brain suspension containing $10^{6.3}$ LD_{50} of an ME-7 type scrapie agent. Five H and five N mice were anesthetized lightly with sodium pento-barbital, then inoculated intracerebrally (IC) with $10^{5.1}$ LD_{50}. A similar number of mice were inoculated IP or IC with a five percent normal brain preparation. Two mice were removed at random from the IP inoculated groups, 28 and 90 days after inoculation. Scrapie agent titers of pooled tissues from spleen and mesenteric lymph nodes were determined in Swiss Webster ICR mice by endpoint dilution using the Spearman Karber method.

Mice were observed daily for clinical signs of disease. Stage I, used to designate early clinical signs, was represented by rough hair coat (except nudes), lethargy, and a huddling posture in the center of the cage. Affected mice became progressively more debilitated. Stage III was reached when mice adducted their hind legs when suspended by their tails, or were unable to remove themselves when hung by their hind legs on the cage lip. Stage III mice were killed and their spleens and brains removed for infectivity assay. Three mice, randomly chosen from each group, were used to determine the scrapie agent titer from pooled tissue suspensions.

A three-way analysis of variance with an n of 48 was used for statistical evaluation. Multiple mean comparison was done using the least significant difference (LSD) test. Both statistical tests were conducted at an α level of .05.

RESULTS AND DISCUSSION

Three-way analysis of variance indicates that there were significant differences for time to Stage I and to Stage III, and the interval between them (Speed). Table 1 shows the LSD comparison of means for time in days to Stage I, Stage III and Speed for the various groups tested. It can be seen that the biggest differences are in mice inoculated IP. Germfree/-euthymic IP inoculated mice took on the average 213.5 and 248.5 days to reach Stage I and Stage III, respectively, while defined flora/euthymic IP inoculated mice reached State I in only 168.2 days and Stage III in 190.4 days. These differences in time to Stage I and Stage III suggest there is either a difference in the transport of the scrapie agent to the brain, or in its replication kinetics. These differences could be due to the influences of the bacterial flora on cells with which the scrapie agent first interacts after parenteral infection. The more phagocytic cells (macrophages) of the defined flora/euthymic mice could localize more of the inoculum in the spleen. However, this seems unlikely because the scrapie agent titers in spleen at 28 days post inoculation are similar among IP inoculated groups. Alternatively, the effect of having a bacterial flora or not could change the number or types of receptors (4) on the cells with which scrapie initially interacts. Altered cell associations could cause a change in the localization of the inoculum, thus altering the pathogenesis of disease.

The presence or absence of a bacterial flora, the mouse phenotype, and the route of inoculation interact to influence the progression of clinical signs. Typically, progression from Stage I to III takes about three weeks (5). The progression of clinical sings is paralleled by an increase in the scrapie agent titer in brain of about one $\log_{10}$ per week (3). Table 1 shows that the mean time for the groups to reach Stage III is about 21 days, however, there is a tendency for nude mice to progress more rapidly. These differences in speed indicate that there are either different replication rates, or that there are factors other than scrapie agent brain titer which contribute to clinical signs. Kimberlin and Walker have reported that the concentration of the scrapie agent in brain is related to the severity of clinical signs (6). Further studies measuring brain titers during the clinical course of disease are necessary to determine if the differences in time to Stage I and Stage III in the various groups were due to differences in the replication rate of the scrapie agent. However, since the scrapie agent titers in brain at Stage III were similar and the speed that mice progress is variable, this suggests that there are different replication rates among the groups, an increased susceptibility, or an enhanced ability to survive with equivalent scrapie titers in brain. Additionally, there appears to be another important consideration in explaining these results.

The variability in the length of the incubation periods could be due to differences in the transport of agent into the central nervous system (CNS). Entry of the scrapie agent to the CNS is thought to occur principally by axonal transport from spleen afferent nerve fibers into the spinal

Table 1. Time in Days to Stage I, Stage III and Speed of BALB/c Mice Inoculated with Scrapie Agent

LSD for Time to Clinical Signs (Stage I)

DF H IC[a] 118.30[b]	GF H IC 126.50	DF N IC 135.78	GF N IC 145.17	DF H IP 168.20	DF N IP 196.50	GF N IP 203.80	GF H IP 213.50

LSD = 16.30[c]

LSD for Time to End-Stage (Stage III)

GF H IC 147.67	DF H IC 151.43	DF N IC 160.78	GF N IC 164.67	DF H IP 190.40	DF N IP 204.33	GF N IP 213.80	GF H IP 248.50

LSD = 18.20

LSD for Speed (Time in Days) to Stage III from Stage I

DF N IP 7.83	GF N IP 10.00	GF N IC 19.50	GF H IC 21.17	DF H IP 22.20	DF N IC 25.00	DF H IC 33.13	GF H IP 35.00

LSD = 14.44

[a]DF = defined flora; GF = germfree; H = euthymic; N = nude; IC = intracerebral; IP = intraperitoneal.

[b]Mean time in days to determination for the group, ordered in increasing magnitude.

[c]Least significant difference value that means must differ by, to be considered significant at the 0.5 α level. Data was computed on an N of 48. Values underlined are not different from each other.

247

cord and brain (5). Differences in incubation periods may be due to alteration in either the movement within the spleen to the afferent nerve or differences in transport within the axon. The latter possibility seems unlikely. However, differences in access to afferent nerve fibers in the
splenic capsule is compatible with differences in localization of the infecting inoculum as effected by bacterial flora and mouse phenotype. An alter-
nate explanation for the possible difference in transport of the scrapie
agent may involve blood cells. Since there are differences in lymphoid
cell populations in athymic (7) and germfree (8) mice, scrapie associations
with this cell type could also vary. While there is no evidence that blood
cell associated transport of the scrapie agent occurs, this possibility
cannot be completely dismissed.

The complex interaction among route of inoculation (IP vs IC), mouse
phenotype (H vs N) and the presence or absence of a bacterial flora (DF vs
GF) that alters the incubation periods in murine scrapie is depicted in
Figure 1. This interaction is most evident in mice that are inoculated IP,
probably because events that ensue after IC inoculation are not as sensitive
to outside influences since virus is inoculated directly into the target
organ. Given that the presence or absence of a bacterial flora and mouse
phenotype, significantly affect the length of the incubation period of mice
inoculated IP with the scrapie agent, this type of experimental approach
could allow the identification of the cell(s) which are involved in extraneural murine scrapie pathogenesis. This can be done by cell reconstitution
experiments. Spleen cells from defined flora, euthymic mice can be passively
transferred to irradiated germfree, euthymic mice and the time to Stage I
and Stage III determined for recipient mice. Should passively transferred
cells confer the donor's incubation period on the recipient, a simple removal
of individual cell types could indicate which cell(s) is(are) involved in
early events in extraneural scrapie pathogenesis.

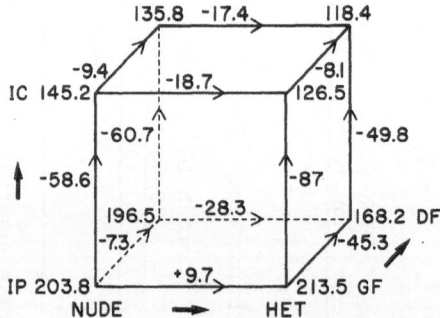

Fig. 1. Three-way interaction of route of inoculation,
mouse phenotype (N or H) and bacterial flora
(GF or DF). Mean time to Stage I for each group
is shown at the vertices. The top of the cube
represents mice inoculated IC, the bottom IP.
Mice that were maintained in a GF isolator are
shown as the front face of the cube while DF mice
are depicted on the back face. The left side of
the cube signifies N mice and right side, H.
Therefore, 203.8 is the mean time for Stage I for
GF, IP, N mice and 213.5 for GF, IP, H mice with
+ 9.7 indicating the difference between the means.
This cube is a convenient medium for viewing the
effect of changing one variable on the pathogenesis
of murine scrapie.

REFERENCES

1. R. H. Kimberlin and P. G. Cunnington, Reduction of scrapie incubation time in mice and hamsters by a single injection of methanol extraction residue of BCG, FEMS Microbiol. Lett. 3:169 (1978).
2. L. B. Allen and K. W. Cochran, Acceleration of scrapie in mice by target organ treatment with interferon inducers, Ann. N.Y. Acad. Sci. 284:676 (1977).
3. G. W. Outram, The pathogenesis of scrapie in mice, in: "Slow Virus Diseases of Animals and Man," R. H. Kimberlin, ed., North-Holland, Amsterdam (1976).
4. A. G. Dickinson and G. W. Outram, The scrapie replication-site hypothesis and its implications for pathogenesis, in: "Slow Transmissible Diseases of the Nervous System," Vol. 2, S. B. Prusiner and W. J. Hadlow, eds., Academic Press, New York (1979).
5. R. H. Kimberlin and C. A. Walker, Pathogenesis of mouse scrapie: patterns of agent replication in different parts of the CNS following intraperitoneal infection, J. R. Soc. Med. 75:618 (1982).
6. R. H. Kimberlin and C. A. Walker, Pathogenesis of murine scrapie: effect of route of inoculation on infectivity titers and dose response curves, J. Comp. Path. 88:39 (1978).
7. G. Sainte-Marie and F. Shiong Peng, Structural and cell population changes in the lymph nodes of the athymic nude mouse, Lab. Invest. 49:420 (1983).
8. B. Woodward, A stereological ultrastructural study of peritoneal macrophages from germ-free and conventionally-reared mice, 192:157 (1978).

AGE AND GENDER RELATED CHANGES IN NORMAL LEVELS

OF CIRCULATING HUMAN IMMUNE CELLS

Alan A. Waldman, William R. Oleszko, Edith Zang,
Celso Bianco and Johanna Pindyck

The Greater New York Blood Program
New York Blood Center, New York, New York

INTRODUCTION

During the last few years there has been an increase in interest in the nature and function of circulating human immune cells. This has been paralleled by increased availability of monoclonal-based reagents which react with specific cell surface markers, allowing rapid and sensitive detection of different functional cell types.

With the realization that diagnosis of immune competence might be of great importance in prediction of susceptibility to diseases, such as acquired immune deficiency syndrome (AIDS), it becomes necessary to have data concerning the normal level of circulating immune cells in individuals, and concerning the extent of acceptable variation in these values. These data have not been readily available.

Recently, we have begun to examine the circulating immune cell content of healthy normal blood donors as part of a program designed to establish the immune status of our donor population. The initial results of the study demonstrate that the expected values for levels of circulating immune cells in a healthy adult vary and that the variation is predictable and dependent on the age, gender, and history of viral infection of the individual.

MATERIALS AND METHODS

Sample Population

All samples were obtained from healthy blood donors who not only passed the standard medical history, but also attested that they were not a member of a group with increased risk of exposure to AIDS.

Sample Analysis: Cellular Content

Blood was anticoagulated with potassium EDTA and stored overnight at room temperature before being analyzed for cellular content. Complete blood counts were performed using automated cell counters (J. T. Baker, Inc.) and leukocyte differentials were made on Wright stained smears.

For flow cytometric analysis, samples were first exposed to specific fluorescein-labeled monoclonal antibodies directed against known cell surface

markers on lymphocytes (Becton Dickinson and Coulter), and then treated
with with an NH$_4$Cl-based lysis buffer to remove erythrocytes (Ortho, Inc.).
The extent of selective staining was determined by examination of the
stained preparation using a flow cytometer (FACS IV, Becton Dickinson).

Sample Analysis: Serologic Assays

Serum from a second, matched aliquot of blood was also available for
each donor sample examined for cellular content. The serum was assayed for
the presence and level of IgG antibodies directed against cytomegalovirus
(CMV), using a commercially available fluorescent test (FIAX, IDT Corporation) and for the total level of the circulating immunoglobulins IgG, IgA
and IgM (ICS, Beckman Instruments).

RESULTS

In the first phase of the study, basic screening results were obtained
for almost 1,000 normal, healthy blood donors (627 males, 369 females) with
an age distribution approximating that of the entire donor base. In summary,
the following observations were made concerning the level of circulating
immune cells:

a) For males, the mean percent of lymphocytes bearing the markers for
T helper, inducer cells (T h,i) increased continually with age of the donor
while the mean percent of lymphocytes bearing markers to T suppressor, cytotoxic cells (T s,c) remained relatively stable;

b) For females, the mean percent of T h,i also increased continually
with age, and in addition, the mean percent of T s,c declined substantially;

c) The increase in T h,i for females was greater than that for males,
as was the decrease in T s,c; and

d) The net effect of these paired changes was clearly seen in the
mean ratio for T h,i to T s,c, with females having on an average a higher
ratio for each group, as well as a much more rapid rate of increase than
did males (p <0.005).

These large and dramatic changes in balances of T h,i and T s,c occurred
in the absence of any obvious change in the average level of total circulating white blood cells (WBC) or in the average WBC differential for granulocytes or lymphocytes. This was true both for males and for females.

Exposure to, and infection by, cytomegalovirus (CMV) is very common
(1). With increasing age, fewer of the donors exhibited a low (undetectable)
level of IgG antibodies to CMV, and more exhibited a high (greater than 140
fluorescent units) level of antibody to CMV. If one redistributed the data
concerning the percent of T h,i and T s,c on the basis of level of antibody
to CMV as well as on the basis of age and gender, one would obtain for both
males and females a slightly lower mean percentage of T h,i and clearly
elevated mean percentage of T s,c in individuals with high titers of anti-CMV
compared to individuals with undetectable anti-CMV.

To confirm and extend these initial findings, we examined in greater
detail a second set of donors pre-selected as males or females between 17
and 30 years or 50 and 65 years of age. The results of these studies are
presented in Table 1, 2, and 3.

For both males and females (Table 1), the following parameters were
found to be essentially constant between the younger (<30) and the older
(>50 groups):

252

Table 1. Values for Circulating Immune Cells and Markers*

Parameter	Males		Females	
	17–30 y	50–65 y	17–30 y	50–65 y
Number Analyzed	40	41	41	40
Cellular Assays:				
WBC (x 10 /mm)	6.3 (1.7)	6.9 (2.3)	6.4 (2.0)	6.5 (0.8)
Lymphocytes (x 10 /mm)	2.7 (0.8)	2.7 (0.8)	2.6 (0.8)	2.9 (0.9)
Lymphocyte Differential				
total B (%)	9 (3)	8 (3)	9 (1)	8 (4)
total T (%)	77 (5)	78 (4)	79 (5)	79 (5)
T h,i (%)	44 (6)	50 (10)	46 (7)	52 (7)
T s,c (%)	25 (6)	24 (9)	25 (4)	23 (7)
T h,i/T s,c	1.9 (0.6)	2.5 (1.4)	2.0 (0.6)	2.6 (1.0)
Serologic Assays:				
Antibody to CMV				
positives (%)	15	63	15	71
positives (titer)	95 (27)	117 (78)	83 (44)	220 (145)
IgG (g/dl)	1.1 (0.2)	1.0 (0.2)	1.0 (0.2)	1.0 (0.3)
IgA (g/dl)	0.2 (0.1)	0.2 (0.1)	0.2 (0.1)	0.2 (0.1)
IgM (g/dl)	0.1 (0.1)	0.1 (0.1)	0.2 (0.1)	0.1 (0.1)

*Data presented as mean (S.D.)

    a)   total WBC;
    b)   total lymphocytes;
    c)   total B cells;
    d)   total T cells; and
    e)   the levels for IgG, IgA, and IgM.

On the other hand, the following parameters varied:

    a) T h,i (which increased);
    b) T s,c (which decreased);
    c) the ratio of T h,i to T s,c (which increased); and
    d) the percent positive for anti-CMV and the titer of such anti-CMV antibodies (which both increased).

These data are in agreement with those previously obtained, and extend the "constants" in the circulating immune cells to include the percentage of total T and the number of total T cells.

The true extent of the variation in T h,i, T s,c, and T h,i/T s,c ratio is not adequately reflected by the means presented in Table 1. A more useful presentation of these data are found in Tables 2A and 2B, which show the distribution of the values. A marked shift to higher levels of T h,i, a spread in values for T s,c, and a net marked spread and shift in the ratio T h,i/T s,c are clearly visible.

A similar distribution of these values in which the effect of previous exposure to CMV is taken into account, is presented in Table 3. As can be seen, individuals with a high titer of anti-CMV antibody have essentially

Table 2. Distribution of Values for Immune Cells*

A > Males

Age Group	% T helper, inducer			
	<30	31-50	51-70	>71
17-30 (n=40)	0	90	10	0
50-65 (n=41)	5	51	44	0

Age Group	% T suppressor, cytotoxic				
	<15	16-20	21-25	26-30	> 31
17-30 (n=40)	2	20	42	20	15
50-65 (n-41)	27	15	29	7	22

Age Group	Ratio: T h,i/T s,c			
	<1.0	1.1-2.0	2.1-3.0	>3.1
17-30 (n=40)	10	65	20	5
50-65 (n=41)	17	32	24	29

B > Females

Age Group	% T helper, inducer			
	< 30	31-50	51-70	>71
17-30 (n=41)	0	76	24	0
50-65 (n=40)	0	38	62	0

Age Group	% T suppressor, cytotoxic				
	< 15	16-29	21-25	26-30	> 31
17-30 (n=41)	2	15	44	34	5
50-65 (n=40)	8	40	28	12	12

Age Group	Ratio: T h,i/T s,c			
	< 1.0	1.1-2.0	2.1-3.0	> 3.1
17-30 (n=41)	2	66	24	7
50-65 (n=40)	2	30	35	32

*Data presented as percent in each group having noted value.

the same T h,i, a spread to higher T s,c, and therefore a shift to lower T h,i/T s,c ratios. This pattern agrees with data from our earlier studies.

Preliminary data from studies designed to examine if the trends of change observed continued for individuals older than 65 years indicated that that both the mean values and the distribution of values yielded the expected pattern, with all cellular parameters measured constant except for T h,i (which increased), T s,c (for which the values spread to lower levels and perhaps separated into two groups) and the ratio of T h,i/T s,c (which increased yet further).

CONCLUSIONS

The results of our studies clearly demonstrate that there is a predictable pattern of change in the balance of active T lymphocytes. The extent of these changes, of a mean increase of T h,i, of a mean decrease of T s,c, and of a sharp and continuous increase in the value of T h,i/T s,c, are

Table 3. Effect of Presence of Anti-CMV Antibody on Values in Individuals 50–65 Years of Age*

Anti-CMV Titer	% T helper, inducer			
	<30	31–50	51–70	>71
undetectable	0	41	59	0
high (> 140)	4	48	48	0
	% T suppressor, cytotoxic				
	<10	11–20	21–30	31–40	>41
undetectable	2	20	42	20	15
high (> 140)	27	15	49	7	22
	Ratio: T h,i/T s,c				
	<1.0	1.1–2.0	2.1–3.0	3.1–4.0	>4.1
undetectable	0	33	30	18	18
high (> 140)	13	30	29	17	0

*Data presented as percent in each group having noted value; for undetectable, n=27; for high n=23.

related to the age and gender of the individual, and continue throughout all ages studied (17–75 years of age).

In addition, the actual value of these parameters, but not the patterns of change themselves, are modulated by the viral history of the individual, as judged by the circulating level of anti-CMV antibodies.

It is hoped that studies such as ours will provide baseline normal ranges, which can be applied to clarify and to predict an individual's immune status. In addition, these data lay the groundwork for future research into into the mechanisms underlying the normal senescence of the immune system (2,3).

REFERENCES

1. E. Gold and G. A. Nankervis, Cytomegalovirus, in: "Viral Infection of Humans: Epidemiology and Control," 2nd Edition, A. S. Evans, ed., Plenum Press, New York (1982).
2. J. W. Williams, Hematology in the aged, in: "Hematology," 3rd Edition, W. J. Williams, E. Beutler, A. J. Erslev, and M. A. Lichtman, eds., McGraw-Hill, New York (1983).
3. M. L. Weksler, Immune senescence in man, in: "Immunology and Aging," N. Fabris, M. Nijhoff, New York (1982).

EFFECT OF REAGENT SOURCE, PROCESSING TECHNIQUES, AND SAMPLE

STORAGE ON DETERMINATION OF CIRCULATING HUMAN IMMUNE CELLS

William R. Oleszko and Alan A. Waldman

Greater New York Blood Program
New York Blood Center
New York, New York

INTRODUCTION

It is generally agreed that an accurate evaluation of an individual's immune status should include information concerning the number and nature of the circulating immune lymphocytes. In order for the testing laboratory to correctly supply this data to treating physicians for use in reliable diagnosis of alterations of the immune system, and thus changes in their patient's immune status, it is necessary that testing methods be standardized and comparable from one test site to another.

It has been reported that there can be substantial variation in results on the same blood sample, and that such variations are related both to actual changes in the test samples during storage as well as to artifacts introduced during the processing attending the different methodologies of cell isolation and staining (1-3). It has become clear that in order to develop standard procedures, it will first be necessary to understand the effect of the equipment used and each variable in the processing and storage of blood on the obtained analytical results.

The following report presents data from studies we conducted to clarify what effect, if any, there would be on assay results due to the use of different flow cytometers, reagents from different commercial sources, and/or the variation of procedures used in the processing and storage of whole human blood.

MATERIALS AND METHODS

Whole blood samples, drawn in potassium-EDTA, were processed and analyzed either fresh (less than four hours after collection) or after storage (16 to 20 hours). Blood samples were selected at random from those accessing the laboratory. Samples were obtained from normal donors, as well as from various study populations with suspected immunodysfunction or immunodeficiency. As detailed below, lymphocytes were enumerated following selective staining with monoclonal antibodies against specific cell surface antigens.

Methods of Staining

Direct: Fluorescein-labeled test and control antibodies (see Table 1, direct panels 1 and 2) were prepared and used according to manufacturers'

Table 1. Reagent Panels

	Direct Reagents			Indirect Reagents
Specificity of Stain	Panel 1		Panel 2	Panel 1
	B-D	Ortho	Coulter	Coulter
total T	--	OKT11-F+ OKT3-F	CCT11-F	CCT11
pan T	--	OKT3-F	--	CCT3
T helper, inducer	Leu 3a-F+ Leu 3b-F	--	CCT4-F	CCT4
T suppressor, cytotoxic	Leu 2a-F	--	CCT8-F	CCT8

recommendations to yield cells bearing surface fluorescence. Direct stain-ing reagent sources include Becton Dickinson (B-D), Coulter Immunology and Ortho Diagnostics.

Indirect: Test monoclonal antibodies, control antibodies and goat anti-mouse Ig labeled with fluorescein (see Table 1, indirect panel 1) were obtained from Coulter Immunology. These reagents were prepared and used according to the manufacturer's recommendations, in a two-step procedure. The first step exposed leukocytes to specific monoclonal reagents, and the second step identified, by fluorescence, cells with specific surface-bound mouse anti-human antibodies.

Sample Processing and Staining Protocols

"Stain and Lyse" Protocol: Aliquots of whole blood were incubated with monoclonal antibody reagents. After incubation, tubes were brought to room temperature and erythrocytes were lysed by treatment with ammonium chloride (according to the protocol of Ortho Diagnostics). Unless otherwise noted this was the procedure used for the experiments.

"Lyse and Stain" Protocol: Separate aliquots of whole blood samples were exposed to ammonium chloride (Ortho Diagnostics) to lyse erythrocytes, washed, and then exposed to monoclonal staining reagents. Tubes were then handled according to reagent manufacturers' recommendations.

"Gradient Isolation and Stain" Protocol: Mononuclear cells, isolated on Ficoll-Hypaque density gradients (4), were washed in phosphate buffered saline, and exposed to monoclonal antibody reagents and handled according to reagent manufacturers' recommendations.

Sample Analysis

In all of the above protocols, after processing and staining, sample tubes were stored briefly in the dark at 4°C until analysis by flow cytometry. All determinations of the percentage of lymphocytes exhibiting an intensity of fluorescence greater than control antibody background levels were performed using a FACS IV (Becton Dickinson), except for comparison analysis of the FACS IV with the EPICS C (Coulter Electronics) or the Spectrum III (Ortho Diagnostics). In all cases lymphocytes were identified by

Table 2. Instrumentation and Reagent Comparison*

Comparison	(n)	Acceptable Values	Not-Acceptable Values (CR)	
Instrumentation				
FACS IV/EPICS C	(32)	total T	T h,i	(1.10)
		pan T	T s,c	(1.09)
		T h,i/T s,c		
FACS IV/SPECTRUM III	(40)	total T	T h,i/T s,c	(1.11)
		pan T		
		T h,i		
		T s,c		
		total B <ND>		
Reagent Panels				
Fresh Blood	(12)			
direct 1/direct 2		all markers		
direct 1/indirect 1		all T markers	total B	(1.24)
direct 2/indirect 1		all T markers	total B	(1.27)
Stored Blood (24°C)	(12)			
direct 1/direct 2		all markers		
direct 1/indirect 1		all markers		
direct 2/indirect 1		all markers		
Fresh/Stored Blood (24°C)	(12)			
direct 1		all T markers	total B	(1.38)
direct 2		all T markers	total B	(1.35)
indirect 1		all T markers	total B	(1.18)

*Data presented relative to acceptable values for all T markers of ± 5% and for total B markers of ± 10%.
Abbreviations: all T markers = total T, pan T, T h,i, T s,c, and T h,i/T s,c ratio; <ND> means not done.

their characteristic low and wide angle light scatter pattern, from which fluorescence was determined.

Data Presentation

Summaries of the analysis of data are presented in Tables 2 and 3. To analyze the effect of each variable being examined on the enumeration of lymphocyte subpopulations, data were generated from individual blood samples for each specific monoclonal reagent. The data from two different conditions were then compared in ratio format. In general, it is the resultant Comparative Ratios (CR) which are presented.

As an example, below is the equation of the CR for an experiment examining the effect of storage on a single blood sample:

$$CR = \frac{\% \text{ T3+ lymphocytes from single fresh blood}}{\% \text{ T3+ lymphocytes from single stored blood}}$$

Table 3. Preparative Methodologies and Blood Storage*

Comparison	(n)	Acceptable Values	Non-Acceptable Values (CR)	
Stain and lyse	(8)			
fresh/stored (24°C)		pan T	total T	(0.94)
		T h,i		
		T s,c		
		total B		
		T h,i/T s,c		
fresh/stored (4°C)		all markers		
Lyse and stain	(8)			
fresh/stored (24°C)		all markers		
fresh/stored (4°c)		total T	T h,i	(1.07)
		pan T	T s,c	(1.07)
		T h,i/T s,c	total B	(1.13)
stored: 24°C/4°C		total T	T h,i	(1.10)
		pan T		
		T s,c		
		Total B		
		T h,i/T s,c		
Stain and lyse/lyse and stain	(12)			
fresh blood		all markers		
stored blood (24°C)		all markers		
stored blood (4°C)		all T markers	total B	(1.11)
Stain and lyse/gradient isolation and stain	(4)			
fresh blood		pan T	total T	(0.94)
			T h,i	(0.85)
			T s,c	(0.93)
			T h,i/T s,c	(0.91)
			total B	(1.79)
stored blood (24°C)	(13)	total T	T h,i	(0.89)
		pan T	T s,c	(1.09)
			T h,i/T s,c	(0.82)
			total B	(2.66)

*Data presented relative to acceptable values for all T markers of ±5% and for total B markers of ±10%. Abbreviations: all T markers = total T, pan T T h,i, T s,c, and T h,i/T s,c ratio; <ND> = not done.

RESULTS

Instrumentation

In order to determine if the use of different flow cytometers resulted in similar enumeration of lymphocytes, the same blood samples were analyzed on pairs of instruments, either the FACS IV and the EPICS C, or the FACS IV and the Spectrum III, and the obtained data were compared. A summary of the analyzed results is presented in Table 2.

Whole blood samples, stored overnight (24°C), were processed using reagents from panel 1 and the "stain and lyse" protocol. Each flow cytometer was operated by trained and experienced personnel, and special care was taken in the determination of the lymphocyte population which was "gated" and analyzed for fluorescence.

Neither the EPICS C nor the Spectrum III generated data which were completely comparable to the data generated by the FACS IV for the same sample tubes. Comparative ratios generated from the comparison of FACS IV and EPICS C data, which were not within our range of acceptance, were those of the T helper, inducer (T h,i) and the T suppressor, cytotoxic (T s,c) cells. Lower proportions of T h,i (CR of 1.10) and T s,c (CR of 1.09) positive staining cells were determined using the EPICS C then the FACS IV. However, these differences balanced out, such that the resulting T h,i/T s,c ratios were almost identical for the data generated from both instruments.

The Spectrum III, on the other hand, consistently generated values for T h,i and for T s,c, which were acceptable on an individual basis, but were at opposite ends of our range of acceptable values. The resulting T h,i/T s,c ratios were found not acceptable (CR of 1.11).

Reagent Panels

We next attempted to determine the extent to which enumeration of lymphocyte subpopulations changed as a result of the commercial source of the reagents. The specific reagents used in each reagent panel are listed in Table 1. The results of several experiments are summarized in Table 2, in which the reagents were compared using identical blood samples. Blood samples, in addition, were prepared and assayed before and after overnight storage.

Analysis of these data indicates that the resulting CR values for all T cell markers were within our predetermined range of acceptability (± 5%), regardless of whether the blood samples were assayed fresh or after overnight storage at 24°C. The values for total B cells, however, did not compare as well. The results obtained on fresh whole blood for the indirect panel 1 total B reagent (CCB1), matched neither the direct panel 1 (Leu 12-F) (CR of 1.24) nor the direct panel 2 (CCB1-F) (CR of 1.27) reagent.

This underestimation of total B, using the CCB1 reagent, was attributed to the lack, until recently, of the appropriate idiotype control monoclonal reagent from Coulter Immunology. In the absence of such a control, a non-monoclonal mixture of normal mouse immunoglobulins (normal MsIg) recommended by Coulter Immunology was used, which we found did not act as an accurate flow cytometric control for determination of total B cells. Recent availability of the appropriate idiotype control monoclonal reagent from Coulter Immunology has corrected this problem.

Next, additional data were obtained using these same blood samples to determine the effect of overnight storage, at 24°C, on whole blood for each individual reagent panel. While the T cell values obtained were all well within our acceptable range, values for total B cells were consistently underestimated, beyond acceptable limits (± 10%). This analysis, summarized in Table 2, led to the further examination of the effect of whole blood storage conditions on results obtained with several commonly used preparative methodologies.

Preparative Methodologies and Blood Storage

The relative effects of various blood preparation and storage procedures on the enumeration of lymphocytes from the same whole blood samples, prepared and assayed both fresh and after overnight storage, were examined using "direct panel 1" reagents. Analysis of the data generated is summarized in Table 3.

The data for all markers, except for a slight variation in total T (CR of 0.94), were virtually identical, regardless of storage temperature, when the "stain and lyse" protocol was used. When fresh and stored blood samples were compared using the alternative "lyse and stain" methodology, storage at 4°C had a real, if only slight effect, lowering the proportion of cells staining for T h,i (CR of 1.07), T s,c (CR of 1.07), and total B (CR of 1.13). When the data were reanalyzed to compare the effect of the two different storage temperatures, only the proportion of T h,i (CR of 1.10) positive cells were found lower, in blood stored at 4°C. Additionally, the T h,i/T s,c ratios generated from fresh and stored blood samples prepared by this methodology were the same.

The effect of storage temperature was also determined on the same blood samples, in conjunction with the comparison of the "stain and lyse" protocol and the "lyse and stain" protocol. Similar values for all markers were obtained with the exception of a very slight decrease in the total B (CR of 1.11). Such an effect (loss) on B cell marker positive lymphocytes in stored (24°C) blood was also demonstrated for each reagent panel used (Table 2).

Other, more marked effects of overnight storage (4°C) of whole blood on lymphocyte enumeration have been reported in systems based upon gradient isolation of lymphocytes (3). We therefore felt it was necessary to determine the extent to which utilization of the "gradient isolation and stain" protocol affect lymphocyte enumeration. The starting material, whole blood, was prepared and assayed either fresh or after overnight storage at 24°C. The results of analysis of several experiments, presented in Table 3 indicated that Ficoll-Hypaque gradient fractionation of whole blood before staining did not yield results similar to those obtained by direct staining and ammonium chloride treatment on the same blood samples. These differences were even more pronounced if the blood had been stored at 24°C before processing. Only values for pan T in fresh blood, and for total T and pan T in 24°C stored blood were within the range of acceptance. The greatest effect was the massive loss of total B cells after gradient isolation, relative to the whole blood method. Gradient isolation of lymphocytes resulted in a loss of greater than 40% of B cells from fresh blood (CR of 1.79) and a loss of greater than 60% from stored blood (CR of 2.66). Additionally, marked alterations were noted for T h,i and T s,c values and the generated T h,i/T s,c ratios, all of which were outside of our acceptable range for both the fresh blood (CR of 0.91) and stored blood (CR of 0.82).

CONCLUSIONS

The evaluation of an individual's immune status requires detailed information concerning the nature of the circulating immune cells. Frequently, blood samples cannot readily be assayed soon after they are drawn, and the potential for incorrect results due to storage prior to analysis is quite real. One of the main objectives of this study is to determine the most appropriate condition for overnight blood storage and processing, i.e. the conditions which will least affect the resulting enumeration of lymphocyte subsets. We also wished to compare the data generated from blood samples prepared with reagents and analyzed by flow cytometers from different manufacturers.

Based on our observations, we conclude that flow cytometric analysis of blood samples exposed to monoclonal antibodies is best performed using a whole blood "stain and lyse" protocol. If performed appropriately, the analytical results will not be dependent upon the equipment used, among the three machines tested.

In addition, it is apparent from our results that blood samples should be processed either immediately after collection or storage should be at room temperature, if it must occur.

REFERENCES

1. J. E. Grunow, R. A. Lubet, M. J. Ferguson, and M. E. Gaulden, Preferential decrease in thymus dependent lymphocytes during storage at 4°C in anticoagulant, Transfusion 16:610 (1976).
2. B. J. Weiblen, K. Debell, and C. R. Valeri, Acquired immunodeficiency of blood stored overnight, New Eng. J. Med. 309:793 (1983).
3. B. J. Weiblen, K. Debell, A. Giorgio, and C. R. Valeri, Monoclonal antibody testing of lymphocytes after overnight storage, Office of Naval Research Technical Report No. 83-12 (1983).
4. A. Boyum, Separation of leucocytes from blood and bone marrow, Scand. J. Clin. Invest. 21:Sup. 97 (1968).

V. IMMUNE RESTORATION IN VIRUS INFECTIONS

IMMUNORESTORATION OF IMMUNODEFICIENCY BY BIOLOGICAL RESPONSE MODIFIERS

Robert K. Oldham

Institute for Biological Therapy
University of British Columbia
Vancouver, British Columbia

INTRODUCTION

It is well known that there are many mediators which are important in
the generation and execution of immune responses. These mediators, when
generated by lymphoid cells or when acting on lymphoid targets, have been
termed lymphokines and those acting on non-lymphoid targets have been named
cytokines. The combination term "lymphokine/cytokine" has been used to
refer to the general class of soluble substances mediating biological responses in cell-cell interactions. These substances are distinct from,
although similar to, hormones which are generally secreted by cells within
the endocrine system acting on a remote target.

With the era of genetic engineering and the use of techniques in molecular biology to isolate, purify and characterize lymphokines/cytokines, the
new science of molecular medicine is upon us (1). In the laboratory and
with rapid translation to the clinic, scientists are isolating gene products
from mammalian cells, characterizing the gene coding for these products,
and through genetic engineering producing these products in large amounts
for preclinical and clinical testing. Unlike the lymphokines/cytokines
previously available, these products are being produced as nearly 100% pure
reagents and as such, they can be used very directly as medicinals in man
and domestic animals. Given the scientific capabilities in molecular medicine that are now available, it has been postulated that lymphokines/cyto-
kines will be developed which can correct a variety of immune deficiency
states. Crude and, more recently, purified preparations of lymphokines/cyto-
kines have been utilized in an attempt to correct congenital and acquired
immunodeficiency states and for the treatment of a variety of inflammatory,
autoimmune and neoplastic disorders. The purpose of this paper will be to
discuss some of the complexities inherent in this area and to consider some
of the difficulties and possibilities in developing lymphokines/cytokines
as medicinals for use in immunodeficiency disorders.

It is beyond the scope of this chapter to discuss the complexity of
the immune response. However, as is illustrated in Figure 1, even when
simplified, the immune response involves a variety of competing and complementary actions mediated by a large number of soluble mediators. One could
draw a diagram much more complex than Figure 1 to illustrate the known pathways associated with each component of the immune response (T-cells, B-cells,
NK-cells, macrophages, antibody, etc.). In addition to the complexity of

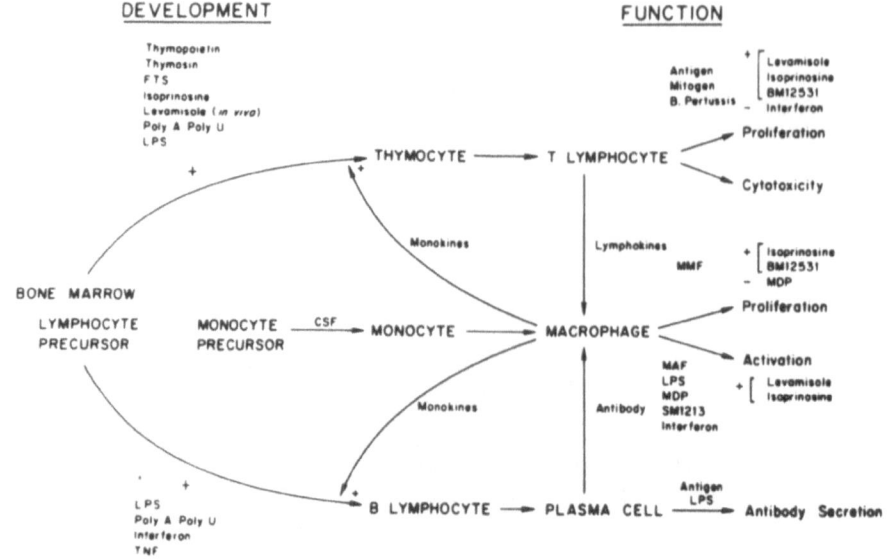

Figure 1. A Schematic Diagram of the Immune Response System

the processes surrounding each of the cell types, there is the further complexity of interactions between these cell types, the enhancement of one
aspect of the immune response may lead to a compensating suppression as the
body attempts to achieve homeostasis after any perceived disturbance.
Finally, as is illustrated in Figure 2, stimulation of any one cell to release mediators, or for that matter, with the injection of any one mediator
there is generally the release of multiple, secondary and tertiary mediators.
These may have enhancing or suppressive effects important to the immune
response being altered by the original lymphokine/cytokine. Thus, one theme
of this chapter will be to emphasize that the inherent complexity of the
immune response will make it difficult for any one mediator to be highly
effective. Unpredictable effects, in addition to those that are being
anticipated through the use of that mediator, are also potential problems.

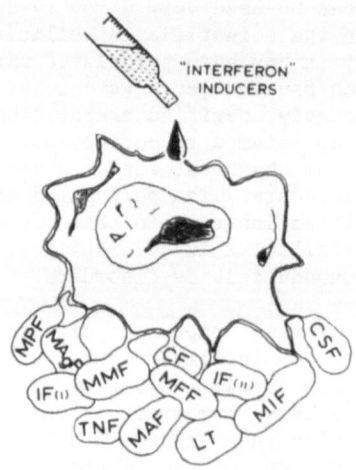

Figure 2. Inducers of interferons and other lymphokines

Table 1. Testing of RPMI 1788 Derived Lymphokines

Prep Code	MIF µg/ml for 20% I	MAF % Kill 400 µg/ml	Interferon Iu/mg protein RIA	Interferon Iu/mg protein Plaque	Chemotaxis Activity at 5 µg/ml	Endotoxin ng/mg
10786A	6.0	15%	12,100	4,000	+	3.3
10786B	1.0	44%	21,760	6,300	+	4.6
10786C	6.0	36%	17,590	2,150	+	6.2
579.2	0.2	20%	<50	<25	NT	13.6
4882	0.06	NT	3,400	1,250	NT	6.0

Another aspect of the issue is the rather high biological activity of these mediators. Lymphokines/cytokines can be active at picogram levels or less. They may have a specific major activity intrinsic to that molecule which can be exploited clinically. The isolation of the major effect of the mediator and an understanding of immunodeficiency states in such a way as to utilize the major effect of the mediator for treatment represents a real hope for the use of these mediators in the treatment of human disorders. Unfortunately, it is now apparent that many human immunodeficiency disorders are multifactorial and may require a complex therapy. Given the complexity of the immune response and given the high specific activity of these molecules in certain restricted areas, a clear understanding of the immunodeficiency state will be necessary to properly exploit the use of these mediators in clinical medicine.

LYMPHOKINES/CYTOKINES: PRECLINICAL TESTING

Lymphokines/cytokines have been known for several decades. Generally, they have been generated by the stimulation of normal lymphocytes or macrophages. These processes of stimulation, thought relatively costly and inefficient, have been used to generate supernatants from which a variety of factors have been identified with respect to their biological activity. The ultimate purification and isolation of factors from these supernatants was enormously difficult and very costly. The possibility of developing medicinals through these processes was rather remote. Some studies were done in preclinical models and in the clinic with relatively unpurified supernatants, but the field of lymphokines/cytokines was advancing very slowly because of the difficulties associated with isolation of the relatively small amount of these molecules from supernatants. Within the last decade, the technology for growing mammalian cells in vitro has improved considerably. Growth factors and nutrients needed for the growth of lymphoid and nonlymphoid cells have improved our ability to isolate short term and long term cultured cell lines. These processes have yielded a source of lymphokines and cytokines quantitatively, if not qualitatively, superior to the use of stimulated lymphoid cells. For example, one of the major interferons being utilized in clinical trials, lymphoblastoid interferon (Wellferon) is derived from the continuous lymphoblastoid cell line, Namalwa, after appropriate stimulation by virus. The cell lines may produce lymphokines/cytokines either with stimulation or constitutively. The Roswell Park Memorial Institute (RPMI) cell line, RPMI 1788, has been extensively used as a source for a variety of lymphokines/cytokines. As is shown in

Table 2. Antigen Nonspecific Mediators, Unrestricted by MHC

Helper Factors
LAD (lymphocyte activating factor – IL-1)
NMF (normal macrophage factor)
BAF (B-cell activating factor)
TRF (T-cell replacing factor)
MP (mitogenic protein)
TDF (thymus differentiation factor)
Transferrin
MF (mitogenic (blasogenic) factor)
NSF (nonspecific factor)
TDEF (T-cell-derived enhancing factor)
TEF (thymus extracted factor)
Complement components
DSRF (deficient serum restoring factor)

Suppressor Factors
Inhibitor(s) of DNA synthesis
AIM (antibody inhibitory material)
IDS (inhibitor of DNA synthesis)
LIF (lymphoblastogenesis inhibition factor)
FIF (feedback inhibition factor)
MIFIF (MIF inhibition factor)
SIRS (soluble immune response suppressor)
LIFT (lymphocyte inhibiting factor-thymus)
IRS (immunoregulatory α-globulin)
Chalones
IF (interferon)
AFP (α-fetoprotein)
LDL (low density lipoproteins)
CRP (C-reactive protein)
Fibrinogen degradation products
NIP (normal immunosuppressive protein)
LMWS (low molecular weight suppressor)
HSF (histamine-induced suppressor factor)
TCSF (T-cell suppressive factor)

Factors Acting on Inflammatory Cells
MIF (migration inhibitory factor)
MCF (macrophage chemotactic factor)
MSF (macrophage slowing factor)
MEF (migration enhancement factor)
MAF (macrophage activating factor)
MAF (macrophage aggregation factor)
MFF (macrophage fusion factor)
PRS (pyrogen releasing substance)
LIF (leukocyte inhibition factor)
NCF (neutrophil chemotactic factor)

PAR (products of antigenic recognition
BCF (basophil chemotactic factor)
ECF (eosinophil chemotactic factor)
ESP (eosinophil stimulation factor)
LCF (lymphocyte chemotactic factor)
LTF (lymphocyte trapping factor)

Factors Acting on Vascular Endothelium
SRF (skin reactive factor)
TPF (thymic permeability factor)
LNPF (lymph node permeability factor)
LNAF (lymph node activation factor)
AIPF (anaphylactoid inflammation promoting factor)
IVPF (increased vascular permeability factor)

Factors Acting on Other Cells
Interferons
TMIF (tumor cell migration inhibition factor)
OAF (osteoclast activating factor)
Fibroblast chemotactic factor
Pyrogens
FAF (fibroblast activating factor)

Growth Stimulating Factors
BCGF (B cell growth factor)
BCDF (B cell differentiation factor)
MGF (macrophage growth factor)
MF (mitogenic (blastogenic) factor)
LIAF (lymphocyte-induced angiogenesis factor)
CSF (colony stimulating factor)
TDF (thymus differentiation factor)
Thymopoietin, thmosin
TCGF (T-cell growth factor – IL-2)
IL-3 (interleukin 3)
EGF (epidemial growth factor)

Direct-Acting Factors
Lysosomal enzymes
CTF (cytotoxic factors
MTF or MCF (macrophage toxic cytotoxic factor)
SMC (specific macrophage cytotoxin)
MCF (macrophage cytolytic factor)
ACT (adherent cell toxin)
Chromosomal breakage factors
Microbicidal factors
LT (lymphotoxin)
PIF (proliferation inhibitory factor)
CIF (cloning inhibition factor)
IDS (inhibitory of DNA synthesis)
Transforming factors
TNF (tumor necrosis factor)

Adapted from B. H. Waksman, Overview: biology of the lymphokines, in: "Biology of Lymphokines," (ed.) Academic Pres (1979).

Table 1, we have been able to detect at least four biological activities, in addition to endotoxin, from preparations of the RPMI 1788 cell line (courtesy Organon Laboratories, Netherlands). Different preparations from the cell line contain strikingly different amounts of these activities. Thus, cultured cell lines may represent a good source for lymphokines/cytokines and these molecules can be purified by standard methods used in protein biochemistry. A further step along this process has included the use of the cell line genomic material as a source for the gene which can ultimately be used, through genetic engineering, to produce the desired protein in a bacterial or mammalian cell host.

It has been postulated that over 100 mediators in the lymphokine/cytokine class exist if one uses the various reports of biological activities from the supernatants of stimulated cells and/or cell lines (2). Some of these mediators are listed in Table 2 (by no means an exhaustive list).

There are those who believe that many of these biological activities can be carried out by fewer molecules than the number of substances that have been named. While it has been demonstrated that certain lymphokines/cytokines, such as gamma interferon, may have a multiplicity of activities, some of which are similar to those previously thought to be carried out by separate mediators (antiviral activity, antiproliferative activity, macrophage activation, etc.); it is also clear that there are other molecules which may carry out some of these same activities and not be part of gamma interferon. I postulate that there are many more than a hundred of these mediators and that many of the mediators named today will turn out to be families of compounds coded for by multiple genes very often with postranslational alterations that can further broaden their biological activity. Our current model is the family of compounds known as interferon. There are over twenty known varieties of alpha interferon, coded by more than fifteen different genes, in addition to beta interferon and gamma interferon which comprise this family. Although every mediator may not be part of such a large and complex family, it does seem probable that many will represent one activity of a family of compounds and not be as singular as currently imagined (3).

A major difficulty in the understanding of lymphokines/cytokines has to do with the assessment of their biological activities. The first step is an assay which can be used to characterize and quantitate a particular mediator. In fact, to even have a name for a particular biological activity, an assay must be developed. Thus, many of the mediators are named by virtue of biological activity in an assay rather than being isolated, purified molecules. Preliminary to translating these biological activities to medicinal compounds for use in man, there is the need to develop appropriate testing mechanisms in preclinical models. In the Biological Response Modifiers Program of the National Cancer Institute, we developed a preclinical screening system in an attempt to characterize the biological activity of immunomodulators and lymphokines/cytokines (4,5). While this system of evaluation is by no means complete and while this system is evolving as an understanding of these molecules and their biological activities evolve, this system does provide a standardized frame of reference in which a variety of these substances can be tested. A general outline of this program is shown in Table 3. The cellular aspects have been divided arbitrarily into the four cell types shown at the top of the table and the testing has been carried out chronologically as illustrated vertically first in vitro and then in vivo. A more complete explanation of the screening program has been published (6). The initial data from compounds tested in the screening program have been enlightening. It is already clear that all compounds do not do everything nor do many of the immunomodulators tested do absolutely nothing. Most show some evidence of selectivity with respect to the activation, enhancement or suppression of immune responses. As is shown for four

Table 3. Preclinical Screening of Biological Response Modifiers

Progression	Macrophages	NK Cells	T-Cells	B-Cells
In vitro activation in vitro testing	In vitro activation for 24 hr, 72 hr cytotoxicity assay of (^{125}I)IUdR tumor cells and 18 hr ($[^{3}H]$ln) tumor cells	In vitro activation for 24 hr, 4 hr cytotoxicity assay $\alpha(^{51}Cr)$-YAC	MLR allogeneic MLTR-CMC allogeneic	
In vivo activation—in vitro testing	Inject BRM i.v.; harvest AM and test for tumoricidal activity	Inject BRM i.v.; measure NK activity in vitro IF stimulation	Immunization αTSTA CTL	Stimulation of specific anti-body production
In vitro activation—in vivo testing		Prevention of metastasis in 3 week old mice (fibrosarcoma)	Immunization αTSTA, s.c. challenge, Alteration of tumor growth in UV-irradiated mice after immunization	
Mechanism	Kinetics of activation Induction of hypo-responsiveness	Kinetics of activation Induction of hypo-responsiveness		

Table 4.

Assay of Immunomodulation	F5	MVE-2	Poly ICLC	MDP
T-cell blastogenesis	+	–	–	+
Allogeneic MLR stimulation	+	–	–	+
Allogeneic MLTR-CMC activation	+	–	–	+
Syngeneic MLTR-CMC activation	+	NT	NT	NT
Immunoadjuvant for specific CTL	+	+	+	+
Immunoadjuvant for tumor challenge	+	+	+	+
In vitro NK cell activation	–	+	+	–
In vivo NK cell activation	–	–	+	–
In vivo NK cell immunoprophylaxis	–	+	+	–
In vitro macrophage activation	–	+	+	+
In vivo macrophage activation	–	+	+	+
Interferon stimulation	–	+	+	NT

of these compounds in Table 4, rather selective activation occurred. Thymosin fraction 5 (F5) predominantly stimulated T-cell responses while MVE-2 and Poly ICLC were most active on NK cells and macrophages. By contrast, nor-MDP had little activity on NK cells, but was quite stimulatory of both T-cells and macrophages. When these compounds were tested in immunotherapy preclinical models (Table 5), similar selectivity in vivo was seen. Thus of the nine compounds tested in the four model areas, it is clear that selectivity of activity was seen for each of these compounds.

As these immunomodulators and lymphokines/cytokines move into clinical testing, it will be of great interest to see if the selectivity observed in the preclinical testing model translates to selectivity in the treatment of human diseases. Insufficient data are available at the moment to correlate human therapeutic trials with these preclinical activities. However, the preliminary data would appear to support the concept of T-cell stimulation by the thymosins both in the preclinical model and in man, and there is some very limited indication that MVE-2 and Poly ICLC may stimulate macrophages and NK cells in both systems. There are many complexities with respect to the purity of the preparations being used, the pharmacology in man, the bioavailability and trafficking of the compound in vivo and a variety of other factors which may affect these correlations. A very important principle in the testing of these compounds in the preclinical models and in their application to man is that there are certain factors that are important in performing these evaluations and assays (Table 6). Unless these factors and others that may only be apparent later are understood, spurious results with respect to preclinical and clinical correlations may result. These factors are also important in correlating the activities of immunomodulators between laboratories. Standardization of assays and reagents is very important. It seems likely that many of the disparaties that are currently being observed may relate to some of the issues discussed above (6).

INTERLEUKIN 2

The interferons have received a great deal of attention and are quite far along in both preclinical and clinical testing. Alpha interferons are antiviral molecules with a multiplicity of actions. Beta interferon appears also to be largely antiviral. Both of these biologicals have antiprolifera-

Table 5. Comparison of BRM Induced Immunotherapy

	MVE-2	OK-432	Poly ICLC	MTP-PE	A/D BgL IFN	Thymosin F5	Lentanin	NED-137	Nor-MDP
Non-specific immunoprophylaxis	Pos.	Pos.	Pos.	STA	Pos.	Neg.	Neg.	Neg.	Neg.
Specific immunoprophylaxis	Pos.	Pos.	Pos.	Pos.	Pos.	Pos.	STA	Neg.	Pos.
Immunotherapy of experimental metastases	Prolongation of survival	STA	Pos.	Pos.	Pos.	Pos.	STA	Neg.	Pos.
Immunotherapy of spontaneous metastases	Neg.	Neg.	Pos.	Pos.	STA	Pos.	Neg.	Neg.	Pos.

Table 6.   Specific Characteristics of BRM Assays

1.   Endotoxin free reagents

2.   SPF animals

3.   Virus/mycoplasma free, tumors/animals

4.   Sequential injections/single assay

5.   Suboptimal assay

6.   Appropriate controls

tive and immunomodulatory effects in addition to their antiviral effects. The third interferon, gamma interferon, is similar to the interleukins and other lymphokines/cytokines in the sense that it has many other activities in addition to its antiviral activity. It may well be that some of these other activities will be more important and will predominate in the use of this biological as a medicinal. However, gamma interferon aside, the first lymphokine to be available for extensive testing in the clinic is Interleukin 2 (IL-2). Since the discovery of T-cell growth factor (now commonly called IL-2), its development has gone through the phases described earlier in this chapter. That is, initial experiments were carried out with crude IL-2 from cell supernatants. Like the interferons, IL-2 activity is manifest in a variety of biological assays, but the predominant activity on T-cells is illustrated in Figure 3. IL-2 was then isolated in quantity from cell lines and it was observed that IL-2 was produced selectively by certain cell lines and not produced by others (Table 7). This selectivity of production probably relates to the degree of gene activation and may provide a clue as to which cell line should be used for the isolation of the gene and its translated message. This has been done for IL-2 and the cloned, highly purified protein product is now in clinical trials. Purified

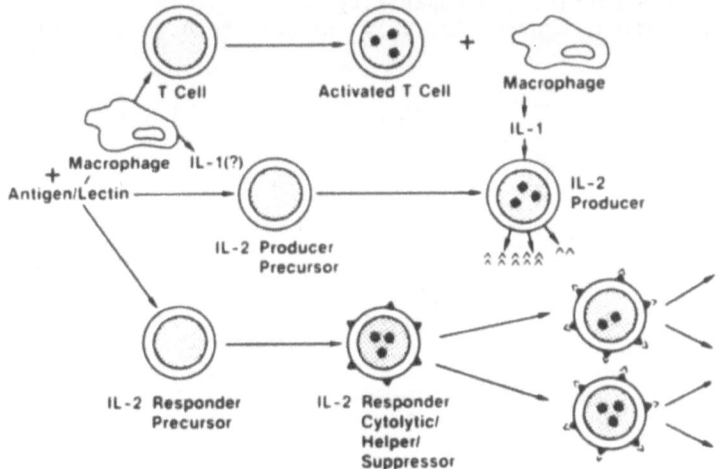

Figure 3.   IL-1/IL-2 Activity on T Cells (Adapted from
Rosetti. F. - BRMP Lymphokine Retreat)

Table 7. Screening of Human Lymphoma – Leukemia Cells for Constitutive Production of IL-2

Cutaneous T-Cell Lymphoma	IL-2 Activity (^{3}H–TdR cmp)
HUT 102	13,000 ± 3,800
HUT 78	5,600 ± 1,700
CTCL-2	3,600 ± 980
Y4TE	300 ± 70
Standard IL-2	18,000 ± 780

Cell Lines with No Activity

T-Cell Leukemia	B-cell Lymphoma – Leukemia	Non T, Non B Neoplasias
CCRF-CEM	RAMOS	NALM-1
CCRF-HSB2	RAJI	NALM-16
Molt-4	DAUDI	ML-1-3
8402	RPMI-1788	U937
T-45	RPMI-8866	KG-1
PEER-1	LPN2	K562
HPB-ALL	BJAB	HL-60
HPB-MLT	EG-3	DHL-2
JM		KM-3
SKW3		REH
TALL-1		NALL-1

Adapted from F. Rossetti, BRMP Lymphokine Retreat

IL-2 can activate T-cells (Table 8) generated through an in vitro mixed leukocyte culture (MLC). IL-2, in common with interferon and many other immunomodulators, stimulates NK activity in vitro and in vivo. Table 9 illustrates the NK activation capability of recombinant IL-2 (IL-2 courtesy of Cetus Corporation, Emeryville, CA). As will be discussed in other

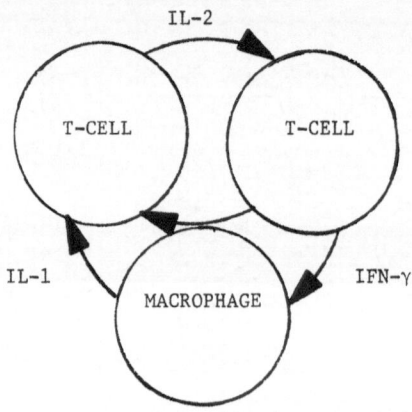

Figure 4. Interrelationship of Interleukin Lymphokines

Table 8. In Vitro Effects of Purified IL-2 on Cell-Mediated Cytotoxic
Responses Developed in 6-Day MLC[a] (1)

A. J. V. - PBL (Nezelof's Syndrome)

| Effector Cells | E:T Ratio | % Cytotoxicity (^{51}Cr Release) Target Cells | |
		Pool PHA[b]	K562
J. V. PBL (before MLC)	50:1	2	28
(J. V. PBL) · (pool x)[c]	50:1	No viable cells recovered	
(J. V. PBL) · (pool x) + IL 2	50:1	21	45

[a]Cytotoxic responses of patients J. V., A. F., and a normal individual
after 6-days in vitro mixed lymphocyte culture in the presence and absence
of exogeneous IL 2.
[b]Pool PHA denotes day three PHA lymphoblasts from a pool of PBL from ten
normal individuals.
[c]x denotes 4000 rads irradiation

(1) N. Flomenberg, K. Welte, R. Mertelsmann, R. O'Reilly, and B. Dupon,
Interleukin 2-dependent natural killer (NK) cell lines from patients
with primary T-cell immunodeficiencies, J. Immunol. 130:2635 (1983).

Table 9. IL-2 Stimulation of NK Activity

| | | In Vitro[1] | In Vivo[2] | |
			IV	IP
Medium Control		0	4	3
Poly I:C		62	9	8
Recombinant IL-2[3]	0.1 U/ml	5		
	1.0 U/ml	6		
	10.0 U/ml	15		
	100.0 U/ml	43		
Recombinant IL-2	10 U/mouse		3	4
	100 U/mouse		4	11
	1,000 U/mouse		3	13
	10,000 U/mouse		2	44

[1]Spleen cells incubated with IL-2 - 4 hr NK assay
[2]Peritoneal exudate cells - 4 hr NK assay
[3]Courtesy Biogen Corporation

chapters in this book, the predominant action of IL-2 is to stimulate T-cells and this lymphokine can be used in vitro as a growth factor in the isolation and characterization of antigen specific clones of cytotoxic T-cells. Similarly, it has been useful in the stimulation of NK cell clones. The current hope is that IL-2 can be used to generate such cells and the cells themselves can then be used in adoptive, perhaps specific, immunotherapy. IL-2 supplements may be needed to prolong these cells' activity in vivo. Early trials assessing the toxicity and biological activity of IL-2 alone when given to rodents and to man are underway (discussed by other authors in this book.)

As illustrated for interferon by Dr. Stewart (Chapter 26), IL-2 has a multiplicity of biological activities and the interactions with a variety of cell types and other mediators will be important in its ultimate in vivo activity. Figure 4 is a simplistic diagram illustrating the interaction and overlap of gamma interferon, IL-1 and IL-2 in T-cell macrophage interactions. Given the actual complexity of these interactions and given the apparent multiplicity of defects present in the acquired immunodeficiency syndrome (AIDS), it does not seem highly probable that IL-2 alone will totally correct the immunodeficiencies associated with this complex syndrome.

However, given the T-cell defect therein, it does seem reasonable to attempt to reconstitute T-cell function in these individuals with IL-2 and/or cells in an attempt to protect them from the many infections to which they are susceptible. The complexity of this clinical syndrome may ultimately require the use of multiple mediators in specific ratios if one is to attempt total reconstitution of such a complex immunodeficiency state. Perhaps there are immunodeficiencies which exist in man which are more singular and if those immunodeficiency states relate to a certain T-cell population, IL-2 with its ability to stimulate T-cells in vitro and in vivo may prove useful in reconstituting that immunodeficiency state (7).

THE INTERFERONS: A LESSON LEARNED

As is illustrated in Figure 5, there are several types of interferon and each has now been made by both recombinant and nonrecombinant technologies. For the alpha interferons, clinical testing is very far along with phase I trials being virtually complete and phase II trials well underway (8,9). Early phase III trials to utilize alpha interferon in combination with other modalities or in place of other modalities have now begun. What have we learned from the use of this mediator in clinical trials? Initially, alpha interferon was visualized as an antiviral molecule since that was the biological activity used to define the molecule. Further testing indicated

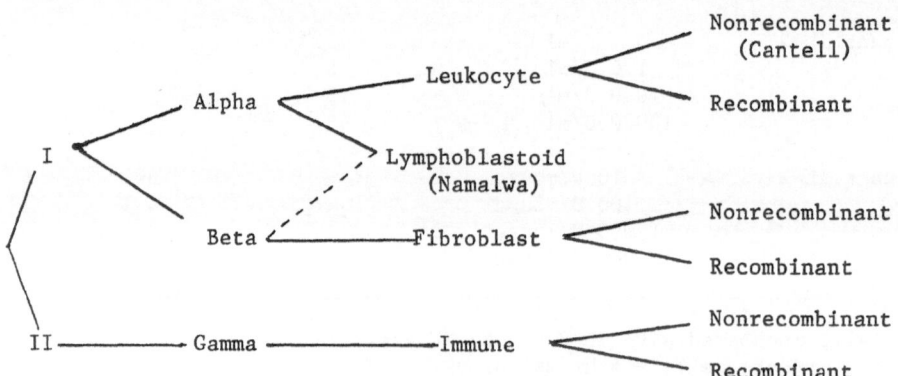

Figure 5. Interrelationship of Interleukin Lymphokines

Table 10.   Phase II Recombinant Leukocyte A Interferon Trial

	Evaluable Patients	Complete Responses	Partial Response	No Response	Progression
Favorable NHL	25	2	14	3	6
Unfavorable NHL	6	0	2	0	4
CLL	8	0	3	2	3
MF	11	0	8	1	2

that it might have some activity as an antitumor agent and there were indications that it could have both antiproliferative and immunomodulatory capabilities. Thus, even during the initial phases of development, three predominant activities (antiviral, antiproliferative and immunomodulatory) were apparent. Each of these activities is in itself complex with selectivity of action of the alpha interferon preparations having been observed in each of the three areas. That is, an interferon is not equally antiviral, antiproliferative or immunomodulatory for all cell populations. Additionally, different alpha interferons display different levels of biological activity. Although there were those who predicted that interferon would be a "wonder drug" in the treatment of viral disorders and malignancies, it is now abundantly clear that the alpha interferons, like many other anticancer compounds, have rather selective actions in certain tumors and have little clinical activity in others (9). In our hands, alpha interferon of the recombinant type (courtesy of Hoffman-La Roche; Genetech, Inc.) has induced regressions in greater than 60 percent of patients with "favorable" histology, non-Hodgkin's lymphoma and in patients with cutaneous T-cell lymphomas (10,11). Less activity has been seen in the unfavorable histology lymphomas and in chronic lymphocytic leukemia (Table 10). The clinical activity for this alpha interferon was rather remarkable in light of the fact that these patients were resistant to multiple drug chemotherapy and to radiotherapy. They had aggressive, advancing disease for which an effective anticancer regimen was needed. For over half of these patients, alpha interferon proved to be an effective anticancer biological inducing partial and complete regressions with a median duration of response in excess of eight months. Several patients became unresponsive to low doses of interferon and were induced into further partial remissions with higher doses of the biological (11). These data would seem to indicate that the predominant mechanism of action for this alpha interferon in these patients under these conditions was antiproliferative. This is an example of the utilization of one of the biological activities of lymphokine/cytokines for exploitation as medicinals. Although tested across a broad dose range, the immunomodulatory effects of this alpha interferon did not appear to correlate with the clinical activity of the biological. This is not to say that alpha interferon will not have significant immunomodulatory activities which may be of use clinically. However, for lymphoma these data do seem to indicate that the predominant mechanism of action for this recombinant interferon was antiproliferative. This is an example of isolating one of the biological activities and exploiting it in a specific clinical circumstance.

There are now data to support the conclusion that alpha interferons have activity in a variety of human cancers (Table 11). In several of these tumors, in a manner similar to the lymphomas, more interferon appeared to

Table 11.   Interferon Phase II Studies

Tumor Type	Interferon	Dose	CR & PR Total	Reference
Renal	α-Cantell	3 mu daily	5/19	Quesada[1]
Renal	α1-Recombinant	50 mu tiw	2/19	Krown[6]
Renal	α1-Recombinant	2-20 mu daily	2/16	Quesada[7]
Melanoma	α-Lymphoblastoid	2.5 mu/m^2 daily	1/17	Retsas[2]
Melanoma	α1-Recombinant	50 mu/m^2 x 3 wk	7/31	Cregan[4]
Myeloma	α-Cantell	3-9 mu daily	6/10	Gutterman[3]
Lymphoma	α-Cantell	3-9 my daily	6/11	Gutterman[3]
Kaposi[1]	various	Low dose<10 mu/m^2 d	1/17	Hersh[5]
		High dose>20 mu/m^2 d	14/34	Hersh[5]
Hairy Cell Leukemia	α-Cantell	3 mu/m^2 daily	7/7	Hersh[5]
CML	α-Cantell	3 mu/m^2 daily	16/22	Hersh[5]

[1]Data for summary by Dr. Evan Hersh presented in Vienna, 1983 summarizing data from Rios et al. (unpublished), Kron (5/12 NEJM) and Volberding (ASCO Abstract #C-206).

References:

[1]Quesada, Cancer Res. 43:940 (1983).
[2]Retsas, Cancer 51:273 (1983).
[3]Gutterman, Annals 93:399 (1980).
[4]Cregan, Cancer (in press, 1983).
[5]Hersh, presented, Vienna (1983).
[6]Krown, ASCO Abstract #225 (1983).
[7]Quesada, AACR Abstract #759 (1983).

be superior to less in inducing or reinducing clinical responses (9,12). However, we have all observed cases where responses have occurred with rather small doses of the interferon. In fact, in our studies, we have seen partial responses at 100,000 units and at ten million units of interferon in two separate patients with melanoma. This wide dose range indicates that the interferon may work in one circumstance by one mechanism of action and in another by a different mechanism of action. Such observations should be kept in mind in the continued testing of the interferons and other lymphokines/cytokines for clinical activity. Table 12 illustrates tumors for which antitumor activity of alpha interferon is reasonably clear. The activity in acute leukemias, though present, has not been clinically meaningful. In breast cancer, the Cantell preparations have been more active than the recombinant alpha interferons. For the other tumors in Table 12, clinical activity has been seen with a variety of interferons in a variety of doses and schedules. It now will be important to compare the interferons with other active agents and to determine the effect of interferon when used in a complementary way with existing active anticancer agents.

Table 12. Antitumor Activity of Alpha Interferon

Non-Hodgkin's Lymphoma

Renal Cell Carcinoma

Mycosis Fungoides

Chronic Lymphocytic Leukemia

Breast Carcinoma

Myeloma

Acute Leukemia

Kaposi's Sarcoma/AIDS

Osteosarcoma

Laryngeal Papillomatosis

Bladder Papillomata

MONOCLONAL ANTIBODY IN IMMUNODEFICIENCY STATES

The testing of monoclonal antibody as a medicinal is in a much earlier phase than the testing described above for the interferons (13,14). Basically, the very early observations of toxicity and biological activity are just being made in man and rest on a rather thin preclinical base. The specificity of monoclonal antibodies will require the major testing ground to be man with respect to both biological activity and toxicity. While there are many trials in progress for the use of monoclonal antibody as a direct tumortargeting agent and as the selective component of immunoconjugate, antibodies can also be envisaged as biologicals which may be useful in the treatment of immunodeficiency states. It is now known that certain lymphocyte subsets can be suppressive and/or overactive in clinical disorders. It is also known that monoclonal antibodies can be used to rather specifically deplete or delete such lymphocyte subsets. For T-cells alone there are now a variety of antibodies defining surface antigens (Table 13). As a clinician identifies immunodeficiency states in man where a specific T-cell subpopulation is overactive, the possibility of using monoclonal antibody, with cells, with complement or as an immmunoconjugate will exist. Already there are preliminary data to indicate that monoclonal antibodies can be used to deplete T-cell subsets which may have important therapeutic consequences (15). Particularly for the autoimmune disorders which can be interpreted as immunodeficiency states, the use of monoclonal antibodies for selective alteration of subpopulations may be important. Unfortunately, the laws of physics may apply equally in biology. That is, for every action there is a reaction and the use of monoclonal antibody in an attempt to deplete certain subpopulations will prompt compensatory responses, both cellular and humoral, by the individual in reaction to this therapy. Our findings in chronic lymphocytic leukemia and in cutaneous T-cell lymphoma are not accompanied by a severe immunodeficiency state as currently defined. Thus, with the use of monoclonal antibody there is an augmentation and stimulation of antiglobulin responses in the body's attempt to eliminate the mouse monoclonal antibody which was injected. By contrast, in chronic lymphocytic leukemia where B-cell immunodeficiency exists, no such antiglobulin response has thus far been encountered. These kinds of observations may prove useful in designing therapeutic strategies with monoclonal antibodies in the treatment of immunodeficiency states (17).

Table 13. Identification of Cell Surface Antigens of T-Lymphocyte
Subsets by Monoclonal Antibodies

Antibody	Distribution	Antigen Size	Synonyms
OKT 1	Pan-T 10-60% Thymocytes	65-69,000	Leu-1, T101, 10.2
OKT 3	Pan-T 60% Thymocytes	19,000	Leu-4
OKT 4	Helper/Inducer	62,000	Leu-3
OKT 5	Cytotoxic/suppressor	76,000 (30K, 32K)	Leu-2
OKT 8	Cytotoxic/suppressor		
OKT 6	70% Thymocytes	49,000	NA1/34
OKT 9	10% Thymocytes	190,000 (94K)	5E9
OKT 10	5% T Most thymocytes precursor myeloid Bone marrow B lymphocytes		
OKT 11	Pan-T		
B1	Pan-B		
BA 1	Pan-B Granulocytes		

From our data and from the data of others using monoclonal antibody in clinical trials, it is now clear that these mouse antibodies can be administered to man reasonably safe with interesting biological consequences (Table 14). These preliminary results would seem to indicate that antibody therapy for cancer, autoimmune disorders and selected immunodeficiency states is practical although much remains to be learned about the clinical efficacy of antibody. On the issue of mouse monoclonals being immunogenic in man, it is apparent that human monoclonals will also be immunogenic at a lower level by virtue of idiotype reactions.

The idiotype story provides the most specific approach to the treatment of certain immunodeficiency states. The principles utilized by Miller and Levy in the treatment of lymphoma (18) will be applicable to immunodeficiency or "autoimmune" states as well. When there is lymphoid cell population which is present in excess or which is overactive, the immunoglobulin determinant idiotype on the surface of the T-cell can be used as the immunogenic entity to create anti-idiotype antibody. This anti-idiotype antibody is selectively active only on the cells bearing the idiotype. Thus, one has the capability to generating reagents highly selective in their activity and theoretically useful in the treatment of disorders where a specific specific subpopulation bearing a specific idiotype needs to be eliminated. Idiotypic immunoglobulin can be created through a variety of methods (Table 15) and anti-idiotypic antibody can be generated through a variety of techniques (19). Although these techniques are currently rather laborious and costly, it is probable that improvements in the technology of monoclonal

Table 14. Results of Monoclonal Antibody Serotherapy Trials

_____

1. Dosages from 1 mg to 1,500 mg can be given with minimal side effects.

2. Intravenous therapy can be given rapidly (15 minutes) or over several
    hours without immediate side effects.

3. A rapid drop in the leukemic blast cell count in the peripheral blood
    generally occurs immediately, but returns to pretreatment levels within
    hours.

4. Sustained reduction of leukemic blast cell count in the peripheral
    blood can occur with repeated dosages of antibody given biweekly over
    several weeks.

5. Bone marrow leukemic cells were not decreased (Ritz et al., _Blood_ 58:78
    (1981)).

6. Skin lesion and enlarged lymph nodes dramatically responded to MoAB
    serotherapy (Miller and Levy, _Lancet_ ii:226 (1981)).

_____

antibody generation, and more specifically of monoclonal anti-idiotypic
antibody generation, will provide mechanisms for the more rapid generation
of these reagents soon. Thus, the more selective treatment of certain
immunodeficiency disorders is on the horizon.

CANCER AS AN IMMUNODEFICIENCY STATE

     There are data to indicate that many cancer patients have discrete or
more general defects in their immune capabilities. Many investigators have
postulated that these immune defects have preceded the cancer and are causative in cancer etiology. While this remains a controversial subject, empir-
ical trials to activate or alter immune responses in patients with cancer
have been attempted (20). Lymphokines/cytokines are now being tested in
cancer patients in an attempt to understand their toxicities and their biological activities. Unfortunately, as was discussed earlier for AIDS, cancer
is undoubtedly a complex problem in biology. Even within specific cancer
types there may be considerable variation from patient to patient as to the
role the immune system may play in the generation of the malignancy and in
its subsequent growth and development. The use of biological compounds to
affect one component of this interaction would not seem likely to be successful in changing dramatically the tumor host interaction. As for the immuno-

Table 15. Sources of Idiotypic Immunoglobulin

_____

1. Circulating paraprotein

2. Extraction

3. Direct stimulation

4. Homohybrids or heterohybrids

_____

deficiency factor, it may be possible in selected patients with certain malignancies to identify a predominant immunodeficiency. That is, one may be able to identify a specific defect in the immune response, correctable by the use of a biological reagent. In that circumstance, the use of a biological may prove beneficial to the patient. There is much to be learned from the area of transplantation immunology in this regard. The clear example of tumor regressions after the withdrawal of immunosuppressive therapy in patients who have developed malignancies after transplantation is an interesting lead. As our understanding of the induced immunodeficiency and the secondary regression of the tumor with the withdrawal of immunosuppressive therapy improves, the hope for using biologicals in an analogous way will gain credence. The current trials using biologicals in cancer patients should be seen as rather crude attempts to derive some very preliminary information about the toxicity and biological activity of these compounds rather than definitive methods of biological therapy. From these early observations, one can proceed with a more rational utilization of lymphokines/cytokines as medicinals. For example, the antiproliferative activity of the interferons in lymphoma is now apparent. This was not apparent early in the interferon trials for lymphoma. In fact, many postulated that the interferon was working through correction of some poorly defined immunodeficiency in these patients. Now that it is clear from the preliminary trials that an antiproliferative activity is the important mediator for the antitumor activity of alpha interferon in lymphomas, rational trials designed to explore dose and schedule and the interaction of interferon with other antitumor approaches are now possible. The interferons have provided a model for what we can learn from these preliminary clinical trials. Investigators should approach IL-2 and the subsequent lymphokines/cytokines available for clinical trials with a similarly open mind and aspire to go in the direction the data might lead with respect to the design of secondary and tertiary trials. This may prove a superior strategy for the use of these biologicals as opposed to the a priori design of clinical trials based on investigators or groups of investigators' assumptions of the clinical activities of these compounds.

REFERENCES

1. R. K. Oldham, Biologicals and biological response modifiers: fourth modality of cancer treatment, Cancer Treat. Rpt. 68(1):221 (1984).
2. B. H. Waksman, Overview: biology of the lymphokines, in: "Biology of Lymphokines," eds., Academic Press (1979).
3. R. K. Oldham, G. N. Thurman, J. E. Talmadge, et al., Lymphokines, monoclonal antibodies and other biological response modifiers in the treatment of cancer, Cancer 1(54) (Supp. 11):2795 (1984).
4. R. K. Oldham, Biological response modifiers program, J. Biol. Resp. Modif. 1:81 (1982).
5. I. J. Fidler, M. Berendt, and R. K. Oldham, The rationale for design of screening assays for the assessment of biological response modifiers for cancer treatment, J. Biol. Resp. Modif. 1:15 (1982).
6. J. E. Talmadge, R. K. Oldham, and I. J. Fidler, Practical considerations for the establishment of a screening procedure for the assessment of biological response modifiers, J. Biol. Resp. Modif. 3:88 (1984).
7. N. Flomenberg, K. Welte, R. Mertelsmann, et al., Immunologic effects of interleukin 2 in primary immunodeficiency diseases. IV. J. Immunol. 130:2644 (1983).
8. S. A. Sherwin, J. A. Knost, S. Fein, et al., A multiple dose phase I trial of recombinant leukocyte A interferon in cancer patients, JAMA 248:2461 (1982).
9. R. K. Oldham and R. V. Smalley, The role of interferon in the treatment of cancer, Proceedings of the Workshop in Interferon, in press (1984).

10. K. A. Foon, S. A. Sherwin, P. G. Abrams, et al., Recombinant leukocyte A interferon: an effective agent for the treatment of advanced non-Hodgkin's lymphoma, N. Eng. J. Med. 311(18):1148 (1984).

11. P. A. Bunn, Jr., K. A. Foon, D. C. Idhe, et al., Recombinant leukocyte A interferon: an active agent in advanced cutaneous T-cell lymphomas, Annals Int. Med. 101(4):484 (1984).

12. J. M. Kirkwood and M. S. Ernstoff, Interferons in the treatment of human cancer, J. Clin. Oncol. 2:336 (1984).

13. R. K. Oldham, Monoclonal antibodies in cancer therapy, J. Clin. Oncol. 1:582 (1983).

14. R. K. Oldham, K. A. Foon, A. C. Morgan, et al., Monoclonal antibody therapy of malignant melanoma: in vivo localization in cutaneous metastasis after intravenous administration, J. Clin. Oncol. 2(11): 1235 (1984).

15. A. B. Cosimi, R. B. Colvin, R. C. Burton, et al., Use of monoclonal antibodies to T-cell subsets for immunologic monitoring and treatment in recipients of renal allografts, N. Eng. J. Med. 305:308 (1981).

16. K. A. Foon, R. W. Schroff, P. A. Bunn, et al., Effects of monoclonal antibody therapy in patients with chronic lymphocytic leukemia, Blood 64(5):1085 (1984).

17. R. W. Schroff, K. A. Foon, S. B. Wilburn, et al., Human antimurine immunoglobulin responses in patients receiving monoclonal antibody therapy, Cancer Res. 45(2):879 (1985).

18. R. A. Miller, D. G. Maloney, R. Warnke, et al., Treatment of B-cell lymphoma with monoclonal anti-idiotype antibody, N. Eng. J. Med. 306:517 (1982).

19. S. L. Giardina, R. W. Schroff, C. S. Woodhouse, et al., Detection of two distinct malignant B-cell clones in a single patient using anti-idiotype monoclonal antibodies and immunoglobulin in gene rearrangement, (submitted, 1984).

20. R. K. Oldham and R. V. Smalley, Immunotherapy: the old and the new, J. Biol. Resp. Modif. 2:1 (1983).

ENDOGENOUS IMMUNOMODULATORS FROM HUMAN LEUKOCYTES AS AGENTS

FOR IMMUNORESTORATION IN PATIENTS WITH AIDS

A. Arthur Gottlieb, Jeffrey F. Farmer, and
Toru Nishihara

IMREG Inc., and the Department of Microbiology-Immunology
Tulane University School of Medicine
New Orleans, Louisiana

In previous reports, we have called attention to a group of endogenous immunoamplifiers present in human leukocyte dialysates (1,2). Two of these immunoamplifiers which we designate as IMREG-1 and IMREG-2 augment delayed hypersensitivity to recall antigens, and enhance the production of lymphokines by lymphocytes of the T helper/inducer phenotype. The immunologic properties of leukocyte dialysates have been studied for many years since their discovery by Dr. Lawrence in 1954 (3). In our judgment, IMREG-1, IMREG-2 and a group of similar molecules in the dialysate which we have identified may well account for some of the immunologic properties of these dialysates. These substances need to be clearly distinguished from specific "transfer factor(s)." The most critical functional distinction between "transfer factor(s)" and the IMREG immunoamplifiers is that the action of the latter is dependent on the presence of an antigen to which the recipient individual or cells have been previously sensitized. Since AIDS patients have a profound deficit in T helper function (4,5) we thought it worthwhile to explore the effect of the immunoamplifier IMREG-1 in patients with this condition, and we describe our results in this chapter.

The IMREG-1 immunoamplifier is prepared from leukocyte dialysates obtained from healthy individuals according to methods which have been previously reported by our group (1,2). In highly purified form, IMREG-1 prepared from 4×10^6 leukocytes can be diluted 10^6 fold and at that concentration significantly accelerates and enhances delayed type hypersensitivity reactions to recall antigens (Figures 1 and 2). It is important to note that the particular antigenic sensitivities of the donor used to prepare the leukocyte dialysates is irrelevant--the immunoamplifier prepared from a tuberculin (PPD) negative donor is fully capable of augmenting delayed hypersensitivity to PPD in an individual who is PPD reactive.

In a prior report (2), we described the ability of the immunoamplifier, IMREG-1, to enhance the production of the migration-inhibitory lymphokines MIF and LIF by T4-enriched cells over and above the levels of these lymphokines produced by these cells in response to an antigenic or mitogenic stimulus alone. The same phenomenon can be shown for interleukin-2. In the study shown in Table 1, peripheral lymphocytes, purified on ficoll-hypaque gradients, are incubated with phytohemagglutinin in the presence of various concentrations of IMREG-1. The culture supernatants arerecovered and tested for interleukin-2 (IL-2) activity on CTLL-2 target cells according to the method of Gillis et al. (6).

In Table 1, the results of studies on four normal subjects are displayed. The production of interleukin-2 (IL-2) in response to the dosages of PHA shown is evaluated as a function of the addition of IMREG-1, an undiluted preparation of which contains the immunoamplifier derived from 4×10^8 leukocytes/ml. We observed that for every test subject and at nearly every dose of PHA, there is an enhancement by IMREG-1 of the amount of IL-2 produced in response to PHA alone.

By treating the PBLs of a healthy individual with monoclonal OK T8 antibody and complement, it was possible to show that the effect of IMREG-1 is exerted on the T4 (helper) lymphocyte subset (Table 2). T8 enriched populations assayed simultaneously did not produce significant IL-2 under any conditions. In studies not shown here we were able to demonstrate that IMREG-1 has no effect on IL-2 production in the absence of a stimulus such as mitogen or antigen. Table 3 presents the results of our studies of the effect of IMREG-1 on interleukin-2 production by lymphocytes, obtained from asymptomatic individuals at high risk for AIDS, and challenged with PHA, while Table 4 illustrates the results of similar studies on PBLs derived from symptomatic patients with the AIDS Related Complex (ARC). In the

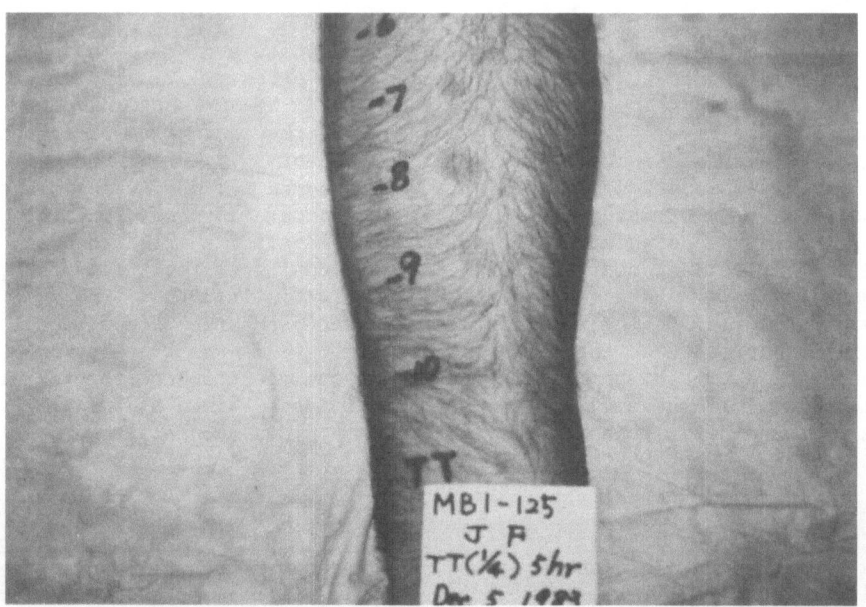

Figure 1. Leukocyte modulator was prepared and stored as a stock solution containing modulator derived from 4×10^8 leukocytes/ml. Fifty μl aliquots of this stock solution were dispensed into vials, lyophilized and reconstituted in 0.5 ml normal saline. This defines a 10^{-1} dilution of the original stock solution. Serial ten fold dilutions of this preparation were made in normal saline. In this figure, 0.05 ml of tetanus toxoid (Fluid, containing 2 Lf/ml) was separately combined with 0.1 ml of the 10^{-6}, 10^{-7}, 10^{-8}, 10^{-9}, and 10^{-10} dilutions of the original modulator preparation and injected intradermally at the sites designated -6, -7, -8, -9, and -10. The same amount of tetanus toxoid (0.05 ml of 2 lf/ml) + 0.1 ml of normal saline was injected intradermally at the site designated TT. The photograph was taken at five hours after injection. Note the reactions at the -7, -8 and -9 sites.

symptomatic high-risk group, basal interleukin-2 production, in response to PHA, varied across a broad range, but could be amplified in every case by addition of IMREG-1. In the three patients with ARC (Table 4) the production of IL-2 in response to PHA was subnormal and could be amplified significantly in two out of three cases. Patient RB was of particular interest in that his basal interleukin-2 production was nil and no improvement was observed in the presence of IMREG-1. This patient was given IMREG-1 subcutaneously (4 x 10^5 leukocyte equivalents) at approximately monthly intervals. After the fourth cycle of therapy, his basal interleukin-2 production rose to significant levels (Table 5) and the addition of IMREG-1 in vitro augmented his interleukin-2 production. This patient received additional doses of IMREG-1 as shown in Table 5. His basal interleukin-2 level rose to normal and modulation of his IL-2 production by IMREG-1 in vitro was considerable. After the last cycle of IMREG-1 (11/11/83), the patient was able to mount a 32mm x 24 mm reaction to tetanus toxoid, an antigen to which he had been completely unreactive eight months earlier. Patient RF also received more than one cycle of IMREG-1. His interleukin-2 production was not followed due to low cell yields, but he also regained his ability to mount a delayed hypersensitivity reaction to tetanus toxoid, after two doses of IMREG-1, having been completely unresponsive to this antigen before treatment.

In a separate study, the mitogen (PHA) responsiveness of PBLs from three patients with AIDS and Kaposi's sarcoma were studied following a single

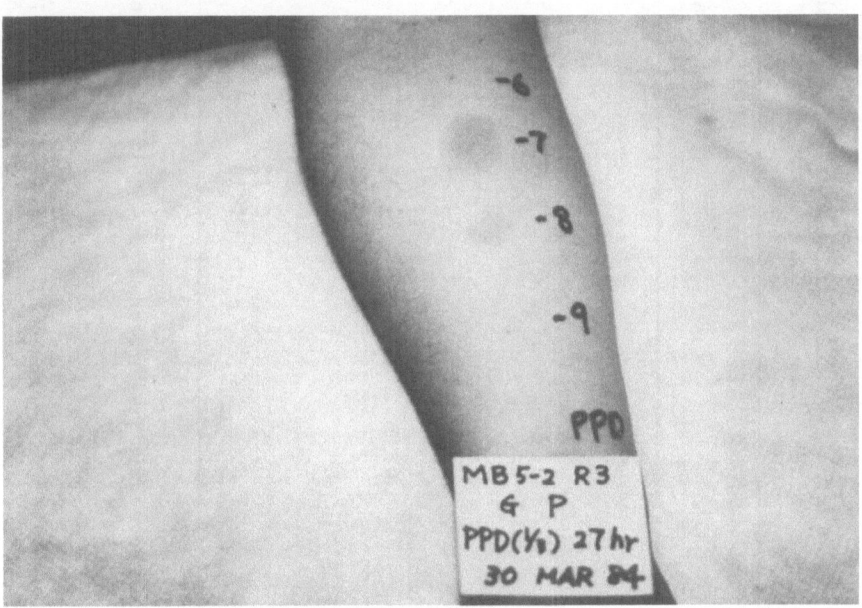

Figure 2.   Leukocyte modulator was prepared as indicated in the legend to Figure 1. 0.05 ml of Tuberculin PPD (1/3 dilution of 5 TU/0.1 ml in normal saline) was separately combined with 0.1 ml of the 10^{-6}, 10^{-7}, 10^{-8}, and 10^{-9} dilutions of the original modulator preparation and injected intradermally at the sites designated -6, -7, -8, and -9. 0.05 ml of the diluted PPD preparation plus 0.1 ml of normal saline was injected at the site designated PPD. The photograph was taken 27 hours after injection. Note the reactions at the -7 and -8 sites.

Table 1. Modulation by IMREG-1 of Production of Interleukin-2 by PHA-Stimulated Normal PBLs.

Donor #	PHA (μg/ml)	− IMREG-1	Units/ml of IL-2 produced with indicated dilution of IMREG-1[a]		
			+1/500	+1/1000	+1/2000
1	0.25	0	0.004[c]	0.0019[c]	0.0025[c]
	0.5	0.38	0.59[c]	0.68[c]	0.79[c]
	1.0	1.62	2.38[c]	2.29[c]	2.14[c]
	0.25	0.0002	0.0003	0.293[c]	0.0039[c]
2	0.5	3.39	3.90[c]	3.67	3.91[c]
	1.0	11.6	11.8[c]	11.8	13.0[c]
	0.25	4.46	NT[b]	4.3	4.4
3	0.5	8.30	NT	9.2[c]	9.0[c]
	1.0	8.30	NT	10.4[c]	16.8[c]
4	0.25	0.12	0.30[c]	0.35[c]	0.63[c]
	0.5	2.18	2.22	2.70[c]	2.23

[a] IL-2 measured in 24 hour culture supernatants. In this and subsequent tables, undiluted IMREG-1 contains modulator derived from 4×10^8 leukocytes in 1.0 ml normal saline

[b] NT = not tested

[c] indicates IL-2 level in presence of IMREG-1 significantly different from PHA alone (p at least < 0.05).

Table 2. Modulation of Normal PBL PHA-induced IL-2 by IMREG-1: Effect of Enrichment for T Cell Subsets

Cell Type	PHA (µg/ml)	-IMREG-1	+1/500	+1/1000	+1/2000	+1/4000
C'control	0.125	0.004	0.008	0.013[+]	0.01[+]	0.015[+]
	0.25	1.16	0.90	1.08	1.51[+]	2.70[+]
	0.5	4.72	5.35[+]	6.69[+]	5.20	5.48[+]
	1.0	6.70	6.94	8.32[+]	6.65	6.82
T4 enriched*	0.125	0.007	0.003	0.015[+]	0.038[+]	0.037[+]
	0.25	1.40	2.15[+]	2.13[+]	2.14[+]	2.17[+]
	0.5	5.35	6.07[+]	6.27[+]	5.72	5.76
	1.0	6.71	7.96[+]	7.83[+]	6.49	6.41

*Prepared by depletion with OKT8+C'; residual contamination with T8+ cells less than 0.1% by FACS analysis. T8 enriched cell populations, assayed simultaneously, did not produce significant IL-2 at any of the PHA concentrations employed.

[+]indicates IL-2 level in presence of IMREG-1 significantly different from PHA alone (P at least <0.05).

Table 3. Modulation by IMREG-1 of Interleukin-2 Production by PHA-Stimulated PBLs
from Asymptomatic Individuals at High Risk for AIDS

| | % of Lymphocytes | | | | | PHA (μg/ml) | Units/ml Interleukin-2 Produced at 24 Hours with Indicated Dilution of IMREG-1[a] | | | |
	T3	T4	T8	Leu 11a	T4/T8		-IMREG-1	+1/500	+1/1000	+1/2000
HC	89.7	57	21.3	10.8	2.68	0.5	1.1	1.1	1.82	0.94[+]
						1.0	6.6	12.2[+]	13.1[+]	9.9[+]
TN	ND	32.6	29.9	ND	1.09	0.25	0.19	0.30*	0.35*	0.63*
						0.5	2.18	2.22	2.70	2.23
JG	78.5	41.3	31.9	11.4	1.29	0.5	0.09	0	0.103*	0.176*
						1.0	0.21	0.76*	1.24*	0.48*
MR	59.8	38.8	27.3	20.5	1.42	1.0	0.075	0.15[+]	0.45[+]	0.10

[+]Significant at p < 0.05 level

*Significant at p < 0.01 level

[a]PBLs were incubated with PHA in the presence of the indicated dilutions of immunomodulator

Table 4. Modulation by IMREG-1 of Interleukin-2 Production by PHA-Stimulated PBLs from Symptomatic Patients with Prodromal AIDS

| | | % of Lymphocytes | | | | PHA | Units/ml Interleukin-2 Produced at 24 Hours with Indicated Dilution of IMREG-1[a] | | | |
	T3	T4	T8	Leu 11a	T4/T8	(μg/ml)	IMREG-1	+1/500	+1/1000	+1/2000
MC	69.5	13.8	41.9	0	0.33	0.25	0.44	0.70[+]	0.39	0.39
						0.50	1.52	2.12[+]	2.3[+]	2.3[+]
						1.0	2.08	3.71[+]	3.71[+]	3.84[+]
RB√	ND	16	43	ND	0.37	0.25	0	0	0	0
						0.50	0	0	0	0
						1.0	0	0	0	0
RF	ND	9.8	68.1	ND	0.14	1.0	0.06	0.08	0.09	0.21*

[+]Significant at p < 0.05 level

*Significant at p < 0.01 level

√See Table 5 for later studies

[a]PBLs were incubated with PHA in the presence of the indicated dilutions of immunomodulator

Table 5. In Vitro Modulation of PHA-Induced Interleukin-2 Production by IMREG-1

Prodromal AIDS Patient RB

Date*	PHA (μg/ml)	Modulator Dosage^x	Units/ml Interleukin-2 Produced at 24 hours in Presence of Indicated Dilution of Modulator			
			−IMREG-1	+1/500	+1/1000	+1/2000
08/01/83	0.5	4 x 10^5	0.004	0.01[+]	0.017[+]	0.027[+]
08/02/83	1.0		0.68	0.69	0.69	0.78
10/11/83		4 x 10^5				
10/31/83	1.0	4 x 10^5	0.28	0.55[+]	1.37[+]	0.60[+]
11/08/83	1.0		0.05	0.05	0.13[+]	0.04
11/11/83	0.5		0.14	0.62[+]	0.51[+]	0.77[+]
	1.0		1.76	1.83	2.86[+]	2.57[+]

*At other time points tested, no IL-2 was induced by PHA alone, and the addition of IMREG-1 did not result in appearance of IL-2 activity in culture supernatants.

[+]Difference between PHA alone, PHA and IMREG-1, significant at $p < 0.05$.

^{x}Amount of modulator derived from indicated cell numbers

dose of IMREG-1. As shown in Figure 3, PHA responses increased significantly in all three cases, following administration of IMREG-1.

Finally, we had a unique opportunity to study the effect of IMREG-1 in a patient with AIDS with Kaposi's sarcoma who had a healthy identical twin. The patient was first seen in early August 1983, at which time his PHA responsiveness and IL-2 production were minimal and he had documented widespread Kaposi's sarcoma. At the time indicated in Figure 4, he received a first transfusion of isologous leukocytes from his identical twin brother whose T4 cell number, PHA responsiveness and IL-2 production to PHA were normal. In addition, he received a dose of IMREG-1 derived from 4×10^5 leukocytes. There was an increase in PHA responsiveness from the initial transfusion, but this was not further increased by the first dose of IMREG-1. His immune function continued to fall back to baseline over a period of four days, at which time a second isologous leukocyte transfusion was given along with three sequential doses (4×10^5, 4×10^6, and 4×10^5 cell equivalents) of IMREG-1. Following this maneuver there was a striking increase in the patient's PHA responsiveness and an increase in his T4/T8 ratio which was attributable to an absolute increase in T4 cells. These parameters reached a peak and began to decline. The patient was clinically stable at this time. A third isologous transfer without IMREG-1 resulted in no improvement in any immune parameters.

These results are reflected in the IL-2 data which were accumulated over the course of treatment of this patient with IMREG-1 (Table 6). The time points at which isologous leukocytes and IMREG-1 were given are shown

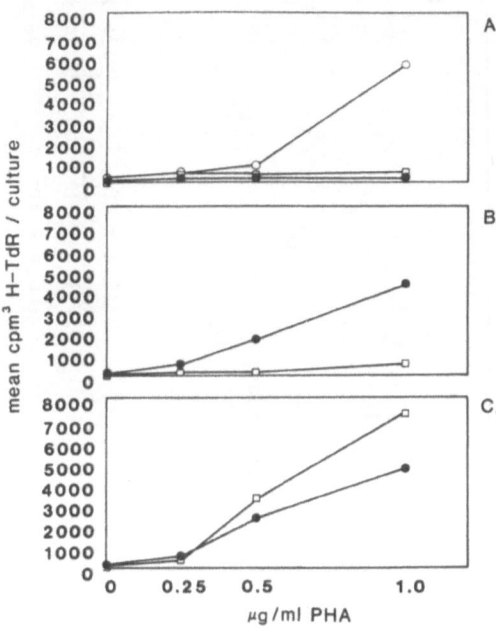

Figure 3. Effect of IMREG-1 on the PHA response of frank
            AIDS lymphocytes. (A) Patient JF, samples taken
            pre-modulator (● - ●), 3 days (◻ -◻) and 7 days
            (0-0) post-IMREG-1. (B) Patient RC, samples taken
            pre-modulator (◻ -◻) and 3 days post-IMREG-1
            (● - ●). (C) Patient TM, samples taken 6 (◻ -◻)
            and 9 (● - ●) days post-IMREG-1. A baseline
            sample was not obtained in this case.

Table 6. Time Course Study of PHA-Induced IL-2 Production and In Vitro Modulation by IMREG-1. Frank AIDS Patient DT

Date	Modulator Dosage**	Units/ml IL-2 in 24 hours culture supernatants* from cells exposed to 1 µg/ml PHA and indicated dilution of modulator			
		PHA Alone	+1/500 IMREG-1	+1/1000 IMREG-1	+1/2000 IMREG-1
08/03					
09/02	Isologous cells	0	0	0	0
9/12	4×10^5				
9/13		0	0	0	0
9/16	Isologous cells				
9/17	4×10^5				
9/18	4×10^6				
9/19	4×10^5	1.1×10^{-5}	1.34×10^{-4}	3.7×10^{-5}	0.25×10^{-5}
9/21		1.4×10^{-5}	1.94×10^{-4}	3.57×10^{-3}	0.554×10^{-3}
9/29		4.6×10^{-2}	1.96×10^{-1}	1.96×10^{-1}	1.96×10^{-1}
9/30	Isologous cells				
10/06		5.9×10^{-3}	4.2×10^{-2}	7.5×10^{-2}	2.96×10^{-2}

*All values refer to IL-2 induced with 1 µg/ml PHA. For the purpose of comparison, cells derived from the patient's identical twin brother produced 2.81 U/ml IL-2 on 9/12.
**Amount of modulator derived from indicated cell numbers.

in this table. We observed no IL-2 production or modulation of IL-2 production by IMREG-1, until after the second cycle of isologous cells and IMREG-1. When isologous cells alone were given, as in the third transfer, no improvement in IL-2 production was observed.

These results indicate that we have identified an important endogenous immunoregulator, IMREG-1 which enhances lymphokine production by T4 cells in response to antigenic or mitogenic stimulation. In the present study, IMREG-1 was evaluated in ARC and frank AIDS patients, with similar findings. Administration of IMREG-1 with tetanus toxoid was found to induce positive skin test response to this antigen, while TT alone induced no significant DTH in these patients. However, enhanced DTH was not observed unless patients had been exposed to the modulator at least once previously, suggesting

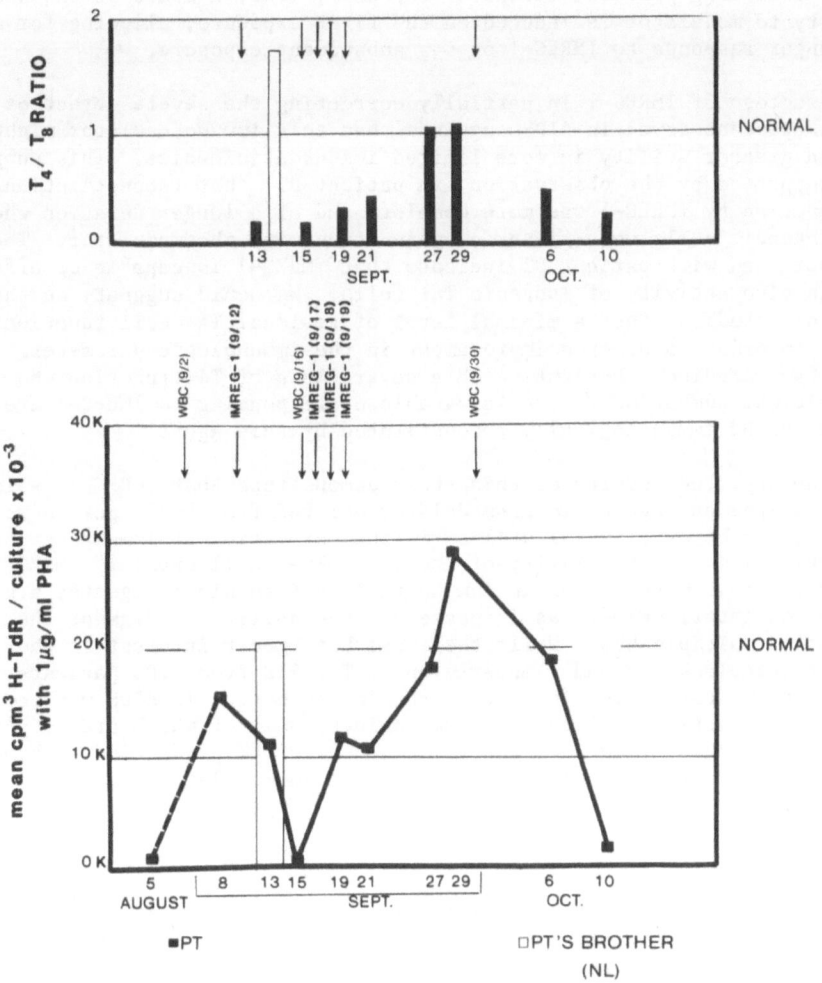

Figure 4.   Time course study with frank AIDS patient DT. The effect of IMREG-1 on the T4/T8 ratio (upper panel) and the PHA response (lower panel) of patient lymphocytes was examined during a treatment course consisting of WBCs from an identical twin, given with or without IMREG-1 as noted in the figure. On 9/12, 9/17, and 9/19 the patient received 4 x 10^5 leukocyte equivalent of IMREG-1, while on 9/18 he received 4 x 10^6 leukocyte equivalents of the immunomodulator.

297

that IMREG-1 induces alterations in systemic immunity in these individuals even in absence of a demonstrable effect on DTH, and that these changes allow for enhanced reactivity to IMREG-1 on subsequent administration. These results are similar to those observed in vitro for IL-2 production.

Following in vivo administration of IMREG-1, several reproducible changes in the in vitro reactivity of patient lymphocytes were observed. PHA-induced proliferation and IL-2 production increased significantly as early as 24 hours after receiving IMREG-1, and this increase in immune reactivity did not require previous exposure to IMREG-1, as was the case with DTH. Additionally, while patient lymphocytes were initially refractory to the ability of IMREG-1 to augment IL-2 production in vitro, the response of lymphocytes to modulation of LK production improved significantly following in vivo administration of IMREG-1. This increased sensitivity to the action of modulator may be responsible for the ability of IMREG-1 to increase DTH responses following previous modulator exposure, i.e., a state of enhanced sensitivity to modulator is induced on the first exposure, allowing for a much stronger response to IMREG-1 on its subsequent exposure.

The success of IMREG-1 in partially correcting the severe defect of immune function observed in AIDS suggests that this immunomodulator might be of even greater utility in more limited immunodeficiencies. This supposition is supported by the observation, in patient DT, that reconstitution of immune function by IMREG-1 was more complete and of a longer duration when normal syngeneic cells were given in conjunction with the modulator. The results obtained with patient DT indicate that IMREG-1 is capable of affecting the in vivo activity of isogenic T4+ cells. We would suggest, on the basis of our studies, that a minimal level of residual T4+ cell function is required, in order to observe improvement in the immunologic parameters which we have studied. Patients with a severe loss of T4+ function who lack a critical number of T4+ cells capable of responding to IMREG-1 are not likely to be immunologically reconstituted by this agent.

In summary, the results of this study demonstrate that IMREG-1, a low molecular weight endogenous immunomodulator derived from human peripheral leukocytes, may be of clinical utility in the correction of immune deficiency attributable to impaired activity of the T4+ helper cell subset. IMREG-1 is likely to prove more useful in immune therapy than single agents, e.g., interferon or interleukin-2, as it possesses the ability to augment the production of multiple LKs. While there has been great interest in the effects of interleukin-2 and γ interferon on T cells from AIDS patients in vitro, effective correction in vivo of the immune defect in AIDS may require the coordinated activity of several lymphokines, some of which are as yet unidentified. IMREG-1 may be a general enhancer of LK production in human T4 cells and further clinical trials of this immunomodulator appear warranted.

REFERENCES

1. A. A. Gottlieb and S. B. Sutcliffe, In vivo modification of delayed-type human leukocytes: partial purification of components causing amplification of response, Clin. Exp. Immunol. 50:424 (1983).
2. A. A. Gottlieb, J. L. Farmer, C. T. Matzura, et al., Modulation of human T cell production of migration inhibitory lymphokines by cytokines derived from human leukocyte dialysates, J. Immunol. 132:256 (1984).
3. H. S. Lawrence, The transfer in humans of delayed skin sensitivity to streptoccocial M substances and to tuberculus with disrupted leukocytes, J. Clin. Invest. 34:219 (1955).
4. M. S. Gottlieb, R. Schroff, H. M. Shanker, et al., Pneumocystis carinni pneumonia and mucosal candidiasis in previously healthy homosexual

men: evidence of a new acquired cellular immunodeficiency, <u>N</u>. <u>Eng</u>. <u>J</u>. <u>Med</u>. 305:1431 (1981).

5. H. Masur, M. A. Michelis, J. B. Greene, et al., An outbreak of community-acquired pneumocystis carinii pneumonia: initial manifestation of cellular immune dysfunction, <u>N</u>. <u>Eng</u>. <u>J</u>. <u>Med</u>. 305:1431 (1981).

6. S. Gillis, M. M. Ferm, W. Ou, et al., T. Cell growth factor: parameters of production and a quantitative microassay for activity, <u>J</u>. <u>Immunol</u>. 120:2027 (1978).

INTERFERONS AND THEIR ROLES IN VIRUS INFECTIONS

William E. Stewart II

Department of Medical Microbiology and Immunology
University of South Florida College of Medicine
Tampa, Florida

INTRODUCTION

Interferons (IFNs) were originally identified by virologists who were looking for a virus-induced virus-inhibitory factor (1) and this induction-action relationship seemed to suggest that interferon's reason for being was to inhibit viruses. This simple relationship was quite comforting for several years, but it then started to get more complex by the observations that IFNs could induce a number of alterations in cells besides inhibition of virus replication (2). Such "non-antiviral activities" of IFNs (3) were for several years dismissed as attributable to impurities in the usually relatively crude IFN preparations, but eventually it was substantiated that IFNs are potent inducers of a number of seemingly unrelated "pleotypic alterations" in various cells (4).

Thus, as illustrated in Table 1, depending on the particular inducer-action relationship one is studying, one could really wonder about IFN's true role or purpose. If one were looking for a virus-induced factor that inhibited viruses, or a mitogen-induced factor that inhibited cell division, or an immune recognition-induced factor that modulated immune responses, each factor could be given an ethnocentrically appropriate name and still be an interferon by definition (5). Indeed, certain lymphokines that have been assigned immunomodulatorily appropriate names have been shown to be IFNs, e.g., macrophage activation factor = IFN gamma (6).

So much recent emphasis has stressed IFNs as antitumor agents and so much work in the last three or four years has concerned IFNs' immunomodulatory activities, that I have even encountered comments by immunologists to the effect that IFNs are actually immunoregulatory substances that just happen to have antiviral activities. Therefore, I shall here briefly and selectively review some information on IFNs as antiviral agents and shall emphasize their contributions to both virus resistance and pathogenesis. It should become clear from this discussion that IFNs are important in resistance to and recovery from virus infections, but they also contribute significantly to the production of viral diseases.

INDUCTION OF INTERFERONS BY VIRUSES

IFNs were originally induced by viruses, but a wide variety of other substances are equally effective at triggering their production by cells.

Table 1.   Interferons as Viewed by Induction-Action
           Relations

Inducer	Activity
Viruses	Antiviral
Mitogens	Cell growth inhibition
Immune responses	Immunomodulations

Indeed, it is probably a shorter list of agents that do not induce IFNs
than those that do so. IFNs are induced by an extensive list of viruses in
all vertebrates that have been tested; thus, IFNs have been induced in dozens
of species of fish, amphibians, reptiles, birds and mammals (2).

In the human system, literally dozens of different IFN forms have been
identified: two beta IFNs; three gamma IFNs and 20 or more alpha IFNs,
including both non-glycosylated and glycosylated native forms (7). In most
cases, these virus induced IFNs are stimulated by the virus genome or its
replicative forms, giving rise to alpha and/or beta IFNs. In some cases,
however, such as in sensitized cells, the viral proteins alone can serve as
IFN inducers, giving rise to the production of gamma IFNs. Thus, the character of the IFNs produced early and late in a virus infection, as well as
those produced during primary and secondary infections are different, changing from alpha/beta to gamma types of IFNs.

ROLES OF IFNS IN PATHOGENESIS OF VIRUS INFECTIONS

IFNs can be produced locally very early in virus infections, as in
rhinovirus and coronavirus infections of the nasal mucosa (8), or they can
be produced locally very late in virus infections, as in rabies or St.
Louis encephalitis virus infections of the CNS (9,10). Also, IFNs can be
produced systemically in generalized virus infection such as measles,
mumps, etc., with interferonemia coincident with the secondary viremia.
Therefore the possible involvements of the IFNs must be considered at many
stages of virus infections, from the portal of entry, the secondary foci,
the circulatory system and in the terminal target tissues.

Quite often, detectable amounts of IFNs are not produced in local or
systemic virus infections, but this does not eliminate their roles in the
virus resistance of the organism. Indeed, Gresser and his associates (11)
have shown that both the pathogenicity and the pathogenesis of many virus
infections can be drastically altered by pretreatment of animals with anti-
IFN antiserum prior to virus infection (Table 2). Obviously, therefore,
even if undetectable levels of IFNs are produced in virus infections, they
can significantly augment resistance mechanisms to virus infections.

MECHANISMS OF IFN-INDUCED VIRUS RESISTANCE

The mechanisms of antiviral activities induced by IFNs must be considered
at both the cellular and the organism levels.

At the cellular level, IFNs action against viruses are myriad. Depending on the particular virus examined, the amounts of IFNs, the types of
IFNs and the stages of replication studied, IFNs can:

Table 2. Endogenous IFN Restriction of Virus Infections:
Demonstration with Anti-IFN Antibodies

Virus Infection	Effect of Anti-IFN Pretreatment
Encephalomyocarditis	Increased fatality; altered pathogenesis (visceral lesions)
Vesicular stomatitis	Shortened intranasal to CNS incubation period
Semliki forest	Shortened incubation period; increased fatality
Herpes simplex	Increased infectivity (several $logs_{10}$)
Molony sarcoma	Earlier, larger, longer-lasting tumors; several $logs_{10}$ increase in tumor-inducing potency

1. Reduce the efficiency of virus attachment/penetration

2. Inhibit uncoating of virus within cells

3. Block primary transcription

4. Inhibit virus messenger RNA translation through induction of enzymes (protein kinase and 2'-5' oligoadenylate synthetase)

5. Interfere with virus progeny assembly/maturation

6. Prevent the release of mature virus progeny from cells

Additionally, IFNs can inhibit virus infections via the many "non-antiviral activities" they induce. Thus, IFNs can, at the organism level:

1. Induce febrile responses which can inhibit virus replication by several mechanisms (e.g., elevation of body temperature above virus optimum; activate endonucleases)

2. Enhance phagocytosis, thus promoting clearance of viremia

3. Activate immune killer cell elements to lyse virus infected cells

4. Sensitize infected cells to antibody-dependent immunolysis

5. Induce other lymphokines (IL-2, TNF, etc.) which can facilitate immuno-removal of virus-infected cells, either alone or in synergy with IFNs.

Thus, in terms of resistance to virus infections, IFNs' mechanisms must be considered both at the molecular level and at the organism level (12,13).

CONTRIBUTIONS TO IFNs TO VIRUS PATHOGENESIS: IFN SIDE-EFFECTS

It is now clear that IFNs can contribute more than beneficial effects to virus infections. It was demonstrated several years ago (11) that IFNs

Table 3. IFN-Induced Disease: Chronic LCM Virus

Newborn mice + LCM	=	Chronic low levels of LCM virus
	=	Chronic low levels of IFN
	=	Liver necrosis
	=	Glomerulonephritis
	=	Runting syndrome
Newborn mice + LCM	=	High levels of LCM virus
	=	No detectable IFN
+ anti-IFN	=	No liver necrosis
	=	No glomeruloenphritis
	=	No runting

could induce damage and death in newborn mice. IFNs also apparently contribute to the production of virus disease and play a causal role in chronic LCM virus infection (Table 3). Thus, chronic IFN production causes the LCM-induced runting syndrome, and neutralization of the IFN induced by the virus prevents this disease (11).

Thus, IFNs presence in virus infections is not uniformly beneficial. Indeed, there was considerable early data showing that crude IFN preparations induced "side effects" in man (14) and recent studies with the various forms of essentially pure natural or recombinant-derived IFNs have shown that IFNs administered systemically can produce several side effects (15,16), some of which can be dose-limiting (Table 4).

Not surprisingly, many of the common prodromal symptoms and circulating IFN levels seen during viremic stages of acute generalized virus infections are similar to the side effects and IFN levels seen at maximum-tolerated doses of patients on IFN therapy.

Even in terms of local utility (as against the common cold), the side effects of IFNs have presented a commercially disturbing situation: the

Table 4. "Side Effects" of Interferons

Route of Administration	Symptoms
Systemic	Flu-like syndrome (fever, malaise, fatigue, headache, nausea, chills, backache)
(intramuscular; intravenous)	Leukopenia (transient)
	CNS toxicity (depression, drowsiness, confusion, loss of smell and taste)
Topical	Nasal stuffiness
	Thickened mucus
(intranasal)	Local inflammation and irritation
	Headache

side effects of intranasally administered IFNs reflect the symptoms of the common cold (Table 4), likely caused in colds by the IFNs induced locally by the viruses.

In terms of antiviral therapy with IFNs late in virus infections, augmentation of IFN levels could be a mixed blessing: eradication of virus from target tissues such as the CNS could be accomplished by the conventional intracellular antiviral mechanisms induced by IFNs; this should be beneficial. However, elimination of virus-infected cells by IFN-induced augmentation of cell-mediated immunolysis of infected brain cells could be detrimental. The best way to sort out the contributions of these various resistance mechanisms induced by IFNs will be to employ various genetically-engineered fused protein hybrid IFN forms that have constant antiviral levels but low or high immunomodulatory potentials. Then it will be possible to better assess the roles of IFNs in virus infections.

REFERENCES

1. A. Isaacs and J. Lindenmann, Virus interference. I. The interferon, Proc. Royal Soc. B 147:258 (1957).
2. W. E. Stewart II, "The Interferon System," Springer-Verlag, Vienna, Austria (1981).
3. W. E. Stewart II, L. B. Gosser, and R. Z. Lockart, Priming: a nonantiviral function of interferon, J. Virol. 7:792 (1971).
4. W. E. Stewart II, E. DeClercq, P. DeSomer, K. Berg, C. A. Ogburn, and K. Paucker, Antiviral and non-antiviral activity of highly purified interferon, Nature 246:141 (1973).
5. W. E. Stewart II, J. E. Blalock, D. C. Burke, C. Chany, J. Dunnick, E. Falcoff, R. M. Friedman, G. J. Galasso, W. K. Joklik, J. Vilcek, J. S. Youngner, and K. C. Zoon, Interferon nomenclature, Nature 286:110 (1980).
6. W. E. Stewart II and D. K. Blanchard, Interferons: cytostatic and immunomodulatory effects, in: "Immunity to Cancer," A. Reif and M. Mitchell, eds., Academic Press, New York (1985).
7. W. E. Stewart II, Heterogeneities of human interferons, in: "Biological Responses in Cancer," E. Mihich, ed., Plenum Publishing Corporation, New York (1984).
8. S. B. Greenberg and Harmon, Clinical use of interferons: localized application in viral diseases, in: "Interferons and Their Applications," P. E. Came and W. A. Carter, eds., Springer-Verlag, Berlin (1984).
9. W. E. Stewart II and S. E. Sulkin, Interferon production in hamsters experimentally infected with rabies virus, Proc. Soc. Exp. Biol. Med. 123:650 (1966).
10. J. P. Luby, W. E. Stewart II, S. E. Sulkin, and J. P. Sanford, Interferon in human infections with St. Louis encephalitis, Ann. Int. Med. 71:703 (1969).
11. I. Gresser, Can interferon induce disease?, in: "Interferon 4," I. Gresser, ed., Academic Press, London (1982).
12. B. Lebleu and J. Content, Mechanisms of interferon action: biochemical and genetic approaches, in: "Interferon 4," I. Gresser, ed., Academic Press, London (1982).
13. W. E. Stewart II, The natural recovery process from acute virus infection, in: "Selective Inhibitors of Viral Functions," W. A. Carter, ed., CRC Press, Cleveland (1973).
14. H. Strander, K. Cantell, G. Carlstrom, S. Ingimarsson, P. A. Jakobsson, U. Nilsonne, Acute infections in interferon-treated patients with osteosarcoma: a preliminary report of a comparative study, J. Infect. Dis. 133:A245 (1976).

15. G. M. Scott, W. E. Stewart II, D. A. J. Tyrrell, K. Cantell, T. Cartwright, and V. G. Edy, Skin reactions to interferon inoculations are reduced but not abolished by purification, J. Interferon Res. 1:79 (1980).

16. D. A. J. Tyrrell, Some thoughts on the clinical exploitation of interferon in infectious diseases, in: "Interferon 4," I. Gresser, ed., Academic Press, London (1982).

EXACERBATION OF THE PATHOGENESIS OF THE DIABETOGENIC VARIANT OF

ENCEPHALOMYOCARDITIS VIRUS IN MICE BY INTERFERON

Cheryl L. Gould, Karyle G. McMannama, Nancy J. Bigley,
and David J. Giron

Department/Program of Microbiology and Immunology,
College of Science and Engineering and School of Medicine
Wright State University, Dayton, Ohio

INTRODUCTION

The D variant of encephalomyocarditis virus (EMC-D) infects pancreatic
beta cells in susceptible mouse strains producing a disease syndrome similar
to insulin-dependent diabetes in humans (5,11). We have recently reported
that EMC-D replicates primarily in the pancreas and spleen of ICR Swiss
male mice, and to a lesser extent in the heart and lung tissues (8). Interferon (IFN) or IFN-inducers have been shown to protect some, but not all,
susceptible mouse strains against the diabetogenic effects of EMC-D (2,3,11).
For example, SWR/J mice respond well to the protective effects of IFN, while
ICR Swiss animals are not protected (3). We have been studying the role of
IFN on the development of virus-induced murine diabetes. Since IFNs have
been shown to be powerful immune modulators (9,10) it was the purpose of
the present study to determine if IFN given after infection by EMC-D had
any effect on the frequency or severity of diabetes in susceptible ICR Swiss
and resistant C57Bl/6 mice. Virus replication in selected tissues was also
determined. The data presented show that IFN exacerbates the severity of
diabetes caused by the virus in ICR Swiss mice and induces the diabetic
state in the otherwise resistant C57Bl/6 animals.

MATERIALS AND METHODS

Virus

The D variant of encephalomyocarditis virus (EMC-D) was propagated and
titrated by methods previously described (7). The virus was passed five
times through L929 (L) cells, twice through BHK 21 cells, and once again
through L cells. The resulting virus stock is diabetogenic, produces large
diffuse plaques in L cells, and does not induce the production of IFN in
vitro. Stock virus was diluted in Hank's balanced salt solution containing
2% calf serum (HBSS). Mice were given a single intraperitoneal (ip) injection (0.2 ml) of the diluted virus at a dose of 800 plaque forming units
(PFU).

Animals

Male ICR Swiss and C57Bl/6 mice were purchased from Harlan Laboratories,
Indianapolis, Indiana and Jackson Laboratories, Bar Harbor, Maine,

respectively. The animals were housed in groups of ten, and at the time of infection were nine weeks of age.

Interferons and IFN-Inducer

Concentrated, practically purified L cell interferon (IFNβ) was prepared by methods previously described (4). The activity of the IFN was determined by the 50% plaque reduction (PR$_{50}$) method using EMC-MM as the challenge agent (4). We have determined that each PR$_{50}$ unit by this method is equivalent to 0.5 NIH (G002-9040511) reference units. Mice were given IFNβ at a dose of 3800 units as indicated. Polyinosinic polycytidylic acid (Poly I:C) was purchased from Sigma Chemical Company, and was given ip in 0.2 ml volumes of HBSS containing 150 μg. These doses were used since previous studies in our laboratory showed that they were sufficient to protect mice against the lethal effects of EMC-MM and production of diabetes by EMC-D (3). Gamma IFN (IFNγ) was kindly provided by Dr. Howard M. Johnson, University of Texas Medical Branch, Galveston, Texas, and was administered at a dose of 80 PR$_{50}$ units per test animal.

Glucose Tolerance Test (GTT)

At seven and 14 days post infection, a nonfasting GTT was done on each of the animals. Each mouse received an ip injection of glucose at a concentration of 2 mg per g body weight. After one hour the animals were bled, and the serum glucose levels determined using a YSI model 23A glucose analyzer. It has been shown that nonfasting glucose levels demonstrate a greater sensitivity to reduction of insulin secretion than does fasting glucose (1). Mice with GTT levels at least three standard deviations (SD) above control means were considered to be diabetic.

Virus Replication in Mouse Tissues

Tissues from ICR Swiss mice were collected seven days post infection, then homogenized and sonicated for 30 sec (Heat Systems Sonicator Model

Table 1. Effect of Interferon on Virus-Induced Diabetes in ICR Swiss Mice

Treatment at Day[a]:		Days Post Infection[b]			
		7		14	
0	4	GTT Mg% Mean ± SD	Diabetic (%)	GTT Mg% Mean ± SD	Diabetic (%)
EMC-D	HBSS	358 ± 137	70	425 ± 181	70
EMC-D	IFNβ	428 ± 158	100[c]	507 ± 217	100[c]
EMC-D	IFNγ	500 ± 127	100[c]	537 ± 124	100[c]
EMC-D	Poly I:C	278 ± 121	70[c]	289 ± 95	70[c]
HBSS	HBSS	147 ± 25	0	191 ± 24	0

[a]Male ICR Swiss mice (10 per group) were given either EMC-D (800 PFU) or HBSS intraperitoneally (IP) at day 0. Four days later the animals received an IP injection of IFNβ (3800 units), IFNγ (80 units), poly I:C (150 μg), or HBSS as indicated.

[b]One hour GTT was done on each mouse at 7 and 14 days post infection. Mice with GTT at least 3 S.D. above control means were considered to be diabetic.

[c]Severe encephalitis evident in these groups of animals.

Table 2. Effect of IFNβ on Induction of Diabetes in C57B1/6 Mice

Treatment at Day[a]		Expt 1		Expt 2	
0	4	GTT Mg%[b] Mean ± SD	Diabetic (%)	GTT Mg%[b] Mean ± SD	Diabetic (%)
EMC-D	HBSS	249 ± 40	0	288 ± 57	0
EMC-D	IFNβ	296 ± 72	30	363 ± 100	50
HBSS	HBSS	232 ± 34	0	211 ± 48	0

[a]Male C57B1/6 mice received either EMC-D or HBSS at day 0 followed by HBSS or IFNβ at day 4 post infection. Dosages were identical.

[b]One hour GTT was done on each mouse 14 days post infection. Mice with GTT at least 3 S.D. above control means were considered to be diabetic.

220F) to free intracellular virus. Cellular debris was removed by centrifugation (2000 g for 15 min), and the clarified fluids were filter sterilized (Millipore, 0.45μ) and stored at -70°C until assayed for PFU content. The relative amount of virus replication in each of the tissues is expressed in terms of replication index (8), which is defined as the number of PFU per g of tissue divided by challenge dose of virus. Virus replication is indicated by indices greater than 1.0.

RESULTS

Effect of IFN on the Induction of Diabetes

ICR Swiss mice were divided into groups of ten mice each. At time 0 test group were infected with EMC-D, while the control group received HBSS. Four days later, the animals were treated with either IFNβ, IFNγ, poly I:C or HBSS as indicated. Glucose tolerance tests were done at days seven and 14 post infection. The data in Table 1 show that, as expected, EMC-D induced diabetes in this mouse strain. Note that treatment of virus-infected animals with IFNβ or IFNγ at day four post infection induced an increased incidence and severity (markedly elevated plasma glucose levels) of the diabetic state. All IFN-treated animals exhibited symptoms of severe encephalitis while infected controls demonstrated little or no overt symptoms. Poly I:C had no effect on the incidence of diabetes and the severity was somewhat reduced, but severe encephalitis was also evident in these animals. Subsequent experiments show essentially the same results.

Two groups (ten mice each) of C57B1/6 mice were infected with EMC-D. Four days later one group received HBSS, the other IFNβ. A third group of animals served as control and was treated with HBSS at both time periods. The GTT was determined on each 14 days post infection. The results of duplicate experiments are shown in Table 2. The data show that mice developed diabetes only when treated with IFN.

Virus Replication in Tissues

The data in Table 3 show that by seven days post infection, EMC-D was absent in the pancreata of infected control ICR Swiss mice, and present, but not apparently replicating in spleen, brain, and heart tissues. When animals were treated with IFNβ or poly I:C, the virus could again be isolated

Table 3. Virus Replication in ICR Swiss Mouse Tissues at Day 7 Post Infection

Treatment at Day[a] 4 post infection	Replication Index[b]			
	Pancreas	Spleen	Heart	Brain
HBSS	0	0.3	0.5	0.5
IFNβ	1.4	0.5	51.3	10.7
IFNγ	0.2	0.3	0.9	1.1
Poly I:C	0.2	0.4	137.2	18.1

[a]Mice were given EMC-D (800 PFU) at day 0. Treatment at day 4 post infection was as described in Table 1.

[b]Replication index is virus PFU per g of tissue divided by the challenge dose of virus.

from the pancreata and replicated significantly in heart and brain tissues. Replication of the virus following the administration of IFN was not as dramatic.

DISCUSSION

The data presented show that administration of IFNβ or IFNγ to (EMC-D)-infected ICR Swiss male mice resulted in an apparent increase in the incidence of severity of the diabetic state. It is also evident that diabetes was induced in resistant C57Bl/6 animals by IFNβ. One possible explanation for the exacerbation of diabetes in ICR Swiss mice is suggested by the data in Table 3 which show that virus replication was reactivated in mouse tissues by IFN and EMC-D could again be demonstrated in the pancreas. However, it is evident that other mechanisms are involved since virus replication was markedly stimulated by poly I:C in heart and brain tissues, with essentially no effect on the development of diabetes. It was noted that all animals treated with IFN or poly I:C exhibited symptoms of severe encephalomyocarditis including generalized weakness, loss of appetite, ruffling of fur, uncontrolled disoriented movements, and hind leg paralysis. In general, virus-infected control animals exhibited no overt signs of illness. The encephalomyocarditis probably reflects the marked replication of the virus in the hearts and brains following the administration of IFN or poly I:C. It has been shown previously that EMC-D does not normally replicate in the brains of ICR Swiss mice, and only to a very limited extent in heart tissue (8).

Possible mechanisms for the reactivation of virus replication are suggested. Previous studies showed that EMC-D replication in cell culture is stimulated by insulin (6). In a recent study, we have determined that a single injection of IFNβ into either ICR Swiss or C57Bl/6 mice results in severe hypoglycemia within four hours (data not shown). This observation suggests that IFN stimulates the release of insulin. In the present study, insulin could have been released from undamaged pancreatic beta cells in response to IFN (glycoprotein). Insulin could have stimulated the replication of EMC-D resulting in additional damage to the beta cells as well as other tissues by as yet unidentified mechanisms.

Another possibility is suggested by a preliminary study in which we have determined that IFN given at day four post infection, significantly decreased the amount of circulating virus-neutralizing antibody present at day seven in both ICR Swiss and C57B1/6 mice (about 60% reduction; data not shown). Interferons are potent immune modulators (9,10) and, in this instance, could selectively decrease the activity of the antibody producing lymphocytes. The reduction in circulating antibody levels may be involved in progression of virus infection and the apparent restimulation of virus replication. Alternatively, the lower levels of circulating antibody may reflect an increase in the formation of virus-antibody complexes due to enhanced viral replication.

It is clear that IFN or poly I:C given after infection by EMC-D alters the course of infection in the two mouse strains studied, resulting in either an exacerbation of the diabetic state, or induction of encephalomyocarditis. The mechanism(s) responsible, remain to be determined.

ACKNOWLEDGMENTS

This work was supported by the Kroc Foundation.

REFERENCES

1. V. Bonnevie-Nielsen, M. W. Steffes, and A. Lernmark, A major loss in islet mass and cell function precedes hyperglycemia in mice given multiple low doses of streptozotocin, Diabetes 30:424 (1981).
2. J. B. Gadzik, A. Naji, and C. F. Barkin, Inhibition of virus-induced murine diabetes by an interferon inducer, J. Interferon Res. 2:59 (1982).
3. D. J. Giron, S. J. Cohen, S. P. Lyons, C. H. Wharton, and D. R. Cerutis, Inhibition of virus-induced diabetes mellitus by interferon is influenced by host strain, Proc. Soc. Exp. Biol. Med. 173:328 (1983).
4. D. J. Giron, R. Y. Liu, F. E. Hemphill, F. F. Pindak, and J. P. Schmidt, Role of interferon in the antiviral state elicited by selected interferon inducers, Proc. Soc. Exp. Biol. Med. 163:146 (1980).
5. D. J. Giron and R. R. Patterson, Effect of steroid hormones on virus-induced diabetes mellitus, Infect. Immun. 37:820 (1982).
6. D. J. Giron, R. R. Patterson, and S. P. Lyons, Alteration of diabetes and interferon induction by the diabetogenic strain of encephalomyocarditis virus through cell passage, J. Interferon Res. 2:371 (1982).
7. D. J. Giron and F. F. Pindak, Propagation of MM virus in L cells, Appl. Microbiol. 17:811 (1969).
8. C. L. Gould, M. L. Trombley, N. J. Bigley, K. G. McMannama and D. J. Giron, Replication of diabetogenic and nondiabetogenic variants of encephalomyocarditis (EMC) virus in ICR Swiss mice, Proc. Soc. Exp. Biol. Med. (in press 1984).
9. I. Gresser, Commentary on the varied biologic effects of interferon, Cell Immunol. 34:406 (1977).
10. G. Sonnenfeld, Modulation of immunity by interferon, Lymphokine Rep. 1:113 (1980).
11. J. Yoon, P. R. McClintock, JT. Onodera, and A. L. Notkins, Virus induced diabetes mellitus. XVIII. Inhibition by a nondiabetogenic variant of encephalomyocarditis virus, J. Exp. Med. 152:878 (1980).

THYMIC HORMONES IN VIRAL INFECTIONS AND AIDS

Nathan Trainin[1], Ygal Burstein[2], Virginia Buchner[2],
Marit Pecht[1], Laura Netzer[3], Zvi Bentwich[3], Rimona Burstein[3],
Ytzhal Berner[4], Ofra Segal[3], and Zeev T. Handzel[3]

Department of Cell Biology[1], Department of Organic
Chemistry[2]-Weizmann Institute of Science; R. Ben-Ari
Institute of Clinical Immunology[3]; Department of Internal
Medicine C[4]-Kaplan Hospital, Rehovot, Israel

INTRODUCTION

Thymic hormones participate in T-cell differentiation in all three lymphoid cell compartments: bone marrow, thymus gland, and peripheral lymphatic system. These hormones play an essential role in the stepwise process of differentiation and maturation of thymocytes and of T-cells in the absence of antigenic stimulation, thus contributing to a balance between subsets of T-helper, T-cytotoxic and T-suppressor cells (1). Viruses, on the other hand, may cause a disarrangement of the lymphoreticular system, the seriousness of which depends on the aggressiveness of the virus involved. Indeed, following infections such as measles, rubella, cytomegalovirus and dengue, the respective viruses have been detected in peripheral circulating lymphocytes (2). During the course of the infection, viruses may destroy lymphoid cells directly or may persist in the lymphoreticular system leading to the alteration of cellular immune functions. These observations, taken together, led us to formulate the hypothesis that thymic hormones may represent a valuable tool in the therapy against a variety of pathogenic viruses. Without aiming at an exhaustive review of this subject, we present our experience with thymic humoral factor (THF) and most of that obtained by now with other thymic hormone preparations, in the struggle against viral infection in humans.

BIOLOGICAL PROPERTIES OF THF

Following our original observations that intraperitoneal implantation of thymus tissue inside cell impermeable diffusion chambers led to significant improvement of the anatomic and functional damage produced by neonatal thymectomy in mice (3), we aimed at isolating and characterizing the soluble product of the thymus gland responsible for this hormone-like type of activity. Since then we have found this activity in the extracts of the thymus of mice, rabbits, sheep and calves (4) and for reasons of convenience we concentrated on calves for further characterization of the hormone. THF is an acidic peptide derived from calf thymuses by a modification of the procedure of Kook et al. (5) involving grinding of the gland, ultracentrifugation, dialysis, ultrafiltration, ion exchange chromatography and high performance

Table 1. Biological Activities of the THF in Mice

---

1. Promotes hematopoiesis
2. Increases the helper effect of T cells in the production of SRBC antibodies and in their reactivity to T-cell mitogens.
3. Raises the competence of T-cells to participate in MLC, GVH and CML in allogeneic or xenogeneic systems.
4. Augments T-cell killing effect against syngeneic tumor cells.
5. Increases the secretion of interleukin-2 by T-cells.
6. Abrogates early thymocyte autoreactivity.

---

liquid chromatography. Amongst the most important biological properties of THF investigated in mice are those shown in Table 1. On the other hand neither direct B-cell activation nor interleukin-1 production by macrophages have been observed with THF. We thus postulated that in addition to its stimulatory effect on the production and differentiation of T-cells, THF has a modulatory function by which it can bring back the balance of the different T-cell subpopulations to normal, when this balance has been impaired (6). Preliminary suggestion of the potential use of THF as an antiviral drug was gathered from the effect of this hormone on lymphocytes damaged by previous exposure to different viruses. Varsano et al. reported that lymphocytes of patients suffering from subacute sclerosing panencephalitis (SSPE) were impaired in their cell mediated immunity and that preincubation of their peripheral blood lymphocytes with THF led to an improvement of their performance in the various assays tested (7). Recently, these observations were confirmed and extended by Handzel et al. (8). Moreover, THF induced an in vitro increase in proliferation of human peripheral blood lymphocytes in response to a challenge with varicella zoster virus (VZV) antigens (9).

The first experimental evidence of an in vivo antiviral effect of THF was brought by Rager-Zisman et al. (10). These authors found a considerable therapeutic effect of THF on mice infected with a potentially lethal dose of Sendai virus administered intranasally. Sendai virus had a striking pathogenic effect in the infected mice expressed as a decrease in total body weight, thymus involution, pneumonia and a low antibody response to the virus. Administration of THF following Sendai virus infection led to a marked improvement in all the parameters studied.

THF AND OTHER THYMIC HORMONES IN THE CLINICS

As shown in Table 2, THF has been administered to approximately 50 patients, mostly children suffering from various viral infections in non-controlled therapeutic trials. THF was administered by daily intramuscular injections in a saline physiological vehicle from seven to fourteen days. Occasionally this schedule was extended up to 28 days. Patients' courses were monitored according to the parameters mentioned in Table 3.

The group with acute severe viral infections recovered clinically within 72 hrs from beginning of THF administration which was followed by reconstitution of total lymphocyte counts and numbers of circulating T-cells. The four patients with SSPE showed an increase in circulating T-cells after the beginning of THF treatment. However, the clinical course varied. There was no change in one case, deterioration was arrested in another, in a third an immediate improvement in the EEG tracing was recorded, and in the fourth patient, a late unexpected remission occurred.

Table 2. Viral Infections Treated with THF

	Disease	No. of Patients
I.	**Primary Severe Viral Infections**	
	Acute Encephalitis	6
	Disseminated Herpes Simplex	1
	Guillain-Barré Syndrome	1
II.	**Subacute Sclerosing Panencephalitis**	4
III.	**Secondary Viral Infections in Malignant Diseases**	
	Varicella Zoster in Lymphomyeloproliferative disorders	29
	Varicella Zoster in Neuroblastoma and Rhabdomyosarcoma	4
	Adenovirus Pneumonitis in ALL	2
	CMV in Histiocytosis X	2
	Measles Pneumonitis in Synovial Cell Sarcoma	1

The majority of the 50 patients treated, suffered (as seen in Table 2) from malignancies complicated by secondary viral infections. The commonest infection was VZV followed by herpes simplex and adenovirus. Clinical signs of the viral infection regressed in an average of three days, which compares favorably with the natural course in similar patients where no immune modulation was attempted. In a few patients THF was administered after failure of treatment with Vidarabine or Acyclovir. A striking increase in cell mediated immunity (CMI) parameters and normalization of the T-cell subset balance was demonstrable in all survivors. In two of the three patients who expired, THF treatment was begun when pulmonary failure was already established due to an extensive viral pneumonitis. It is noteworthy that in most cases the disappearance of signs of infections preceded the reconstitution of impaired CMI which usually followed a certain sequence characterized first by a rise in the number of circulating lymphocytes and T-cells. The next step led to normalization of the various T-cell subsets. Proliferative responses to mitogens were then enhanced and finally, delayed hypersensitivity reactions in vivo reappeared (11,12). The first randomized controlled trial of treatment with THF in a viral disease was performed in Cape Town, South Africa in 20 infants with severe complicated acute measles infection. Ten children with onset of measles rash in the preceding two days and with symptoms of

Table 3. Clinical and Laboratory Parameters Studied in Viral Diseases

1. Progress or regression of viral lesions (vesicles, rashes, pulmonary infiltrates, etc.)
2. Peripheral blood lymphocytic (PBL) counts
3. Total T-cell counts (E-rosettes - OKT-11)
4. T-cell subsets (OKT-3, OKT-4, OKT-8)
5. T-mitogenic responses to PHA and Con A
6. Xenogeneic and GVH of patients' lymphocytes in irradiated rats
7. Dermal delayed hypersensitivity to recall antigens (SK/SD, Candida, PPD)

severe disease, with pulmonary or encephalitic complications or secondary infections were allotted to each group. THF was given for seven days or until the temperature had returned to normal. THF treatment resulted in less morbidity and fewer admissions to the intensive care unit. Objective benefit was evidenced by improvement in the Erythrocyte Sedimentation Rate and a fall in C reactive protein, fewer pulmonary complications and reduced incidence of secondary herpes infection. In addition, an increased ratio of helper to suppressor T-cells (OKT 4:8 ratio) and a greater lymphocyte transformation response to PHA was seen in these children receiving THF. No side effects whatsoever were observed as a result of THF administration (13).

In addition to THF, anti-viral properties of other thymic hormones and factors have been described in experimental systems and in clinical conditions in humans both in vitro and in vivo. Signs of abrogation of viral infections, enhancement of interferon (IFN) production and modulation of natural killer (NK) cell activity were studied.

Thymosin fraction 5 has been reported to increase survival of reovirus-infected mice without affecting their T-cells (14), and to prevent a chronic influenza infection (15). Thymosin's synthetic derivative-DT alpha's capacity to increase IFNγ production by human leukocytes has been shown to be dose-dependent (16).

Thymostimulin (TP-1 or TS) was able to confer anti-viral protection to immunosuppressed patients (17), and to increase anti-herpes simplex antigen proliferation and NK activity concomitantly with a clinical anti-viral effect in a controlled randomized trial in 21 patients (18). A similar therapeutic effect was demonstrated in 13 children with T-cell immune defects (19). TS also increased in vitro IFNγ production by human leukocytes (20).

Thymic serum factor (FTS) increased or decreased NK activity in cancer patients and in mice, depending on the dose administered, on whether they were thymectomized or not, and on strain sensitivity (24).

The FTS-Zn compound ("Thymulin") increased NK cells in tumor bearing, non-amputated mice, but decreased them after amputation of the tumor carrying limb (25).

Recently, a survey of the immune status in 160 asymptomatic male homosexuals (MHS) was performed in Israel (26). Forty percent of them manifested various T-cell impairments, mainly reductions in T-helper cells (T_H) and in the T-helper/suppressor cell (T_H/T_S) ratio as measured by monoclonal antibodies. In addition, about 60% had elevated serum levels of interferon and showed increased IFNα production, resulting in an anti-viral state of these cells (27).

These findings are of special interest in view of the fact that Israel remains a low incidence country for AIDS and that in only two of the examinees lymphadenopathy was found as part of a possible AIDS Related Complex (ARC) (28), all the others being symptom free. Our MHS population was also characterized by relatively stable lifestyles and low sexual promiscuity.

According to criteria of a two Standard Deviation (SD) decrease from normal Circulating T_H (980±220) associated with lymphopenia (< 1000/cmm), or another CMI defect, eleven individuals out of the 160 examined entered a randomized double-blind trial of immunomodulation with THF versus placebo. All received 24 injections divided into two courses of 12 with a week interval. A battery of CMI assays was performed at days 0, 15, and 35 of the trial. Either no change or a decrease in circulating lymphocytes, pan and T-cell subpopulations occurred in the placebo treated group. In comparison, increases in the numbers of circulating total lymphocytes, pan

T-cells and their subpopulations occurred in three out of five individuals of the THF treated group. All these changes were registered at day 35 at the end of the trial. Ratios between means of increments ΔX_{35} and starting values (X_0) for lymphocytes and T-cell populations when comparing between the two groups were significant at $p < 0.05$ as expressed by

$$\frac{\Delta (X_{35} - X_0)}{X_0}$$

in a students' t test. No differences were observed in proliferative responses to PHA and Con A and in MLC reactions between the two groups.

DISCUSSION AND CONCLUSION

The results of the pilot, randomized THF trial suggest the feasibility of modulating the immune impairment commonly found in MHS. However, the long term effect of such a modulation in preventing the development of AIDS in the future has not yet been established. The assessment of the potential value of such an approach is further complicated by the fact that probably only a minority of MHS with immune derangements evolve into ARC or AIDS. Nevertheless, the findings described here offer some hope to the application of modern immunotherapeutic modalities in the benefit of patients with ARC or AIDS in their early stages. Altogether, the data presented indicate that THF is an inducer of T-cell proliferation and leads to repair of CMI by bringing to normal the ratio between helper and suppressor/cytotoxic subsets of T-cells. The antiviral effect of THF could be interpreted either by the recruitment of new, intact T-cells or by the restoration of the ability of infected lymphocytes to exert a direct cytotoxic effect or to produce soluble factors such as IL-2 which are necessary for an intact immune response. In this context, it should be mentioned that THF has not been found so far to induce or to augment the production of IFNγ in cultures of spleen cells of mice either spontaneously or after mitogenic stimulation respectively. Finally, as to the effect of THF on NK cells, more experience is needed to support the observations that THF treated patients tend to a late repair of the NK population when these cells have been damaged by the viral infection.

REFERENCES

1. N. Trainin, M. Pecht, and Z. T. Handzel, Thymic hormones, Immunol. Today 4:16 (1983).
2. E. F. Wheelock and S. T. Toy, Participation of lymphocytes in viral infections, in: "Advances in Immunology," F. J. Dixon and H. G. Kunkel, eds., Academic Press, New York (1973).
3. N. Trainin, Thymic hormones and the immune response, Physiol. Reviews 54:272 (1974).
4. N. Trainin, A. Bejerano, M. Strahilevitch, D. Goldring, and M. Small, A thymic factor preventing wasting and influencing lymphopoiesis in mice, Israel J. Med. Sci. 2:549 (1966).
5. A. I. Kook, Y. Yakir, and N. Trainin, Isolation and partial chemical characterization of THF, a thymic hormone involved in immune maturation of lymphoid cells, Cell Immunol. 19:151 (1975).
6. B. Shohat, Z. Shapira, C. Servadio, and N. Trainin, In vitro induction of T-suppressor lymphocytes in recipients of renal allografts by THF, a thymic hormone, Transplantation 35:68 (1983).
7. I. Varsano, Y. Danon, L. Jaber, E. Livni, B. Shohat, Y. Yakir, A. Shneyour, and N. Trainin, Reconstitution of T cell function in patients with subacute sclerosing panencephalitis treated with thymus humoral factor, Israel J. Med. Sci. 12:1168 (1976).

8. Z. T. Handzel, N. Gadot, D. Idar, M. Schlesinger, E. Kahana, R. Dagan, S. Levin, and N. Trainin, Cell mediated immunity and effects of thymic humoral factor in 15 patients with SSPE, Brain and Devel. 5:29 (1983).

9. N. Trainin, V. Rotter, Y. Yakir, R. Leve, Z. T. Handzel, B. Shohat, and R. Zaizov, Biochemical and biological properties of THF in animal and human models, in: "Subcellular Factors in Immunity," H. Friedman, ed., Ann. N.Y. Acad. Sci. 332:9 (1979).

10. B. Rager-Zisman, Z. Harish, V. Rotter, Y. Yakir, and N. Trainin, Treatment of mice infected with Sendai virus with THF, a thymic hormone, in: "Advances in Allergology and Immunology," A. Oehling, ed., Pergamon Press, Oxford and New York (1980).

11. Z. T. Handzel, R. Zaizov, I. Varsano, S. Levin, M. Pecht, and N. Trainin, The influence of thymic humoral factor on immunoproliferative disorders and viral infections in humans, in: "Advances in Immunopharmacology," J. Hadden et al., eds., Pergamon Press, Oxford and New York (1981).

12. N. Trainin, Z. T. Handzel and M. Pecht, Biological and chemical properties of THF, Thymus (in press).

13. D. W. Beatty, Z. T. Handzel, M. Pecht, C. R. Ryder, J. Hughes, K. McCabe, and N. Trainin, A controlled trial of treatment of acquired immunodeficiency in severe measles with thymic humoral factor, Clin. Exp. Immunol. (in press).

14. D. E. Willey and R. N. Ushijima, The effect of thymosin on murine lymphocyte responses and corticosteroid levels during acute reovirus type 3 infection of neonatal mice, Clin. Immunol. and Immunopathol. 19:35 (1981).

15. Z. D. Savtsova, I. A. Grinevich, I. S. Nikolskii and O. I. Denisenko, Role of immune cytolysis and its thymosin stimulation in experimental influenza, Zh. Microbiol. Epidemiol. Immunobiol. (1982).

16. L. P. Svedersky, A. Hui, L. May, P. McKay, and N. Stebbing, Induction and augmentation of mitogen-induced immune interferon production in human peripheral blood lymphocytes by N-alpha-desacetylthymosin alpha-1, Eur. J. Immunol. 12:244 (1982).

17. P. A. Tovo and P. Nicola, TP-1 therapy in patients with secondary immunodeficiencies, in: "Thymus, Thymic Hormones and T-Lymphocytes," F. Aiuti and H. Wigzell, eds., Academic Press, London (1980).

18. F. Aiuti, M.C. Sirianni, R. Paganelli, A. Stella, G. Turbessi, and M. Fiorilli, A placebo-controlled trial of thymic hormone treatment of recurrent herpes simplex labialis infection in immunodeficient hosts, Int. J. Clin. Pharmacol. Ther. Toxicol. 21:81 (1982).

19. L. Businco, P. Ross, I. Quinti, and R. Perlini, Therapy with TP-1 of viral diseases in immunodeficient patients, in: "Thymus, Thymic Hormones and T Lymphocytes," F. Aiuti and H. Wigzell, eds., Academic Press, London (1980).

20. J. Shoham, I. Eshel, M. Aboud, and S. Salzberg, Thymic hormonal activity on human peripheral blood lymphocytes in vitro. II-enhancement of the production of immune interferon by activated cells, J. Immunol. 125:54 (1980).

21. K. Zaruba, M. Rastorfer, P. J. Grob, H. Jaller-Jemelka, and K. Bollak, Thymopentin as adjuvant in non-responders or hyporesponders to hepatitis B vaccination, Lancet 2:1245 (1983).

22. M. Fiorilli, M.C. Sirianni, F. Pandolfi, I. Quinti, U. Tosti, F. Aiuti, and G. Goldstein, Improvement of natural killer activity and of T cells after thymopoietin pentapeptide therapy in a patient with severe combined immunodeficiency, Clin. Exp. Immunology 45:344 (1981).

23. M. Fiorilli, M.C. Sirianni, V. Sorrentino, R. Testi, and F. Aiuti, In vitro enhancement of bone-marrow natural killer cells after incubation with thymopoietin 32-36 (TP-5) Thymus 5:375 (1983).

24. P. Bardos and J. F. Bach, Modulation of mouse natural killer cell activity by the serum thymic factor, Scand. J. Immunol. 16:321 (1982).

25. D. Kaiserlian, W. Savino, and M. Dardenne, Studies of the thymus in mice bearing the Lewis Lung Carcinoma. II. Modulation of thymic natural killer activity by thymulin (FTS-Zn) and the antimetastatic effect of Zinc, Clin. Immunol. Immunopathol. 28:192 (1983).

26. Z. T. Handzel, E. Galili-Weisstub, R. Burstein, Y. Berner, M. Pecht, L. Netzer, N. Trainin, N. Barzilai, S. Levin, and Z. Bentwich, Immune derangement in asymptomatic male homosexuals in Israel: a "pre-AIDS" condition? Proc. N.Y. Acad. Sci. New York (in press, 1984).

27. S. Levin, T. Hahn, Z. T. Handzel, V. Bergman, N. Barzilai, R. Myer, M. Tinowitz, E. Galili-Weisstub, and Z. Bentwich, Activated interferon system in healthy homosexuals (in press).

28. J. E. Groopman and P. A. Volberding, The AIDS epidemic: continental drift, Nature 307:211 (1984).

SPECIFIC ANTI-INFLUENZA ANTIBODY SYNTHESIS AND AGING:

IN VITRO EFFECTS OF THYMOSIN

Ann L. Moore[1], William B. Ershler[2], Mark A. Socinski[3], and Carolyn J. Greene[4]

Departments of Medicine[1,2,3] and Pharmacology[2] and The Vermont Regional Cancer Center[1,2,3,4], University of Vermont, Burlington, Vermont

INTRODUCTION

Among the wide variety of immune senescent changes that have been investigated, the age-related deficient antibody response to complex antigens (i.e., those that require T-cell interactions such as tetanus toxoid (1) or influenza antigen (2)) are of practical concern. For example, the antibody response to tetanus toxoid and influenza has been shown to be deficient in a substantial portion of otherwise normal, elderly recipients (3,4). In the present study, we have analyzed age-related changes in antibody response to influenza vaccine and tested the capacity for thymic hormones to augment specific antibody synthesis in vitro. To do this we utilized a microculture antibody synthesis enzyme-linked assay (MASELA) (5,6) specifically adapted for influenza antigen. The response to influenza vaccine was diminished in the elderly, but could be augmented in vitro in the majority by the addition of Thymosin.

MATERIALS AND METHODS

Volunteers, Vaccination, and Samples

Sixty-one healthy volunteers were injected with the trivalent influenza vaccine (Fluzone, Connaught Laboratories, Stillwater, Pennsylvania) containing 15 micrograms of hemagglutinin of each of the following strains: A/-Brazil/11/78 (H1N1), A/Phillipines/2/82 (H3N2), and B/Singapore/222/79. Of the 61 volunteers, 31 were young (19-30) and 30 were elderly (65-92 years).

Mononuclear Cell (MNC) Preparation and Characterization

Heparinized peripheral blood was separated by density gradient centrifugation and the MNC fraction was resuspended in "complete" media as described (4-7). Prior to immunization lymphocyte surface marker and functional studies were performed and revealed minimal differences in the study populations.

In Vitro and In Vivo Specific Anti-Influenza Antibody Production

Peripheral blood MNC were cultured in a microculture antibody synthesis enzyme-linked assay (MASELA) as previously described (5,6) and outlined in Figure 1.

Triplicate cultures of 25, 50, 100, or 200 x 10^5 cells in 250 µl of complete media were incubated at 37°C in humidified air with 5% CO_2 for six days. For 28 of the elderly and 30 of the young, parallel cultures were also established in which either Thymosin Fraction 5 (TF5) (at 50 µg/ml, 100 µg/ml, or 200 µg/ml), or Thymosin Alpha 1 (Tα1) (0.01 ng/ml, 0.1 ng/ml, or 1.0 ng/ml) were added to the culture media.

Specific plasma antibody (reflecting in vivo response to vaccination) was measured prior to and three weeks after vaccination in an enzyme-linked immunosorbent assay (ELISA). Serial plasma dilutions were added to influenza antigen coated microtiter plates and the antibody was measured by a method analogous to the final two steps of the MASELA (Figure 1). The areas between the pre- and post-immunization antibody dilution curves are calculated as described (7) for both in vitro production (MASELA) and in vivo production (plasma level).

RESULTS

Volunteers

We found no significant difference in blood counts, percent lymphocytes, or percent T-cells between the young and old volunteers. There was, however, in the elderly, a significantly smaller percentage of circulating T_4 positive (helper) cells (35.9% ± 1.5% elderly; 40.4% ± 0.9% young, p < 0.05). Correspondingly, in that group there was a reduction in the T_4/T_8 ratio (1.34 ± 0.09 elderly; 1.56 ± 0.05 young, p < 0.05). Of note, five of the elderly volunteers had a T_4/T_8 ratio of < 1, whereas none of the young did.

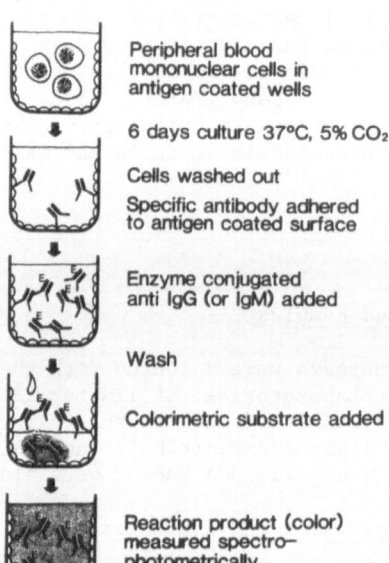

Peripheral blood mononuclear cells in antigen coated wells

6 days culture 37°C, 5% CO_2

Cells washed out
Specific antibody adhered to antigen coated surface

Enzyme conjugated anti IgG (or IgM) added

Wash

Colorimetric substrate added

Reaction product (color) measured spectro-photometrically

Figure 1. MASELA. Microculture antibody synthesis enzyme linked assay (MASELA) for determination of specific antibody synthesis in vitro. Mononuclear cells were cultured in antigen coated microtiter wells and the specific antibody synthesized, secreted into the culture supernatant and adhered to the solid phase antigen is measured by standard enzyme linked immunosorbent assay.

Table 1. Antibody Response after Influenza Vaccine (area)

	Elderly (n = 30)	Young (n = 31)
In vitro synthesis (MASELA)	66.3 ± 13.2	211.2 ± 23.4
In vivo synthesis (Plasma)	72.2 ± 9.5	173.2 ± 15.2

Antibody Studies

As can be seen in Table 1 there was a greater antibody response observed in vitro (MASELA) and in vivo (plasma level) in the young volunteers.

Furthermore, there was a positive correlation between capabilities of in vitro antibody response and the observed plasma response (Figure 2). Of interest, all of the elderly volunteers and eight of the young volunteers had received vaccines in the previous years. Pre-immunization plasma levels were significantly greater for the old and young "booster" group when compared to the young, "non-booster" ($p < 0.025$). Nevertheless, the young "booster" group did achieve a post-vaccination level (in vitro and in vivo) comparable to the "non-booster" immunized young, significantly greater than the old ($p < 0.001$).

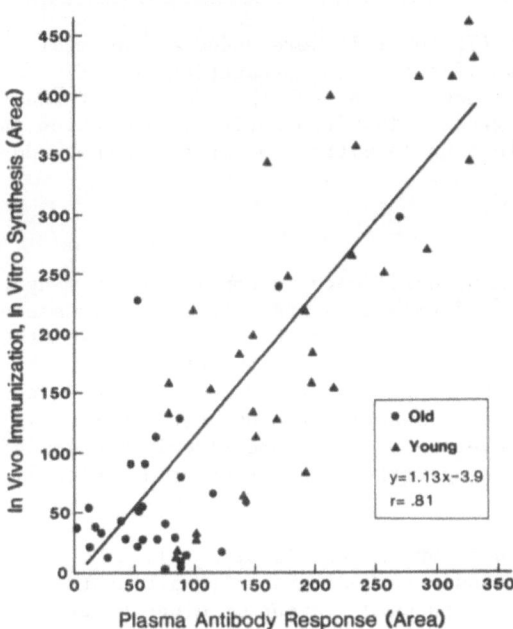

Figure 2. Correlation between plasma antibody levels and in vitro synthesis after vaccination. Greater production in vitro was generally observed in individuals who also responded with higher in vivo (plasma) production ($p < 0.01$).

Table 2. Δ In Vitro Synthesis[‡]
ΔIn Vivo Synthesis

	Young	Elderly
*Thymosin α1	1.25	.79
0.01 ng/ml	1.30 (4)	.91 (15)
0.1 ng/ml	1.30 (4)	.96 (22)
1.0 ng/ml	1.35 (8)	1.18 (49)
*Thymosin Fraction 5		
50 µg/ml	1.35 (8)	.93 (18)
100 µg/ml	1.44 (15)	1.09 (38)
200 µg/ml	1.33 (6)	1.03 (30)

[‡]Value represents the slope of the regression line correlating
in vitro synthesis (by the MASELA) and in vivo synthesis (plasma
antibody level pre- and post-immunization).

*The change in slope when thymic hormone was added to the in vitro
synthesis assay is represented with the percent change in paren-
theses. A positive increment in slope represents greater in
vitro antibody synthesis with the added hormone. Both thymosin
α1 and fraction 5 augmented antibody production in vitro to a
greater extent in the elderly.

The Effect of Thymic Hormones on In Vitro Antibody Production

Thymic hormones (TF5 or Tα1) were added to the media of the lymphocyte
cultures in which specific antibody production in vitro (MASELA) was
measured. As can be seen in Table 2, the addition of the thymic hormone
was associated with greater in vitro antibody production in the elderly,
without striking effect on in vitro production in the young.

DISCUSSION

Age-acquired immune deficiency is considered by many to be causally
related to the increased neoplasia and infectious disease observed in the
elderly population. In addition to the increased susceptibility to infections, immunodeficiency contributes to the greater severity of acquired
infections, such as influenza. For that reason, the United States Public
Health Service recommends annual influenza vaccine for all people over 65
years of age (8). Nevertheless, in some elderly people deficient antibody
responses have been demonstrated and influenza has clearly occurred in vaccinated subjects (3).

The age-acquired immune defect is primarily a "T" cell dysfunction
(9); and antibody response to T-dependent complex antigens such as viral
proteins has been shown to be deficient in elderly subjects. The demonstrated in vitro biologic activity (primarily augmentation) of the thymic
hormone preparations is also consistent with at least some alteration in
T-cell function accounting for the observed decreased antibody response in
our elderly subjects. Thymic hormones are generally considered immunorestorative when T cell deficiencies exist, but have been shown, in general,
to have little in vitro activity in normal immune-competent subjects (10).

In our study, we have shown that specific antibody response to the trivalent influenza vaccine was significantly less in a group of fully ambulatory, healthy elderly volunteers when compared to young controls. This was true even when accounting for that component of the reduced response due to previous immunization and pre-immunization antibody levels. After a fairly extensive in vitro evaluation of immune competence we found that the best prediction of antibody response was the in vitro specific antibody synthesis measured in the MASELA. This correlation would be necessary if one is to use the assay to test, in vitro, the capabilities of biologic response modifiers such as thymic hormones and project the potential clinical efficacy of such intervention. Accordingly, from our studies, it is apparent that in vitro antibody production was less in those people in whom peak plasma levels were also less. It is in these same individuals that it also appears that thymic hormones have their greatest effect in vitro. These findings would suggest that treatment with the thymic hormones as an adjunct to vaccination, may be associated with a more favorable antibody response in certain cases. Whether or not the increased antibody level would result in "protection" in an individual who, at the lower level would not have been protected from influenza infection, is a matter of obvious importance but one that will not be resolved until a large prospective, randomized trial is undertaken.

REFERENCES

1. H. N. A. Willcox, Thymus dependence of the antibody response to tetanus toxoid in mice, Clin. Exp. Immunol. 22:341 (1975).
2. J. L. Virelizier, R. Postelwaite, G. C. Schild, and A. C. Allison, Antibody responses to antigenic determinants of influenza virus hemagglutinin I. Thymus dependence of antibody formation and thymus independence of immunologic memory, J. Exp. Med. 140:1559 (1974).
3. J. Phair, C. A. Kauffman, and A. Bjornson, Failure to respond to influenza vaccine in the aged: correlation with B cell number and function J. Lab. Clin. Med. 92:822 (1978).
4. W. B. Ershler, A. L. Moore, M. P. Hacker, J. T. Ninomyia, P. B. Naylor, and A. L. Goldstein, Specific antibody synthesis in vitro. II. Age-associated thymosin enhancement of anti-tetanus antibody synthesis, Immunopharmacology (in press).
5. W. B. Ershler, A. L. Moore, and M. P. Hacker, Specific in vivo and in vitro antibody response to tetanus toxoid immunization, Clin. Exp. Immunol. 49:552 (1982).
6. A. L. Moore, W. B. Ershler, and M. P. Hacker, Specific antibody synthesis in vitro. I. Technical considerations, J. Immunol. Methods (in press).
7. W. B. Ershler, A. L. Moore, and M. A. Socinski, Influenza and aging: age-related changes and the effect of thymosin on the antibody response to influenza vaccine, J. Clin. Immunol. (in press).
8. Center for Disease Control, Department of Health and Human Sciences, Influenza Vaccines 1982-83, Recommendation of the Immunization Practices Advisory Committee, Ann. Intern. Med. 97:581 (1982).
9. T. Makinodan and M. M. B. Kay, Age influence on the immune system, in: "Advances in Immunology," H. G. Kunkel, F. J. Dixon, eds., Academic Press, New York (1980).
10. A. L. Goldstein, J. L. K. Low, G. B. Thurman, M. Zatz, N. R. Hall, J. E. McClure, S. K. Hus, and R. S. Schulof, Thymosins and other hormone-like factors of the thymus gland, in: "Immunological Approaches to Cancer Therapeutics," E. Michich, ed., John Wiley and Sons, New York (1982).

STUDIES OF BONE MARROW AND SERA OF CATS RECOVERING

FROM LEUKEMIA FOLLOWING PROTEIN A THERAPY

Wing T. Liu, Robert W. Engelman, Liem Q. Trang, Osmond
J. M. D'Cruz, Robert A. Good, and Noorbibi K. Day

Cancer Research Program, Oklahoma Medical Research Foundation
Oklahoma City, Oklahoma and University of South Florida
College of Medicine, Department of Pediatrics/St. Petersburg
at All Children's Hospital, St. Petersburg, Florida

INTRODUCTION

The feline leukemia virus (FeLV) is a contagious retrovirus of cats
that causes leukemia-lymphoma and various neoplastic diseases including
immunosuppression and a regenerative anemia (1). We have shown that FeLV
infected cats with leukemia are hypocomplementemic (2) and have elevated
levels of circulating immune complexes (CICs) (3). More recently, we have
treated some FeLV leukemic cats by ex vivo immunoadsorption therapy using
Staphylococcus Protein A filters (4) and some by intraperitoneal injections
using purified Protein A.

Our results show that about 50% of the cats improved when either treatment was used. During therapy, tumor regressed and marrow and peripheral
blood neoplastic cell populations were reduced. Long-term remission of
disease occurred in 33% of treated cats. Five percent of these cats also
had clearance of viremia.

We show here that long-term remission was associated with first the
appearance of high levels of interferon, associated with the appearance of
a complement-dependent cytotoxic antibody. The cytotoxic antibody was
found to be specific for the membrane protein gp70 of the virus.

MATERIAL AND METHODS

Animals

Pet cats were selected for treatment by ex vivo immunoadsorption (4),
or by injection with purified SPA (Pharmacia Fine Chemicals, Uppsala,
Sweden). The Protein A injections were given I.P. (20 µg/2.75 kg body
weight) twice weekly for 10-12 weeks. Bone marrow and peripheral blood
smears were evaluated prior to treatments and following every tenth treatment. FeLV status was determined biweekly by indirect immunofluorescence
assay (IFA) (5), and enzyme-linked immunosorbent assay (ELISA) as described
previously (4). Pre- and post-treatment serum samples were stored at -70°C
until assayed for interferon (IFN) and cytotoxic antibody.

Feline IFN Assay

Feline IFN was assayed by a modification of the microplaque reduction method (6) using approximately 40 plaque-forming units (PFU) of vesicular stomatitis virus (VSV) per well on FFC-9 cells (Fetal cat fibroblast cell line kindly provided by Dr. N. C. Pedersen, University of California, Davis, California). A concentration of 1 unit/ml IFN was defined as the concentration required to decrease the number of PFU per well by 50%. All serum samples were assayed in duplicate and the IFN titers represent the average of the two determinations. For all IFN assays, Staphylococcal enterotoxin A (SEA)-induced feline IFN, and Newcastle disease virus (NDV)-induced feline IFN were used as reference feline IFNs for monitoring the assays.

In Vitro Induction of Feline IFNs by SEA or NDV

SEA (Microbial Biochemistry Branch, Division of Microbiology, Food and Drug Administration, Cincinnati, Ohio) and NDV (American Type Culture Collection, Rockville, Maryland) were used for the in vitro induction of IFNs (7,8). For SEA-induced IFN, normal cat peripheral blood lymphocytes (PBL), isolated by centrifugation of heparinized blood through Ficoll-Hypaque gradient (Pharmacia), were incubated with SEA (0.5 μg/ml) at a concentration of 5×10^6 cells/ml in 35 mm Falcon (Oxnard, California) culture dishes. Cultures were maintained at 37°C in culture boxes gassed with 10% CO_2, 7% O_2, and 83% N_2 mixture for three days on a rocking platform (8 cycles/min). The supernates from these cultures containing feline IFN were stored in aliquots at -70°C until used. For induction of feline IFN by NDV, FCC-9 cells were grown in minimal essential medium (MEM) supplemented with 10% fetal calf serum (Gibco, Grand Island, New York) and 40 μg/ml Garamycin (Gibco) in 75 cm^2 plastic flasks (Falcon) until the monolayer became confluent. The culture medium was then replaced by 3 ml of MEM containing NDV (approximate titer 2.5×10^4 egg infecting dose EID_{50}). Virus was allowed to be adsorbed for 1 hr before addition of 15 ml of fresh culture medium. The monolayer was maintained for 24 hrs. The culture medium was then centrifuged at 20,000 rpm for 45 min (JA-21 fixed angle rotor, Beckman, California) to remove the virus. The supernate containing feline IFN was stored in aliquots at -70°C until used.

Characterization of Serum IFNs in Cats

Feline IFNs were characterized on the basis of pH 2 and heat lability (56°C for 30 min) (7,9). IFN preparations were lowered to pH 2 with 1 M HCl, incubated at 4°C for 24 hrs, and then raised to pH 7.0 with HEPES buffer (Gibco) prior to the IFN assay.

Reagents for Assay of Cytotoxic Antibody

Buffers. Veronal (barbital)-buffered saline (VBS^{++}), pH 7.4, ionic strength 015μ, containing 0.1% gelatin, 0.15mM $CaCl_2$ and 1 mM $MgCl_2$.

Complement (C). Pooled guinea pig serum (GPS) (Gibco) was used as a source of C for the cytotoxicity assays.

Target cells. FL-74 cells were grown in 75 cm^2 plastic flasks (Falcon), in McCoy's 5A modified growth medium (Gibco) supplemented with 15% heat-inactivated fetal calf serum (Gibco), and 2mM glutamine (Gibco). Penicillin (100 units/ml), Streptomycin (100 μg/ml) and fungizone (0.25 μg/ml) were included. Normal cat peripheral blood lymphocytes (PBL) were obtained by centrifugation of heparinized blood through Ficoll-Hypaque gradients (Pharmacia, Piscataway, New Jersey). The final PBL concentration was adjusted to 2.5×10^6 cells/ml, unless stated otherwise.

Viruses. FeLV ABC/KT (0.94 mg protein/ml) (Pfizer, Inc., Groton, Connecticut) and mouse mammary tumor virus MMTV/C3H (3 mg protein/ml), (Meloy Laboratories, Inc., Springfield, Virginia) were used.

Cytotoxicity Assay for Antibodies to FL-74 Cells

Cytotoxicity assay. FL-74 cells were washed twice in VBS^{++} and suspended to 2.5 x 10^6 cells per ml in VBS^{++}. 100 µl of 1:3 dilution of heat inactivated (56°C for 30 min) cat plasma at 73°C for 30 min. The cells were washed once in VBS^{++}, then centrifuged at 1200 rpm in Model J6B centrifuge (Beckman) for 8 min. The supernate was removed and the cells resuspended in 300 µl of 1:10 dilution of fresh GPS (experimental group) or 300 µl of a 1:10 dilution of heat inactivated (56°C for 30 min) GPS (control group). The reaction mixtures were incubated for 37°C for 60min. Cell viability was determined by vital dye exclusion and by assay of LDH release. PBL from FeLV negative cats were also used as target cells.

Assays for cell viability. Vital dye exclusion and release of LDH (10) with minor modification was used.

Detection of IgG Antibodies Against Membranes of Viable FL-74 Cells by Indirect Immunofluorescence Assay (IFA)

The test plasma was diluted 1:5 with phosphate buffered saline (PBS), pH 7.4. 200 l of diluted serum was incubated with 100 µl of FL-74 cells (3 x 10^7 cells/ml) in PBS at 37°C for 30 min. The cells were washed three times with PBS. The cell pellet was suspended in 100 µl of diluted (1:25 in PBS) fluorescein-conjugated rabbit anti-cat IgG (Antibodies, Inc.), and the mixture incubated at 37°C for 30 min. The cells were washed three times and resuspended in one or two drops of glycerol containing 50% by volume of PBS. A drop of the suspension was placed on a microscope slide and mounted with a cover slip. Immunofluorescent preparations were scored using a Leitz (Dialux 20) microscope (Leitz, Inc., Rheinsberg, Berlin, Germany) under epi-illumination.

Absorption studies. Cat plasma samples positive for cytotoxic antibody to FL-74 cells were absorbed with FeLV or MMTV. Different volumes (30 µl or 50 µl) of undisrupted virus mixed with 300 µl of cat plasma. The absorption procedure was carried out on a rotor (Model 7537, Cole-Parmer Instrument Company, Chicago, Illinois) at 4°C for 16 hrs. The mixture was centrifuged at 20,000 rpm for 45 min (JA-21 fixed angle rotor, Beckman). Activities of the preadsorbed and adsorbed plasma samples were evaluated in parallel by the cytotoxicity assays described above. The specificity of the cytotoxic antibody was also determined by electroblot technique and with monoclonal antibodies (11).

RESULTS

Only cats with advanced FeLV associated disease were treated. Fifty percent of the cats (48 were evaluated) improved objectively. During treatment tumor regressed, marrow and peripheral blood neoplastic cell populations were reduced and hematologic values became normal. Figures 1, 2, and 3 represent a cat with erythroleukemia that had responded to treatment with injections of Protein A (11). Long-term remission of disease occurred in six of 18 cats (33%) and clearance of FeLV viremia occurred in 28% of cats.

Interferon studies. Serum interferon levels of treated cats were as follows: cats responding to treatment had elevated levels of interferon and in some instances were 30-fold over normal levels (11). Cats not

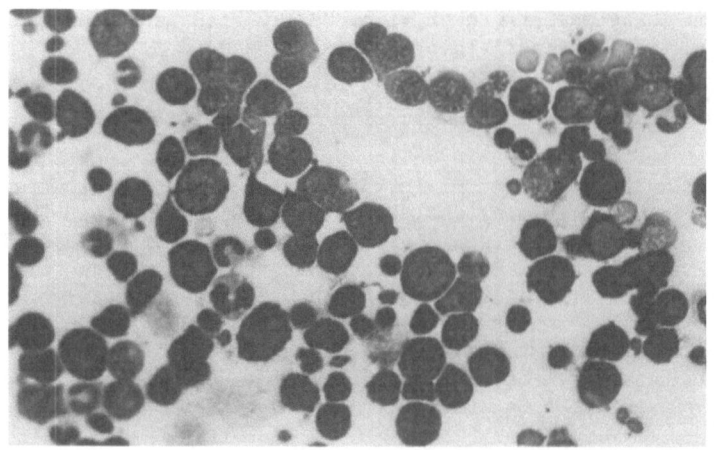

Figure 1. Pretreatment bone marrow cytology of cat 152 with erythroleukemia. Excessive numbers of rubriblasts and prorubricytes and inappropriately few numbers of more mature erythrocytic precursors are present.

responding to treatment had undetectable levels. Healthy cats (two of six) showed moderate transient elevations.

Complement-dependent cytotoxic antibody. Marked elevations of cytotoxic antibody appeared only in sera of those cats that responded to therapy. The cytotoxic antibody was found to be specific for gp70 of the membrane protein of the virus (12).

Relationship Between Interferon Levels, Cytotoxic Antibody and Loss of Viremia

In all cases of successfully treated cats, the increased interferon levels preceded the appearance of cytotoxic antibody and loss of virema (11).

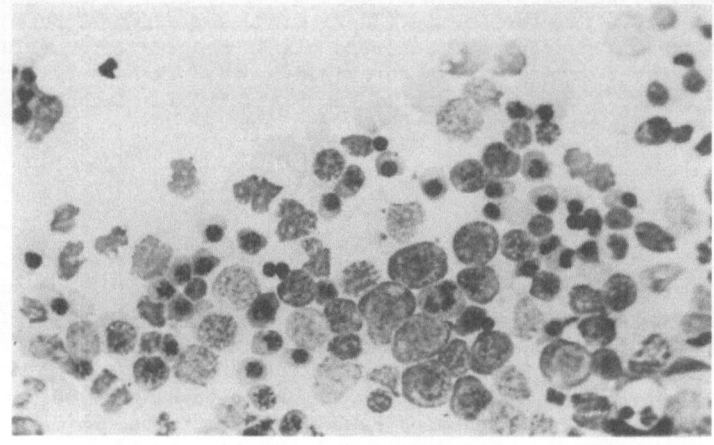

Figure 2. Bone marrow cytology of cat 152 after ten treatments. Numerous megaloblastoid rubricytes and metarubricytes are present and the blast population is reduced from pretreatment numbers.

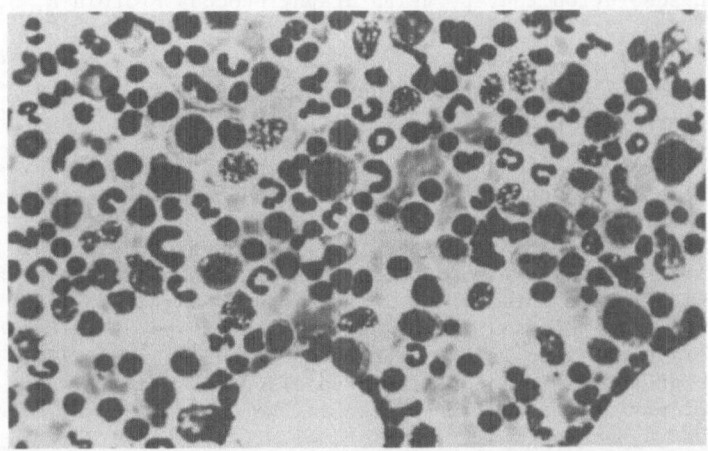

Figure 3. Post-treatment bone marrow cytology of cat 152. A heterogeneous population of cells is present without significant abnormalities.

CONCLUSION

1. Regression of leukemia occurred in about 50% of persistently FeLV infected cats with leukemia following treatment with Staphylococcus Protein A.

2. Fifteen to eighteen percent of cats went into long-term remission.

3. Five percent of cats also became non-viremic.

4. Cats responding to therapy developed high levels of serum interferon followed by the appearance in the circulation of a complement-dependent cytotoxic antibody.

5. The complement-dependent cytotoxic antibody was directed against the gp70 of the membrane protein of FELV (11,12).

ACKNOWLEDGMENTS

This work was supported in part by grants awarded by the National Institutes of Health, grant #CA-34103, and the American Cancer Society, grant #IM-298.

REFERENCES

1. W. D. Hardy, The virology, immunology and epidemiology of the feline leukemia virus, in: "Feline Leukemia Virus," W. D. Hardy, M. Essex, and A. J. McClelland, eds., Elsevier/North-Holland (1980).
2. L. Kobilinsky, W. D. Hardy, and N. K. Day, Hypocomplementemia associated with naturally occurring lymphosarcoma in pet cats, J. Immunol. 122:2139 (1979).
3. N. K. Day, F. O'Reilly, W. D. Hardy, Jr., R. A. Good, and S. S. Witkin, Circulating immune complexes associated with naturally occurring lymphosarcoma in pet cats, J. Immunol. 125:2363 (1980).
4. N. K. Day, R. W. Engelman, W. T. Liu, L. Q. Trang, and R. A. Good, Remission of lymphoma leukemia in cats following ex vivo

immunoadsorption therapy using Staphylococcus Protein A, J. Biol. Resp. Mod. 3:278 (1984).

5. W. D. Hardy, Y. Hirshaut, and P. Hess, Detection of the feline leukemia virus and other mammalian oncornaviruses by immunofluorescence, in: "Unifying Concepts of Leukemia," R. M. Dutcher and L. Chicco-Bianchi, eds., Karger, Basel (1973).

6. J. B. Campbell, T. Grunsberger, M. A. Kochman, and S. L. White, A microplaque reduction assay for human and mouse interferon, Can. J. Microbiol. 21:1247 (1975).

7. M. P. Langford, J. A. Georgiades, G. J. Stanton, F. Dianzani and H. M. Johnson, Large-scale production and physiochemical characterization of human immune interferon, Infect. and Immun. 26:36 (1979).

8. L. Hanna, T. C. Merigan, and E. Jawetz, Inhibition of TRIC agents by virus-induced interferon, Proc. Soc. Exp. Biol. Med. 122:417 (1966).

9. J. S. Youngner and S. B. Salvin, Production and properties of migration inhibitory factor and interferon in the circulation of mice with delayed hypersensitivity, J. Immunol. 111:1914 (1973).

10. C. L. Koski, L. E. Ramm, C. H. Hammer, M. M. Mayer, and M. L. Shin, Cytolysis of nucleated cells by complement: cell death displays multi-hit characteristics, Proc. Natl. Acad. Sci. USA 80:3816 (1983).

11. W. T. Liu, R. A. Good, L. Q. Trang, R. W. Engelman, and N. K. Day, Remission of leukemia and loss of feline leukemia virus in cats injected with Staphylococcus Protein A: association with elevated levels of circulating interferon and complement-dependent cytotoxic antibody, Proc. Natl. Acad. Sci. USA in press (1984).

12. W. T. Liu, R. W. Engelman, L. Q. Trang, K. Hau, R. A. Good, and N. K. Day, Appearance of cytotoxic antibody to viral gp70 on feline lymphoma cells (FL-74) in cats during ex vivo immunoadsorption therapy: quantitation, characterization and association with remission of disease and disappearance of viremia, Proc. Natl. Acad. Sci. USA 81:3516 (1984).

SYNERGISTIC ANTI-TUMOR EFFECT OF AN IMMUNOPOTENTIATOR (PAV)

AND AN INHIBITOR (CIMETIDINE) OF T-SUPPRESSOR CELLS

Eddy Ríos-Olivares, Zilka M. Orraca and Julio I. Colón

Escuela de Medicina de Cayey, Cayey, Puerto Rico and
Puerto Rico Cancer Center, San Juan, Puerto Rico

INTRODUCTION

As our understanding of the complex polyantigenic nature of the human cancer cell expands, it becomes more apparent that it would require the development of a large catalogue of specific vaccines, a large library to fill them, or a battery of monoclonal antibodies for the many types of known and undiscovered human cancer.

One way to overcome this limitation is to potentiate the immune response on a global basis. This approach supplemented with the application of agents with known immunomodulating activity might prove to be a more effective strategy in manipulating the immune system against cancer. It is in this context that the present study was designed to evaluate the combined utilization of two substances with potential immunotherapeutic application.

Polyantigenic vaccine (PAV) consists of a mixture of inactivated bacteria and influenza virus in a peanut oil-arlacel-A-aluminum monoesterate emulsion. PAV has been shown to increase tumor resistance and regression in tumor-bearing mice (1). Also preliminary human data (2) indicate that PAV increased the phytohemagglutinin induced lymphocyte transformation into proliferating lymphoblast.

Cimetidine (C) is an H-2 histamine receptor antagonist that has been used clinically in the United States since 1977 as a potent inhibitor of gastric acid secretion. Recently, cimetidine has been shown to augment the proliferative response of human lymphocytes to mitogens, bacterial antigens, or alloantigens (3) and that it is capable of reducing tumor formation in mice challenged with two types of syngenic tumor (4). Clinical success was reported in patients with malignant melanoma when alpha interferon was administered with cimetidine (5).

MATERIAL AND METHODS

Seventy-seven two-month old female and male mice were divided into 11 groups. Except for the untreated control group, all other groups were implanted intraperitoneally with various amounts of Ehrlich Ascites Tumors (EAT) ranging from 10^5 to 3×10^6 cells/mouse and treated with different regimens of either PAV, C or a combination of both. Treatment for two weeks was given to indicated groups by continuous oral doses of C (Tagamet, Smith-Kline and French Laboratories) and PAV between 0.53 (0.53 mg/day/mouse is equivalent to the recommended human daily dose) and 3.18 mg/day/mouse and/or five 0.1 ml doses of PAV (one every three days) administered intraperitoneally. Cimetidine and/or PAV treatment were started three and four days after tumor implantation respectively. Tumor growth was assessed every three or four days by weighing each mouse. For each modality of treatment, the percent of survival was determined at 30, 60, and 90 days. Average days of survival was calculated by assigning a maximum of 90 days to those mice that were alive at that time.

In separate experiments 100,000 X G-spleen and thymus homogenates, prepared from a pool of 15 mice that were treated daily with 0.1 ml of PAV, were tested on L-929 cell 24 hour monolayers. Cytotoxicity was detected by determining the percent of cells surviving a 24 hour exposure to different homogenate dilutions (undiluted to 1:48). Cytotoxicity was also assessed by measuring inhibition of ^{3}H-thymidine incorporation in L-929 cell 24 hour monolayers by the mouse spleen and thymus homogenates.

The homogenates were also assayed for the presence of interferon. For this purpose, the plaque reducing test was performed utilizing vesicular stomatitis virus and L-929 cells. An internal standard of beta interferon (250 interferon units/ml) was used as positive control. Separate tests were run with acid-treated and with non-acid treated homogenates.

RESULTS AND DISCUSSION

Mice implanted with a low tumor load (10^5 cells/mouse) of EAT showed a significant reduction in tumor growth ($p < 0.05$) in the groups that received

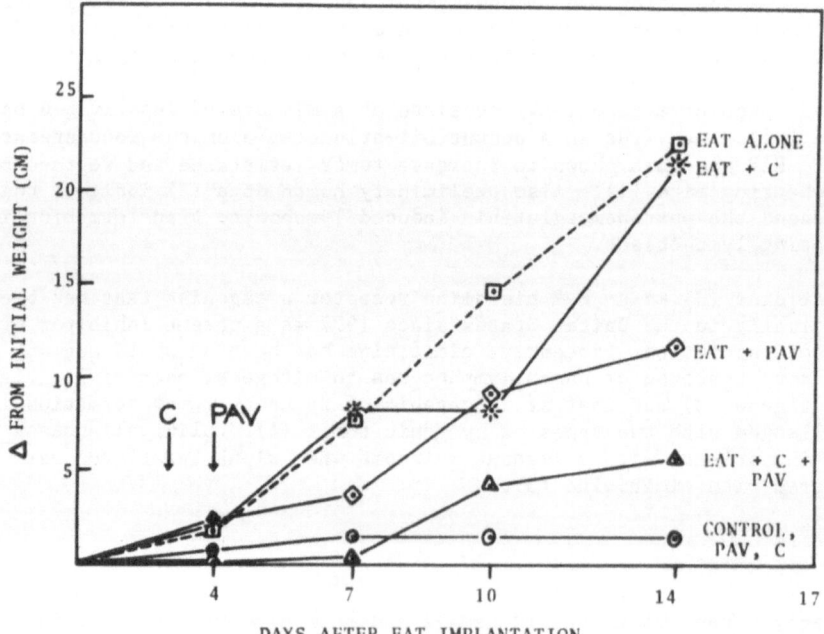

Figure 1. Tumor growth in mice implanted with 3×10^6 EAT cells/mouse and treated with 1.06 mg/day/mouse of cimetidine (c), PAV or a combination of both.

Table 1. Survival of Mice Implanted with 3 x 10^6 EAT Cells/Mouse and
Treated with PAV Different Doses of Cimetidine (C)

| Treatment | No Mice | % Survival | | | X Day Survival (90 Days) |
		30 Days	60 Days	90 Days	
Control	21	100	100	100	90
EAT alone	21	9.5	0	0	23.2
EAT and PAV	21	70	24	19	42.2
EAT + C + PAV 0.53 (a)	7	71.4	42.9	28.6	54.1
EAT + C + PAV 1.06	7	100	57.1	28.6	60
EAT + C + PAV 2.12	7	72	28.6	28.6	50
EAT + C + PAV 3.18	7	43	0	0	32

(a) 0.53 mg/day/mouse = human daily dose

PAV or the combination (PAV + C) when compared to the untreated implanted
group. Cimetidine and PAV when used separately or combined were able to
protect tumor-bearing mice and the survivals obtained when utilizing 1.06
mg/day/mouse of cimetidine were 54%, 74.8%, and 80.4%, respectively. There
were no survivors in the group that received only EAT. The difference between the PAV and PAV + C treated groups was not significant. However, as
the tumor load increased to 5 x 10^5 cells/mouse, differences in mortality
and average day survival among the groups receiving the various therapeutic
regimens became more pronounced.

The response of mice implanted with high tumor dose (3 x 10^6 cells/-
mouse) to 1.06 mg/day/mouse of cimetidine either alone or combined with PAV
are shown in Figure 1. There was no significant difference in the tumor
growth curves in the groups treated with PAV alone compared with those that
received the combination at concentrations of 0.53 and 3.18 mg/day/mouse of
cimetidine. However, a significant reduction in tumor growth ($p < 0.05$) was
detected if the concentration of cimetidine used in the combined therapy
was either 1.06 or 2.12 mg/day/mouse.

The survival data of mice implanted with a heavy load of tumor and
treated with PAV and different doses of cimetidine are presented in Table 1.
The survival and the average day of survival is higher in the group that
received a combined treatment in which the concentration of cimetidine employed was 1.06. The effectiveness of the combined therapy was assessed
using the fractional product method (6). Synergistic effect was found when
the concentrations of cimetidine utilized were 0.53, 1.06, and 2.12 mg/day/-
mouse.

There were no detectable side effects associated with either cimetidine,
PAV or the combination during the period of observation.

Similar in vitro cytotoxic activity was detected in mouse spleen and
thymus homogenates prepared from mice treated with PAV and those groups
treated with the combination of PAV + C. On the other hand, there was no
significant increase in the interferon titer (<100 units) in the treated

groups of mice. Previous attempts to detect significant induction of interferon by PAV in chickens were also unsuccessful.

CONCLUSION

The most important finding to emerge from this study is that there was a definite enhancement of antitumor activity when cimetidine and PAV therapy were combined. When tumor load was small, treatment with PAV alone or the combination were similarly effective in reducing tumor growth and increasing mouse survival. However, as the tumor load increased there were statistically significant differences in the anti-tumor activity between the groups treated with the combination as compared to those groups that received either PAV or cimetidine alone. Synergistic and not additive activity appears to explain the increased anti-tumor effect of the combined therapy. The most effective oral concentration of cimetidine when used in combination with PAV was 1.06 mg/day/mouse.

Our results are in agreement with earlier findings (1,7,8) of the immunotherapeutic value of PAV in the enhancement of the immune response to experimental tumor and with those of the in vitro detection of induced cytotoxic activity.

The failure of the repeated attempts to detect interferon might be explained by either: (1) a regulatory effect of PAV on its production; (2) inactivation by other components present in the spleen or thymus homogenates; and (3) sensitivity of our test system or a combination of these. Nevertheless, our data suggest that other substances(s) with cytotoxic activity might be responsible for the anti-tumor activity observed. This subject will be dealt with in future communications.

REFERENCES

1. J. I. Colon, A. M. Marchand, A. A. Roman, and E. A. Santiago-Delpín, The immunotherapeutic effect of a polyantigenic vaccine in animal tumor models, Bol. Asoc. Med. PR 73:162 (1981).
2. J. I. Colón, A. M. Marchand, M. T. Rodríguez, and D. Valldejuli, Stimulation of phytohemagglutinin blast transformation in cancer patients by a polyantigenic vaccine, in: "Regulation of the Immune Response," P. L. Ogra and D. M. Jacobs, eds., (1982).
3. R. R. M. Gifford, S. M. Hatfield, and J. R. Schmidtke, Cimetidine induced augmentation of human lymphocyte blastogenesis by mitogen, bacterial antigen and alloantigen, Transplantation 29:143 (1980).
4. R. R. M. Gifford, R. M. Ferguson, and B. V. Voss, Cimetidine reduction of tumor formation in mice, Lancet i:638 (1981).
5. S. Borgstrom, F. E. von Eyben, P. Flodgren, B. Axelsson, and H. Sjogren, Human leucocyte interferon and cimetidine for metastatic melanoma, N. Eng. J. Med. 307:1080 (1982).
6. J. L. Webb, "Enzymes and Metabolic Inhibitors," Academic Press, New York (1963).
7. E. Ríos-Olivares, A. M. Orraca, A. M. Marchand, and J. I. Colón, Cell growth inhibiting factor induced by a polyantigenic vaccine, Abstract of ASM 88 (1981).
8. Z. M. Orraca, E. Ríos-Olivares, A. M. Marchand, and J. I. Colón, Inhibition of DNA synthesis in L-929 cells by spleen homogenates of mouse injected with a polyantigenic vaccine, in press.

IMMUNOMODULATION BY A POLYANTIGENIC VACCINE (PAV) IN

PATIENTS WITH ACQUIRED IMMUNODEFICIENCIES

J. I. Colón, J. N. Moreno, M. L. Santaella, K. M. Lang,
A. M. Marchand, M. R. Ortiz, K. D. Bonilla, M. I. Roque,
M. Cortés, F. López-Malpica, P. Mora-Urdaz

Puerto Rico Cancer Center and Departments of
Pathology and Medicine, School of Medicine
and San Juan City Hospital, Medical Sciences Campus
San Juan, Puerto Rico

A polyantigenic vaccine consisting of a mixture of antigens of inactivated bacteria and antigens of influenza virus in a peanut oil-arlacel-A-aluminum monoesterate emulsion (1) increased tumor resistance and tumor regression in tumor-bearing mice (1,2) and induced cell growth inhibiting factors in spleen and thymus of mice (3). This vaccine also stimulated phytohemagglutinin (PHA) blast transformation in cancer patients and in patients with viral infections (4,5). This report is the result of a trial of immunomodulation by PAV in patients with acquired cell-mediated immunodeficiencies.

Patients included in this study belong to high risk groups and presented generalized adenopathy, reversal of the T cell helper-suppressor ratio, cutaneous anergy to PPD, mumps and candida, weight loss and fever. Six patients were included in this open study. Three received two subcutaneous injections of PAV per week, one patient was on a placebo and two did not receive PAV or placebo. All patients were monitored at different intervals for immunomodulation, clinical toxicity and response. Monocytes, B cells and T subsets were monitored with monoclonal antibodies. Enumeration of lymphocyte populations were done with sheep red blood cells using the EAC and E rosette techniques for B and T cells. The blastogenic response was done with PHA stimulation.

The lymphocyte subset analysis and functional assays for patients treated with PAV are shown in Table 1. Treated patients demonstrated normalization of the helper-suppressor ratio, augmentation of T4 (helper) cells, decreased T8 (suppressor) cells and increased blastogenic response.

The lymphocyte counts, subset analysis and functional assays of patients not treated with PAV or on a placebo are shown in Table 2. The suppressor cells increased and the helper cells and the blastogenic response decreased.

The clinical features of the patients are shown in Table 3. All PAV treated patients showed diminution in lymph node size, weight gain, no development of infectious processes and were completely asymptomatic. Of the two patients not treated with PAV, patient #5 developed systemic candidiasis and Pneumocystis carinii pneumonia and patient #6 developed

Table 1. Lymphocyte Subset Analysis and Functional Assays of Patients Treated with PAV

Patient Number	% Total T	% T$_4$	% T$_8$	% Total B	Ratio T$_{4/8}$	PHA** Index
1 02/19/83	–	–	–	–	0.72	8.3
03/03/83	69	18	47	16	0.38	–
03/21/83*	66	28	41	4	0.68	20.8
04/21/83	84	40	42	15	0.95	25.7
08/21/83	60	42	24	9	1.75	43.5
2 04/11/83	77	24	52	11	0.46	31.6
05/03/83*	76	16	62	5	0.26	–
06/28/83	57	16	54	18	0.3	51.5
08/23/83	48	24	40	8	0.6	60.0
03/03/84	–	–	–	–	–	20.6
3 10/24/83*	41	17	27	5	0.63	15.0
01/16/84	80	31	38	11	0.82	12.0
04/04/84	84.3	31.3	53.2	43.3	0.59	22.4
Normal Values	72±8	46±12%	28±8	12±4	1.6±0.74	18±7

* PAV started;   **PHA phytohemagglutinin

Table 2. Lymphocyte Subset Analysis and Functional Assays of Patients Not Treated with PAV

Patient Number	% Total T	% T$_4$	% T$_8$	% Total B	Ratio T4/8	PHA Index
4 04/18/83	73	41	45	4	0.91	21
08/15/83	36	18	18	11	1.00	11
10/24/83	65	19	28	16	0.68	–
12/13/83*	59	13	32	17	0.41	27
01/16/84	41	29	33	14	0.88	26
04/04/84	72.8	25	40	13.3	0.6	60.5
5 10/15/82	–	–	–	–	–	13.0
02/24/83	–	–	–	–	–	11.3
06/27/83	–	–	–	–	0.1	4.7
08/22/83	16	8	20	3	0.4	3.2
10/03/83**	53	0	45	3	0.01	1.3
04/04/84	77	4.9	68.6	28.3	0.1	5.0
6 04/05/83***	–	5	54	–	0.1	41.2
05/02/83	–	–	–	–	–	24.8
09/06/83	–	6	27	–	0.2	40.6
Normal Values	72±8	46±12	28±8	12±4	1.6±0.74	18±7

* Patient started on PAV 11/08/83; ** Patient started on PAV 08/23/83
***Death on 10/83

Table 3. Clinical Features of Patients with AIDS After Treatment with PAV

Pt #	Age	Onset of Illness	Manifestations	Treat-ment	Current Status
1	29	10/82	Lymphadenopathy, fever, weight loss, diarrhea, night sweats, weakness frequent infections	03/83	Diminution in lymph node size, 18 lbs weight gain, asymptomatic
2	22	03/82	Lymphadenopathy, fever, arthralgia diarrhea, weight loss	05/83	Diminution in lymph node size, weight gain (24 lbs) asymptomatic
3	24	08/83	Lymphadenopathy, weight loss	12/83	Asymptomatic, diminution in lymph node size
4	48	03/82	Lymphadenopathy, fever, splenomegaly weakness	12/83	Asymptomatic, diminution in lymph node size
5	55	10/82	Weakness, anorexia, fever, lymph node enlargement, diarrhea, oral and esophageal candidiasis, autoimmune hemolytic anemia, P. carinii	08/83	Febrile on and off, urinary tract infection, no adenopathies
6	23*	05/83	Fever, general malaise weight loss, cytomegalo-virus infection, atypical mycobacteria infection, P. carinii	09/83	Died 10/83

*Female

systemic Mycobacterium intracellulare infection and P. carinii pneumonia. After two weeks on PAV patient #6 died and patient #5 is still alive after seven months treatment. Patient #4, who was on placebo, was put on PAV after showing clinical and immune deterioration. At the present time, after six months on PAV this patient is asymptomatic.

The results of these studies indicate that the administration of PAV to patients with acquired immunodeficiencies lead to a substained augmenta-tion of the lymphoproliferative response to PHA, normalization of the T helper-suppressor ratio, and disappearance of clinical symptoms, with diminu-tion in lymph node size, weight gain and no development of infectious pro-cesses. A clear relationship between clinical response and changes in immune cell parameters was evident. PAV showed no toxicity.

The normalization of the helper-suppressor ratio could be ascribed to a decrease of the suppressor cell population and the increase of helper population in some patients and the increase of helper population in others.

The exact mechanism of the clinical responsiveness in patients with acquired immunodeficiencies remains to be elucidated by further experimental work now in progress.

In summary, the results after six to twelve months of treatment strongly indicate that the immunomodulation and the improvement of lymphoblast reactions shown in vitro coupled with the positive clinical response observed in patients following treatment with PAV is worthy of further exploration as a modality for the treatment of patients with generalized lymphadenopathy, lymphadenopathy wasting syndrome, pre-AIDS or early stages of AIDS.

While this work was in progress the immune systems of 35 patients were evaluated and diagnosed as pre-AIDS or AIDS. Of this group, which received no treatment with PAV 13 died, five are very sick with opportunistic infections and two have Kaposi's sarcoma.

REFERENCES

1. J. I. Colón, A. M. Marchand, A. A. Román-Franco, and E. A. Santiago-Delpín, The immunotherapeutic effect of a polyantigenic vaccine in animal tumor model, Bol. Asoc. Med. PR 73:162 (1981).
2. J. I. Colón, A. M. Marchand, A. A. Román-Franco, and E. A. Santiago-Delpín, Induction of tumor regression by a poly-antigenic vaccine in mice, In Vitro 16:208 (1980).
3. E. Ríos-Olivares, Z. M. Orraca, A. M. Marchand, and J. I. Colón, Cell growth inhibiting factors induced by a polyantigenic vaccine, Abstracts of the Annual Meeting of the ASM 61 (1981).
4. J. I. Colón, A. M. Marchand, M. T. Rodríguez, and D. Valldejuli, Stimulation of phytohemagglutinin blast transformation in cancer patients by a polyantigenic vaccine, in: "Regulation of the Immune Response," P. L. Ogra and D. M. Jacobs, eds., Karger Press, Buffalo (1982).
5. J. I. Colón, A. M. Marchand, M. T. Rodríguez, and D. Valldejuli, Immunoenhancing effect of a polyantigenic vaccine in patients with deficient lymphocyte transformation, Abstracts of the Annual Meeting of the ASM 87 (1983).

VIRUSES, IMMUNITY, IMMUNODEFICIENCY AND CANCER*

Robert A. Good

University of South Florida College of Medicine
Department of Pediatrics/St. Petersburg at
All Children's Hospital
St. Petersburg, Florida

This scientific meeting has been an impressive experience for me for a number of reasons. First, it reminded me that my being captured for a career in immunology occurred in a context of a chance discovery which related to an influence of an immunologic process on virus infection and vice versa. As a graduate student, I was using a Herpes simplex virus infection of the peripheral nerve and anterior horn cells to influence nerve impulse transmission over the two neurone-two axon reflex in rabbits. It was at this time in 1943 that Kolouch introduced me to the plasma cell as a possible antibody-producing cell. Kolouch had observed plasma cell accumulation in the marrow and spleen in a patient with subacute bacterial endocarditis. In subsequent experiments with rabbits he had seen that during anaphylaxis, after repeated intravenous antigenic stimulation, plasma cells accumulated also in the marrow and spleen. He had, thus, postulated that the appearance of plasma cells in marrow and spleen represents an adaptive response of antibody producing cells to antigen injection. But he was worried that the physiologic concomitants of anaphylaxis might be responsible for anaphylaxis. To clarify this issue, I proposed that we produce anaphylaxis by either to two means--passive or active anaphylaxis. When the actively immunized rabbits were given a secondary or challenging injection of antigen to produce anaphylactic shock, a massive proliferation of precursor cells and extraordinary development of plasma cells was launched in the bone marrow and spleen. Not so with passive anaphylaxis. No readily demonstrable plasma cell accumulation was not due to physiologic changes secondary to anaphylaxis but rather to the secondary stimulation with antigen that launched the active anaphylaxis. This was my first immunologic experiment. It was a nice one. It was based on my own idea for evaluation of Kolouch's brilliant hypothesis and it formed the basis of my first independent scientific publication. But the experiment was done in pursuit of Kolouch's general hypothesis concerning plasma cells as the antibody-producing cell and as such as not extremely commanding to me. Because money for research projects was scarce in those days, I did pilot experiments for the plasma cell investigations with rabbits which had been

---

*This chapter is based on the final presentation of the Symposium by the author on April 25, 1984.

infected with and had recovered from acute infection with the herpes simplex virus that I was using for my neurophysiologic inquiries. To my amazement, I discovered that after initiation of an immunologic event, namely active anaphylaxis, it was possible to activate a residual latent virus infection. How that accidental discovery turned me on! There is no question about it, that discovery made me an immunologist instantly and completely committed for life. That was more than 40 years ago now and I have had the privilege of growing up with the field of immunology over the past 40 year period. At that early time, you will recall we knew nothing about the cells, organs or molecules involved in immunity, and in spite of even the great contributions of Metchnikoff, precious little about the other blood cells, e.g., macrophages and polymorphonuclear leukocytes, and their functions in the bodily defense.

The present conference has shown how sophisticated we have become in immunological matters over this forty year span. We now speak knowingly about the function of the thymus, we quantify the subpopulations of T cells and B cells and we analyze the interactions of these populations in quantitative terms and in terms of membrane antigens and receptors for growth factors. We consider the possibility that one of the major cell populations, T cells or macrophages, exerts controlling influences on other cells, e.g., B cells and/or T cells. We recognize and quantify the influence of natural killer cells, killer cytotoxic cells (ADCC) and specific cytotoxic lymphocytes that can destroy infected cells containing virus to which the host has been immunized. We even understand specificity in terms of a detailed knowledge of the chemistry of antibodies and immunoglobulins. We know about T lymphocyte receptors and we can think creatively in terms of gene rearrangements and somatic mutations for both the T cell receptors and antibodies.

Only recently has the molecular mechanism of how T cell specificity is achieved been worked out. The basis for this specificity is a two-chain molecule anchored at the cell surface extending through the cell membrane. This molecule, elusive for so long, looks very much like two light chains tied together by disulfide linkages toward the proximal end and anchored into the cell membrane by hydrophobic stretches at the end of each of its constituent monomers.

My initial discovery suggesting that an immunological event can influence virus expression was, in those early days, wrapped in mystery. It remains so today even though the finding has been confirmed by several others. The finding indicates that though we have learned much about immunity to viruses, we still have much to learn. We need to know more about how viruses influence immune functions, how immune functions influence virus latency, how and whether immune function can influence viral integration into host cells, how immune functions succeed in elimination of viruses from the body and how immune functions influence development of cancer under viral influence. In each of these areas, this conference seemed to say something important.

The temporal setting for our international symposium has been extraordinary. In this context we are at this very moment just beginning to face the threatening disease that directly involves host defense that has appeared during my forty years as an immunologist. Perhaps AIDS is the most threatening medical event to appear even during the past 100 years. It seems to be a new disease—at least new to patients in the United States, if not as I believe, new to the world. It is a lethal infection which destroys the helper-inducer T cells and makes the body vulnerable to all manner of infection. Patients with acquired immunodeficiency syndrome (AIDS) are particularly vulnerable to infection with other viruses like Herpes simplex, EB virus (EBV), and cytomegalovirus (CMV). This disease permits persistent infection and invasion with protozoa-like Pneumocystis carinii, toxoplasmosis, cryptosporidiosis and <u>Giardia lambdia</u>, destructive disseminated fungus infections and opportunistic bacterial infections like <u>Mycobacterium avium intracellulare</u>. Patients with AIDS have an immunodeficiency every bit as profound as those we have seen in children with severe combined immunodeficiency (SCID). Because this immunodeficiency is unrelenting, it is no wonder that it, like SCID, has been a highly lethal disease. Before my colleagues and I introduced bone marrow transplantation as a means to cure SCID, all children who suffered from SCID died of infection or cancer; mostly from infection, but many from cancer. Few survived two years and most died before one year of age. Although I do not think bone marrow transplantation has been sufficiently tested in patients with AIDS and ultimately needs to be imaginatively tested, it seems unlikely that this approach should be effective because the causative agent is still in the picture and with its trophism for T_4 cells demonstrated in this conference, it probably would destroy the T_4 cells of the donor marrow as soon as they are formed from the new bone marrow just as its destroys marrow-derived T lymphocytes of the patients.

Experimentally, however, in my laboratory we have already begun to work with the possibility of being able to identify and, with bone marrow transplantation, to introduce resistance genes which can resist the development of cancer. This approach already can be shown to be working with experimental systems and the approach already permits our introducing resistance to retrovirus-induced malignancies and even to autoimmune diseases in autoimmune-prone mice in which retroviruses are also regularly involved in some way. We are now attempting with marrow transplantation to introduce resistance genes even to chemical carcinogens into the body.

In this conference we heard from Dr. Popovic that not only as we were shown in Tokyo have the French scientists isolated and identified LAV as a potential causative agent in AIDS but American scientists have also identified, isolated and developed in vitro methods for culturing a similar if not identical retrovirus agent from American patients with AIDS. The NCI scientists under Gallo, however, have discovered an immortal T_4 cell line that is not killed by and can thus produce lots of virus for critical analysis. I believe this agent will prove to be the true causative agent of AIDS. It should be emphasized that this virus is not the same retrovirus agent that was earlier being proposed by both the Gallo group and Essex last year as being a virus associated with AIDS. Nor is it the retrovirus which the Japanese led by Professor Hinuma have linked inextricably to adult T cell leukemia. The latter virus is a different virus and it does not cause AIDS but rather it is certainly the cause of adult T cell leukemia. Thus, we now see clearly that there does exist an intimate association of human retroviruses with human cancer just as is the case with many animals. How Robert Huebner would appreciate that association. To establish such a retroviral link to cancer as well as to establish the reality of his oncogenes was his life's work. Both of these formulations we can now be certain are, in fact, associated with human cancer by hard scientific data, and the latter findings fully justify, it seems to me, the goals of Huebner's insistance on an NCI-based crash program for understanding the roles of viruses and oncogenes in human cancer. That crash program I remember came under much heat from many in the scientific community. The current observations show Huebner was right about the threat of oncogenes and also about the probability that retrovirusinduced malignancies are not limited to animals but would also be found to be a reality for humans. These are exciting days in retrovirology. I cannot help but think that Temmin gave up too easily.

But what of the evidence presented in this conference for the link between cancer and the several herpes viruses? The link to cancer of EBV also seems inextricable even though the likelihood is that this relationship probably involves at least one additional influence (before cancer is a consequence). Whatever the event, it involves reciprocal translocation of chromosomes probably associated with activation of C oncogenes. Something must surely happen to abrogate the function of T lymphocytes which ordinarily control proliferation of B lymphocytes that have been immortalized by a virus infection they cannot get rid of.

We also reviewed in this conference the possible causative role of cytomegalovirus as a possible etiologic agent that is responsible for each of the forms of Kaposi's sarcoma. Each of the forms of Kaposi's sarcoma represent a malignancy that involves endothelial cells. This seems clear from the factor VIII marker on these cells. Evidence that Kaposi's sarcoma is a true malignancy is less compelling than is the case with the Burkitt's lymphoma, B lymphomas in primary immunodeficiency patients, B lymphomas that occur in immunosuppressed recipients of marrow transplants or the B lymphomas which sometimes occur in bone marrow transplant recipients. All of these are true cancers, and often, if not always, can be shown to reflect a monoclonal expansion. However, the word is out that Starzl in recent work has found that the way to eliminate trillions of cancer cells when the patient has developed a B cell cancer after organ transplantation is simply to stop suppressing the immune system. Together these findings bring right back to center stage both the viral etiology of cancer and the concept of immunosurveillance originally postulated by Ehrlich, restated first in the modern era by Thomas and then promulgated by Burnet and our group. The surveillance concept has taken a lot of heat in recent years and it is good to see that it had been revived from what Gus Nossal referred to as a moribund state and has been brought back to health by the experiences with patients with AIDS, studies of immunosuppressed transplant patients with cancer and by those patients with primary immunodeficiencies. The crucial analysis which truly establishes the reality of immunosurveillance at least vis-a-vis certain cancers is the elimination of disseminated cancer by restoring immune function. With respect to the primary immunodeficiency diseases it is eminently clear that if you completely correct immunologically any of the forms of severe combined immunodeficiency disease you completely eliminate the very great susceptibility to malignancy in these patients. If you do not correct the immunological deficiency but only partially correct the immunodeficiency cancer occurs in these patients nearly fifty percent of the time.

We also heard in this conference again Lopez's contention that it neither T cell nor B cell immunity that gets patients with AIDS into desperate clinical trouble by making them susceptible to intercurrent or opportunistic infection and to certain cancers but rather that it is defects of other cells including NK cells, monocytic cells and polymorphonuclear leukocytes that play the most telling role. I have repeatedly argued this issue with both Lopez and F. Siegal. I do not question that the cells to which they attribute the major defense represent important bulwarks of the bodily defense. That we pointed out years ago. However, I do know that T cell and/or B cell deficiencies without NK deficiencies or without monocyte or PMN deficiencies can by themselves be sufficient to open the door to both lethal infections and malignancy. What I do not know is that NK deficiencies or monocyte-PMN deficiencies are essential to create the basis for opportunistic infection. It is not the case in the primary immunodeficiencies and I still doubt it is an essential features in AIDS. However, if multiple deficiencies are present and multiple bulwarks have been battered down, things are a lot worse than if only one or two are inadequate. Thus, I feel confident that the T cell deficiency alone with or without B cell deficiency, or even B cell deficiencies alone, and certainly defects of the two systems are sufficient to permit occurrence of a sufficient number of infections to make the deficiencies highly lethal early in life. That such diseases would be more lethal if PMNs, NK cells, primary immunodeficiencies or monocytes are also lacking seems likely and perhaps that is what Lopez is attempting to convey.

344

We held this conference at a time when it has been possible to witness the bodily defense in still another perspective. The Bubble Boy, David, in Houston has just recently died. The lethal termination of a long struggle occurred when doctors made an effort to restore immunological function in David's body by using bone marrow transplantation with marrow purged of T cells using in vitro treatment with monoclonal antibodies. One issue was how this was accomplished. Whether what was done was ideal is a complex issue which I will not argue here. Even though this 11 year old David had SCID, he lived eleven years without immunity. His relatively long life was attributable to maintenance in a relatively microorganism-free environment. It is, however, unlikely that he escaped all those years without being contaminated and one must await detailed description of the microbial flora that was tolerated in this child in the face of SCID. One important bulwark of the bodily defense is that represented by the many kinds of friendly, non-virulent microorganisms that occupy crucial niches within the body and there compete for Lebensraum with other potentially more pathogenic organisms.

We also have considered in this conference quite extensively the FeLV-induced lymphoid cancer which, as with AIDS, may be associated with many other infections, a broad range of immunodeficiencies and a variety of nonmalignant consequences. The considerations in the conference included dramatic evidence of induced regression of the leukemia virus-induced cancer in FeLV-infected cats with disseminated lymphoma or leukemias using ex vivo immunoabsorption. More recently, similar regressions have been produced after parenteral injections of Protein A. Detailed studies are needed of the dramatic influence on virus-induced cancer, which has been induced in these cats. This is particularly true because the organisms causing the disease may be either greatly reduced or eliminated entirely during effective treatment of the cancer. In this regard, a fascinating relationship has been elucidated by Day and her associates, Liu and Engelman.

Recovery from the virus-induced malignant disease has been shown by Liu et al., Day et al. and Engelman et al. to be associated with an interesting sequence of responses that address the cancer as well as the virus infection in one fell swoop. First, after staph protein A treatment, what appears to be gamma interferon is induced to appear in the blood. Then the responding cats develop antibody to a gp-70 envelope glycoprotein of the virus. This antibody exhibits potent cytotoxicity for both the cancer cells bearing the 70 antigen (presumably of the recombinant virus that was formerly called FOCMA) and the virus itself. Thus, both tumor cells and virus are eliminated from the body. If this association proves to be the general case in the cats who are cured of their cancer by injection of Staph protein A, one must speculate on how the interferon response and the cytotoxic anti-70 could work together to eliminate both the infection and the malignancy. I believe a reasonable relationship may have been suggested during Dr. William Stewart's extensive review of the actions of interferon. He talked of the capacity of interferon to interfere with shedding of surface virus antigen, e.g., GP-70, from cells it is influencing. In this way perhaps a more extensive target for the cytotoxic antibody plus complement on the cell surface could be a consequence of the interferons inducing action. In such a context, cytotoxic antibody might be made truly destructive of the nucleated tumor cells, the circulating virus and also the budding virus available at the cell surfaces. Further experiments will be necessary to elucidate details, but it is exciting that in an experimental system endogenous gamma interferon may be intimately associated with the immunologic mechanism means of curing at least one cancer.

The association of immunodeficiency with cancer must also be viewed in the context of Herman Friedman's keynote address. He was discussing the fact that for many years it has been known that oncogenic viruses can depress greatly immunologic functions. Von Pirquet first saw this relationship when he discovered the immunosuppressive action of measles virus. Our laboratories were heavily involved in these efforts at the very first step. Raymond D.A. Peterson and I initially, and then later Peter B. Dent with Peterson and I developed for the first time a model of virus-induced oncogenic immunodeficiency that appears prior to the development of the virus-induced cancer. In 1960 and 1961 and then again in 1962 and 1963, we studied the influence of the Gross passage A viruses on antibody production and showed that a profound, persistent and progressive immunodeficiency is produced in this model which ultimately terminates in the malignancy. Both the immunodeficiency and the oncogenicity are products of the Gross retrovirus superinfection. This is similar to part of the story with AIDS. Here, of course, because of the immunodeficiency produced by the virus is so profound the door is open to influence of other cancer-causing viruses, e.g., EBV, CMV and perhaps also Herpes simplex viruses I and II. The malignancies which develop in the patients with AIDS include Kaposi's sarcoma, which can be closely linked to CMV infection; malignant B cell lymphomas, which are linked to EBV; Hodgkin's disease, in which a virus etiology is suspected but not established; squamous cell cancers, which are possibly linked to the Herpes viruses; and melanomas, not yet linked to any virus so far. In AIDS, the retrovirus, LAV, or HTLV III, produces a profound, persistent and progressive immunodeficiency that makes the patients susceptible to common bacterial infection, fungus infection, protozoal and mycobacterial infections. At least some of the virus infections which occur in these patients may be components in the pathogenesis of certain of their cancers. Pneumocystis carinii, an especially bad actor in these patients continues to be a highly lethal disease because of the profound immunodeficiency it produces in these patients. Because of the immunodeficiency it produces, AIDS is uniformly lethal and thus the most threatening disease to appear on the scene in our time. I, for one, am, however impressed that Kaposi's sarcoma can be induced to undergo dramatic regression in some patients after treatment with interferon as has been shown by the Sloan Kettering group led by Krown Safai et al (60) and by Hersh and his co-workers. I wonder, however, whether treatment of AIDS with any single agent except a potent antiviral or anti-retroviral agent will be truly effective. A combined strategy in which several drugs which exert beneficial effects on the immunity systems of the host and are used together or in sequence may be necessary. Ingenuity in such combined modality therapy may give more promising results than the relatively disappointing results so far obtained by each of the immunomodulators that have been tried so far.

It is important to take this AIDS epidemic seriously because many people are infected by the responsible virus and, as such, are continuing to bear and transmit the causative virus. A prodromal disease, AIDS-related complex, has been shown to exist in persons in the high risk group and this syndrome is already known to be able to progress to AIDS with a significant frequency. Once it has progressed to AIDS, it, like spontaneous AIDS, is a lethal disease.

Dr. Lawrence reviewed the epidemiology of AIDS at the banquet last night and it was conservative estimate that even if a vaccine against LAV or HTLV III were to be developed instantly (which will not happen), at least 40,000-50,000 more cases of AIDS will occur, with all of the mortality from infections and cancer that is to be expected. At the very best, it will take five to ten years to develop a safe and effective vaccine and even then much good fortune will be needed if an effective vaccine is to be developed. I am sure that such a vaccine will eventually become available, but it may take unusual ingenuity because the virus agent involved is trophic for what are probably the most important cells of the entire immunologic system, the T_4 helper-inducer population. Thus, a killed virus, a vaccine made with key virus component antigens, or even an attenuated or genetically

346

engineered live virus will be necessary. Development of such a vaccine will not happen quickly. So we must face the realities of a continuing epidemic that may be slowed by application of prudent public health measures plus development of specific means to detect infected blood and elimination of hazardous preparations of antihemophiliac factor. The epidemic, however, according to the most optimistic estimates, will continue for another five to ten years and matters may get much worse. One question occurs to me in light of Aronson's recent work showing that a hijacked gene is perverted to the use of the virus for managing the cells it infects. In the Simian sarcoma virus infection that causes sarcomas in monkeys the hijacked gene codes for the platelet growth factor. Could it be the very genes essential to turning off immune responses for the mammalian body have been hijacked by the AIDS retrovirus instead of the platelet growth factor. Much evidence compatible with a view like this is breaking out in the most recent literature and relates to the regular immunosuppressive actions of retrovirus infections some of which open the door to cancer.

This epidemic probably originated with appearance of the virus in Africa at least ten years before it turned up in the United States. In Africa it is often spread by heterosexual transmission rather than only among homosexuals and drug abusers. This factor surely carriers ominous implications for the future of the present epidemic if we cannot come to grips with the virus infection or its consequences. If AIDS really is transmitted from males to females and from females to males, then the limitations of the disease to present risk groups will no longer be the case and the lives of all of us will be dramatically influenced. I think we have already seen consequences of an ominous transmission as we view the now convincing evidence that children can catch this disease from their infected and sometimes quite healthy mothers. Yet the children catch highly lethal AIDS. I have been critical of some of the cases which have been included among the roster of patients described by A. Rubenstein, A. Amman and J. Olesky, but I am not critical of the concept that AIDS does occur in children. It really does but we must be highly critical that we have solid evidence of who has AIDS and who has primary immunodeficiency or immunodeficiency secondary to another disease. The most convincing patients it seems to me have not been those children with agammaglobulinemia, hypo-gammaglobulinemia, or dysgammaglobulinemia who have sometimes been described, but rather those with failure to thrive, persistent hepatosplenomegaly and lymphadenopathy associated with combination of hypergammaglobulinemia, antibody deficiency syndrome and deficiencies of T helper cell numbers and functions. With the availability of the new means to quantify antibodies and the availability of virus isolation procedures described in this conference, diagnosis of infants and children with this disease will surely become more scientific.

John Trentin discussed another potentially oncogenic virus which has not yet been proved to be a cause of cancer in man. This is the viruses of the adenovirus group. Trentin thinks these viruses may still represent a threat to cause cancer in man if they occur in just the right or wrong circumstance. Adenovirus represents a human DNA virus that produces a variety of cancers in hamsters and possibly can produce or contribute to production of cancer in man. Those of us who work with marrow transplantation already must have great respect for adenovirus infections. We have encountered this virus as a problem in our immunodeficient patients especially after marrow transplantation and know it can produce devastating destructive inflammation in the immunodeficient patients.

I believe this conference shows we are just beginning to experience substantial fruits to be anticipated from use of methodologies which permit elucidation of the way in which viruses participate to cause both immunodeficiency and the development of cancers. We will, I believe, see the

347

immunobiologic, molecular biologic, cellular biologic and chemical revolution pay off with much great understanding in the years immediately ahead. New information concerning the relationships between virus infection, immunodeficiency, cancer and opportunistic infections are and will continue to be forthcoming. The progress to be anticipated in the next few years should be nothing short of dramatic. A number of human cancers have already been associated with virus infection and the exact molecular role of these viruses in development of these cancers will be rapidly elucidated. Take the hepatitis virus as an example. Maybe the first effective anticancer vaccine will be against hepatic cancer and will be soon demonstrated as hepatitis B infection is prevented by immunization against this virus by the Chinese investigators and Blumberg et al. quite independently. I feel certain that a number of other cancers such as certain forms of breast cancer and some cases of cervical adenocarcinomas may also be linked to viruses in important ways in the years ahead. The observations by Day and Diana Lopez presented here suggest that such may be the case at least for some forms of breast cancer.

This conference has been an eye opener for all of us. We have had a lively exchange, have learned much from each other and we can now each hustle happily back to our laboratories to pursue our new leads. It remains only to thank Dean Szentivanyi for backing this extraordinary interchange and to express our appreciation to Herman Friedman and his associates especially Dr. Steven Specter for bringing us all together and organizing this conference in such a fine way. We want to express our deep appreciation to them all for providing so well for our scientific interactions and making it possible for all of us to have so very much fun.

CONTRIBUTORS

F. Basolo
Institute of Pathological Anatomy and Histology
University of Pisa
Pisa, Italy

Mauro Bendinelli, M.D., Ph.D.
Institute of Epidemiology, Hygiene and Virology
University of Pisa
Pisa, Italy

Zvi Bentwich
R. Ben-Ari Institute of Clinical Immunology
Rehovot, Israel

Ytzhal Berner
Department of Internal Medicine
Kaplan Hospital
Rehovot, Israel

Celso Bianco
The Greater New York Blood Program
New York Blood Center
New York, New York

Nancy J. Bigley
Department of Microbiology and Immunology
College of Science and Engineering and
School of Medicine
Wright State University
Dayton, Ohio

Baruch S. Blumberg, M.D., Ph.D.
Associate Director for Clinical Research
Institute for Cancer Research
Fox Chase Cancer Center
Philadelphia, Pennsylvania

Karl Boatman
Baptist Medical Center
Oklahoma City, Oklahoma

K. D. Bonilla
University of Puerto Rico School of Medicine
San Juan, Puerto Rico

Virginia Buchner
Department of Organic Chemistry
Weizmann Institute of Science
Rehovot, Israel

Rimona Burstein
R. Ben-Air Institute of Clinical Immunology
Rehovot, Israel

Ygal Burstein
Department of Organic Chemistry
Weizmann Institute of Science
Rehovot, Israel

Julio I. Colon, Ph.D.
Professor
Department of Pathology
University of Puerto Rico School of Medicine
San Juan, Puerto Rico

M. Cortes
University of Puerto Rico School of Medicine
San Juan, Puerto Rico

Noorbibi K. Day, Ph.D.
University of South Florida
College of Medicine
Department of Pediatrics/St. Petersburg
All Children's Hospital
St. Petersburg, Florida

Osmond J.M. D'Cruz
Cancer Research Program
Oklahoma Medical Research Foundation
Oklahoma City, Oklahoma

C. Dees
Department of Veterinary Science
University of Wisconsin - Madison
Madison, Wisconsin

Robert W. Engelman
Cancer Research Program
Oklahoma Medical Research Foundation
Oklahoma City, Oklahoma

William B. Ershler
Department of Pharmacology
The Vermont Regional Cancer Center
University of Vermont
Burlington, Vermont

Max Essex
Department of Cancer Biology
Harvard University School of Public Health
Boston, Massachusetts

Jeffrey L. Farmer, Ph.D.
Department of Microbiology-Immunology
Tulane University School of Medicine
New Orleans, Louisiana

Michael Fischbach
The University of Texas Health Science Center
Audie L. Murphy Memorial
Veterans Administration Hospital
San Antonio, Texas

Herman Friedman, Ph.D.
Chairman and Professor
Department of Medical Microbiology and Immunology
University of South Florida
College of Medicine
Tampa, Florida

David A. Fuccillo
National Institute for Neurologic and Communicative
  Disorders and Stroke
National Institutes of Health
Bethesda, Maryland

Robert S. Fujinami
Department of Immunology
Scripps Clinic and Research Foundation
La Jolla, California

Frank Gatchell
Presbyterian Hospital
Oklahoma City, Oklahoma

T. L. German
Department of Veterinary Science
University of Wisconsin - Madison
Madison, Wisconsin

David J. Giron
Department of Microbiology and Immunology
College of Science and Engineering and
School of Medicine
Wright State University
Dayton, Ohio

Robert A. Good, M.D., Ph.D.
University of South Florida
College of Medicine
Department of Pediatrics/St. Petersburg
All Children's Hospital
St. Petersburg, Florida

A. Arthur Gottlieb, M.D.
Department of Microbiology-Immunology
Tulane University School of Medicine
New Orleans, Louisiana

Cheryl L. Gould
Department of Microbiology and Immunology
College of Science and Engineering and
School of Medicine
Wright State University
Dayton, Ohio

Carolyn J. Greene
The Vermont Regional Cancer Center
University of Vermont
Burlington, Vermont

Zeev T. Handzel
R. Ben-Ari Institute of Clinical Immunology
Rehovot, Israel

Gertrude Henle
The Joseph Stokes, Jr., Research Institute
The Children's Hospital of Philadelphia
Philadelphia, Pennsylvania

Werner Henle
The Joseph Stokes, Jr., Research Institute
The Children's Hospital of Philadelphia
Philadelphia, Pennsylvania

Ronald B. Herberman, M. D.
Associate Director
Biological Response Modifiers Program
National Cancer Institute
Frederick, Maryland

Lee Hsu, Ph.D.
Assistant Professor
Department of Medical Microbiology and Immunology
University of South Florida
College of Medicine
Tampa, Florida

Jerry M. Karabin
Department of Microbiology and Immunology
Louisiana State University Medical Center
New Orleans, Louisiana

Kokichi Kikuchi
Sapporo Medical College
Sapporo, Japan

L. Kitchen
Department of Cancer Biology
Harvard University School of Public Health
Boston, Massachusetts

K. M. Lang
University of Puerto Rico School of Medicine
San Juan, Puerto Rico

Dale Lawrence, M.D.
Centers for Disease Control
U.S. Department of Health and Human Services
Atlanta, Georgia

Wing T. Liu
Cancer Research Program
Oklahoma Medical Research Foundation
Oklahoma City, Oklahoma

Carlos Lopez, Ph.D.
Associate Member
Sloan-Kettering Institute for Cancer Research
Cornell Graduate School of Medical Sciences
New York, New York

Diana M. Lopez
Department of Microbiology and Immunology
University of Miami School of Medicine
Miami, Florida

F. Lopez-Malpica
University of Puerto Rico School of Medicine
San Juan, Puerto Rico

Roger M. Loria
Department of Microbiology and Immunology and Pathology
Medical College of Virginia
Richmond, Virginia

Katsuhiko Machida
Oklahoma Medical Research Foundation
Oklahoma City, OK

A. M. Marchand
University of Puerto Rico School of Medicine
San Juan, Puerto Rico

R. F. Marsh
Department of Veterinary Science
University of Wisconsin - Madison
Madison, Wisconsin

Donatella Matteucci
Institute of Microbiology
University of Pisa
Pisa, Italy

Karyle G. McMannama
Department of Microbiology and Immunology
College of Science and Engineering and
School of Medicine
Wright State University
Dayton, Ohio

Søren C. Mogensen
Institute of Medical Microbiology
University of Aarhus
Denmark

Ann L. Moore
Department of Medicine
The Vermont Regional Cancer Center
University of Vermont
Burlington, Vermont

P. Mora-Urdaz
University of Puerto Rico School of Medicine
San Juan, Puerto Rico

J. N. Moreno
University of Puerto Rico School of Medicine
San Juan, Puerto Rico

Lata Nerurkar
Children's Hospital National Medical Center
and George Washington University
Washington, D.C.

Laura Netzer
Department of Cell Biology
Weizmann Institute of Science
Rehovot, Israel

Toru Nishihara, M.D.
Department of Microbiology-Immunology
Tulane University School of Medicine
New Orleans, Louisiana

Meihan Nonoyama
Showa University Institute for Biomedicine in Florida
St. Petersburg, Florida

Robert K. Oldham, M.D.
Institute for Biological Therapy
University of British Columbia
Vancouver, British Columbia

Michael B.A. Oldstone
Department of Immunology
Scripps Clinic and Research Foundation
La Jolla, California

William Oleszko
The Greater New York Blood Program
New York Blood Center
New York, New York

Zilka M. Orraca
Puerto Rico Cancer Center
San Juan, Puerto Rico

M. R. Ortiz
University of Puerto Rico School of Medicine
San Juan, Puerto Rico

Ronald D. Paul
Department of Microbiology and Immunology
University of Miami School of Medicine
Miami, Florida

Robert J. Pauley
Department of Microbiology and Immunology
University of Miami School of Medicine
Miami, Florida

Marit Pecht
Department of Cell Biology
Weizmann Institute of Science
Rehovot, Israel

Johanna Pindyck
The Greater New York Blood Program
New York Blood Center
New York, New York

Richard Pope
The University of Texas Health Science Center
Audie L. Murphy Memorial Veterans Administration Hospital
San Antonio, Texas

Eddy Rios-Olivares, Ph.D., M.P.H.
Professor and Chairman
Department of Microbiology
Escuela de Medicina de Cayey
Cayey, Puerto Rico

William Rodriguez
National Institute for Neurologic and Communicative
  Disorders and Stroke
National Institutes of Health
Bethesda, Maryland

M. I. Roque
University of Puerto Rico School of Medicine
San Juan, Puerto Rico

M. L. Santaella
University of Puerto Rico School of Medicine
San Juan, Puerto Rico

Ofra Segal
R. Ben-Ari Institute of Clinical Immunology
Rehovot, Israel

John L. Sever
National Institute for Neurologic and Communicative
  Disorders and Stroke
National Institutes of Health
Bethesda, Maryland

Lien Shou
National Defense Medical Center
Taipei, Taiwan

Mark A. Socinski
Departments of Medicine
The Vermont Regional Cancer Center
University of Vermont
Burlington, Vermont

Mary Ann South
National Institute for Neurologic and Communicative
  Disorders and Stroke
National Institutes of Health
Bethesda, Maryland

Steven Specter, Ph.D.
Associate Professor
Department of Medical Microbiology and Immunology
University of South Florida
College of Medicine
Tampa, Florida

William E. Stewart II, Ph.D.
Professor
Department of Medical Microbiology and Immunology
University of South Florida
College of Medicine
Tampa, Florida

Andor Szentivanyi, M.D.
Dean of the College of Medicine
Deputy Vice President for Medical Affairs
Chairman and Professor
Department of Pharmacology and Therapeutics
University of South Florida
Tampa, Florida

Judith Szentivanyi, M.D.
Associate Professor
Department of Comprehensive Medicine
University of South Florida
College of Medicine
Tampa, Florida

Norman Talal
The University of Texas Health Science Center
Audie L. Murphy Memorial
Veterans Administration Hospital
San Antonio, Texas

Hideki Teshima
Kyushu University
Fukuoka, Japan

Anthonio Toniolo
Institute of Microbiology
University of Pisa
Pisa, Italy

Nathan Trainin
Department of Cell Biology
Weizmann Institute of Science
Rehovot, Israel

Liem Q. Trang
Cancer Research Program
Oklahoma Medical Research Foundation
Oklahoma City, Oklahoma

John J. Trentin, Ph.D.
Division of Experimental Biology
Baylor College of Medicine
Houston, Texas

William F. Wade
Department of Veterinary Science
University of Wisconsin - Madison
Madison, Wisconsin

Alan A. Waldman
The Greater New York Blood Program
New York Blood Center
New York, New York

Ambrose Wasunna
Kenyatta Hospital
Nairobi, Kenya

Maxine Watson
Oklahoma Medical Research Foundation
Oklahoma City, Oklahoma

Joseph F. Williams
Professor
Department of Pharmacology and Therapeutics
University of South Florida
College of Medicine
Tampa, Florida

Akihiro Yachie
Children's Hospital National Medical Center
and George Washington University
Washington, D.C.

Edith Zhang
The Greater New York Blood Program
New York Blood Center
New York, New York

Jian-Lin Zhang
Department of Medical Microbiology and Immunology
University of South Florida
College of Medicine
Tampa, Florida

Beta-adrenergic subsensitivity
  and allergic tissue injury, 229, 232
  autoimmunity, 233–234
  mechanism of, 217–226
  and viral infection, 217, 219, 220
B-lymphoblastoid cells, 49
  suppressor activity of, 49–57
B-lymphocytes
  age-related concentrations, 253
  and beta-adrenergic suppressor
    system, 215
  in coxsackievirus-B3 infection,
    102
  and cytomegalovirus, 60, 68
  gender-related concentrations, 253
  in MMTV infection, 110, 114, 115,
    116, 119
  response to F-MuLV, 133, 134
  suppression of, 33, 37
  transformed, 27, 28, 43–46, 49–57
  viral effects, 26, 27, 28, 29
Bovine rhinotracheitis, 21
Burkitt's lymphomia, 46, 49, 51 (*See
    also* Epstein-Barr virus)

Cancer
  effect on immune system, 159–161
  effects of immune system on, 160–163
  human breast
    familial, 123, 126
    IgA:IgG ratio in, 123, 124
    MMTV antibodies in, 123, 125, 126,
      127
    presence of gp52 antigen, 123, 124
      126, 127
  vaccine, 155
Cell mediated immunity, 26
  deficiency of, 61, 62
  to herpes simplex virus, 73
  serum factors, 30
  suppression of, 27, 32
  thymic hormonal factor, 313, 315
Cimetidine treatment
  combined with polyantigenic
    vaccine, 335, 336
  doses, 335
  effect on tumor growth, 334
  and increased interferon, 333, 335,
    336
Coxsackievirus B infection
  and acquired immunodeficiency, 104
  animal model studies, 197–198, 201
  and atherosclerosis, 198, 201
  and B-cell proliferation, 101
  cause of immunodeficiency, 101, 103
  effect on lymphoid organs, 102,
    103–104, 197, 198, 201
  genetic predisposition to, 202
  immune responses to, 26, 102–105
  and onset of diabetes, 197–198
  and T-suppressor cell activity, 102

Creutzfeld-Jacob virus
  infection mechanisms, 31
Cytomegalovirus infection
  acquired, 60, 62
  antibody response, 60, 61, 68
  compared to AIDS, 67, 70–72
  congenital, 59–60, 62
  in drug-suppressed patients, 61, 62
  and IgG antibodies, 252, 253
  immune response to, 26, 27, 44, 60,
    61
  immunodepression by, 59
  as opportunistic infectious agent,
    59, 63, 64
  perinatally acquired, 60, 62
  and T-cell concentrations, 60, 61,
    69, 70, 71, 72
    age related, 252–255
    gender related, 252–255
  transfusion acquired, 61, 62
  treatment of, 63
Cytotoxic T lymphocyte
  modified-self, 205
  response, 205

Dengue virus
  immune response to, 26, 27
  infection, 31
Desensitization, tissue
  homologous, 231, 232
  heterologous, 231, 232
  and injury, 232
Diabetes
  and atherosclerosis, 199
  induced by encephalomyocarditis, 307
  interferon activated, 309–310
  interferon enhanced, 308–309
  role of CBV-B in, 198
Down's syndrome
  Australian antigen in, 83–84
  serum-iron levels in, 83

Echovirus, 26
Eosinophilla
  and beta-adrenergic effector system,
    216
Encephalomyocarditis infection
  effect on pancreas, 307
  interferon as enhancer of, 307,
    308–309
  and murine diabetes, 307, 308
  reactivation by interferon, 309–310
Epstein-Barr virus, (*See also* specific
    virus)
  in AIDS, 70, 145
  anti-VCA, 43–45
  and chromosomal translocations, 46
  Daudi cells, 49
  immune response to, 26, 27, 30,
    43–46
  and Kaposi's herpetic eruption, 223